Alcohol Misuse
A European Perspective

edited by

Timothy J. Peters

King's College
London, UK

harwood academic publishers

Australia • Canada • China • France • Germany • India • Japan • Luxembourg
Malaysia • The Netherlands • Russia • Singapore • Switzerland • Thailand
United Kingdom

Emmaplein 5
1075 AW Amsterdam
The Netherlands

British Library Cataloguing in Publication Data

Alcohol misuse : a European perspective
  1. Alcoholism - Europe
  I. Peters, Timothy J. (Timothy John), 1939–
  362.2'92'094

   ISBN 3-7186-5814-3 (hardcover)
           3-7186-5869-0 (softcover)

CONTENTS

Preface   vii

Introduction   ix

Contributors   xiii

1. Trends in alcohol consumption in the EU countries   1
    J. Simpura
2. Racial/ethnic and gender differences in alcohol use and misuse   23
    D.P. Agarwal
3. Alcohol and nutrition   41
    R. Estruch
4. Alcohol and the liver   63
    D. Sherman, J. Koskinas and R. Williams
5. Alcohol misuse and the skin   77
    E.M. Higgins
6. HIV and alcohol abuse   89
    T.J. McManus and P. Weatherburn
7. Alcohol and the brain: neuropathology and imaging studies   99
    K. Mann
8. Musculo-skeletal problems in alcohol abuse   123
    A. Urbano-Márquez and J. Fernández-Solà
9. Alcohol and the pancreas   145
    H. Sarles, J.P. Bernard and C.D. Johnson
10. Alcohol and malignancies   163
    A.J. Tuyns
11. Alcohol-related adverse social consequences within the European Union   181
    E. Österberg
12. Conclusions   195
    G. Edwards and T.J. Peters

Index   199

PREFACE

The risk analysis of alcohol usage is a complex topic involving economic, philosophical, political and toxicological issues. It is therefore essential to review objectively the various degrees of tissue damage consequent upon chronic alcohol misuse. At a time when various arms of the liquor industry, often disguised as Trusts, Groups, Councils and Associations, are attempting to play down these damaging effects and promote the "Beneficial Medical Effects" of usage, independent evaluation of the clinical consequences of chronic ethanol toxicity is vital. This monograph is the result of a peer-reviewing discussion group assessing a series of reports by acknowledged experts in the field of alcohol misuse. These reports have subsequently been revised and form the basis of individual chapters in this monograph.

In preparing the reports, assembling the peer-reviewing group and the preparation and publications of the final chapters the single and sole support of the European Commission is gratefully acknowledged. The concluding summary and proposed Action Plan outlines research directions necessary to investigate further the pathogenesis of tissue damage due to both 'normal' and excessive alcohol usage. Particular reference is made to both the well-known and little-known areas of toxicity, highlighting especially neglected areas of research. In addition, psycho-social problems particularly relevant to European countries are considered.

In the preparation of the monograph the wise, unstinting and invaluable guidance of Griffith Edwards, the expert administrative and secretarial skills of Rosamund Greensted and Jacqui De Groote and the help and advice of Harwood Academic Publishers are gratefully acknowledged.

Professor T.J. Peters

INTRODUCTION

Toward a European Response to Alcohol: Getting Research onto the Map

Griffith Edwards

A MAP OF SOME COMPLEXITY

If so minded, how might one set about drawing a drinking map of Europe? What would the landscape look like if instead of contour lines we marked in per capita alcohol consumption — what plateaux, valleys or mountain ranges would emerge? What symbols should we use to designate areas of great drunkenness, how should we colour in the regions where there is acute as opposed to only minimal political concern, how should we mark in the vineyards or famous breweries or distilleries, or such national monuments as the place where Father Mathew preached his first crusading sermon, Magnus Huss wrote *Alcoholismus*, or where Mendes France drank that famous glass of milk? How shall we indicate the latitudes of temperance and the longitudes of beer festivals? The idea of such a map is intriguing, but had better be left to another day.

The member states which together make up modern Europe certainly comprise a remarkably varied set of drinking terrains. For instance, in the northern areas of the continent, there are countries which have a tradition of spirit drinking, where alcohol is thrown back rather than sipped and is not usually taken with meals, and where drinking to intoxication is viewed as the probable outcome when a group of friends get together with a bottle or two of hard liquor. Per capita consumption in such countries is often quite low, but control measures are restrictive and the temperance tradition strong. Paradoxically, these are frequently the countries which support national institutes for alcohol research and which have established specialised university departments dealing with this topic.

Toward the south of Europe the situation contrasts in many ways with the northern picture. Wine is the traditional beverage, alcohol will often be taken with food or around the family table, and may be regarded as a beneficial item of diet rather than as an intoxicant. Alcohol consumption tends to be high, adverse physical health consequences are endemic, controls lax, and until quite recently governments in such countries would probably have made only small investments in relevant research.

It is also possible to designate a middle band of countries where beer is the favoured beverage, where consumption is again quite high and the few scientists who are interested in alcohol and alcohol problems are likely to lead somewhat lonely professional lives. But to describe Europe as rigidly divided into spirit, wine and beer cultures would be misleading. There are many mixed patterns, different regions or cultures within one country can display varied patterns, and the traditional modes of drinking can change rapidly in the face of trade and economic pressures, or as a result of the mysterious, intangible forces of modernisation. Young people are beginning to drink beer in Italy.

Within this total, shifting field, one fact is outstandingly certain. Across the great expanse of Europe we will still for many years be encountering immensely varied patterns of drinking which have their roots in diverse and ancient cultural and religious traditions and agricultural and industrial contexts, giving rise to different prevalences and patterns of alcohol-related problems, responded to within different social, political and administrative traditions. Europe's experience with alcohol was, is, and for the foreseeable future will be, about heterogeneity. A Finn, a Czech, or an Italian will not conjure up one and the same images when cued by such words as drink, drunk, drunkard, drinking problem, or licensing law. Politicians will see very different constraints and feasibilities cued by alcohol issues, and the media will not all be carrying the same kinds of stories about alcohol in Sweden, Poland and Spain. And meanwhile scientists across a spectrum of European countries will encounter vastly contrasting funding possibilities and career opportunities if they take an interest in drinking problems.

In brief, what even a cursory attempt to delineate a drinking map of Europe must surely point up, is that Europe is not one drinking culture, but a fantastic mosaic of drinking cultures. Perhaps in looking at alcohol we suddenly rediscover something about the deep cultural complexity of our continent. Whatever the particular problem under discussion, to talk of common cause when standing in front of that kind of map will require courage, determination, and a sensitivity toward other people's beliefs and cultures.

ALCOHOL RESEARCH: TOWARD A EUROPEAN DIMENSION

In the new Europe can we expect alcohol issues be given salience and handled intelligently and well and in the interests of the people, or left to whim and chance? If the future is left only to unfettered commercial interests, the map can be expected to evolve over the next few decades toward one high drinking plateau, with all countries drinking up toward the level of those countries which at present constitute the drinking peaks. The consequent economic, health and social costs would be shocking, with Europe seen internationally as a disaster area so far as drinking problems were concerned. Such an extreme scenario is possible but unlikely, but only an extreme optimist would today feel confident that Europe will develop easily and rapidly into a union which handles alcohol issues in exemplary fashion, rationally, and for the public good. WHO has promulgated a well considered European Alcohol Action Plan, but whether governments have the political will to support this plan has yet to be tested.

If Europe is to handle alcohol issues well, one of the necessary inputs to facilitate that development will come from the direct and indirect inputs of the relevant European science. The direct contribution will stem from research which describes the extent of the problem, and which confronts the public and the policy makers with the facts with price tags attached. In addition, there will be a direct contribution from research which can explain rather than just describe the patterns and shifts of drinking and drinking problems across the varied terrain. And research is needed to assess the efficacy of the policies which are being implemented. A direct contribution of another kind will come from a strong research input dealing with biological or genetic issues, and such lines of investigation will have fundamentally important clinical and public health applications.

As to the more indirect benefits to Europe which will flow from a well-founded alcohol research base, under this latter heading the strong, essential, and subtle contribution will be in terms of the impact of science on Europe's culture for decision-making. We must hope that this will be a culture where science counts. No one would be so naive as to assume that science is ever the only input to influence public awareness or political decisions, but we should nonetheless argue for a strong voice for alcohol science in a new Europe.

In stressing the importance to the health of this continent of a European dimension to alcohol research, one should guard against any tendency toward the absurdities of some kind of continental chauvinism as a perverse substitute for old nationalisms. The European science base for alcohol matters, but European science will be a poor thing if it is not part of the wider world endeavour and tested by international standards and expectations.

WHY THIS BOOK IS SIGNIFICANT

This book represents the outcome of a European initiative, and derives from a review exercise and related scientific meeting funded by the European Commission. The authors are drawn from Finland, France, Germany, Spain, and the United Kingdom. In terms of the analysis offered above, this volume might be seen as serving European interests in ways which are both direct and indirect. Directly, it makes important contributions to description of the European situation through its chapter on consumption trends in EU countries (Chapter 1), and with the account which is given of alcohol-related social consequences within the Community (Chapter 11). The chapter on ethnic and gender differences (Chapter 2) starts in an interesting fashion to bridge description and explanation. These three chapters between them constitute a very preliminary essay in map making, but they show what is needed and what can already be said.

The highly informative set of chapters on medical complications of drinking (Chapters 3–6 and 8–10) deal in turn with nutrition, liver diseases, skin disease, HIV risks, musculo-skeletal disorders, the pancreas and malignancies. Between them these statements offer persuasive evidence for the importance of alcohol issues for European clinical research and clinical medicine.

This book also, however, demonstrates the multiple sophistication of the existing European research base which is engaged with this broad array of social and medical topics. A chapter-by-chapter reading of the book confirms that we have the strong beginnings of a European scientific presence which will have the capacity to inform and influence the quality and rationality of policy and public debates on alcohol issues. Thus, as well as there being specific, direct messages and content in the individual chapters, there is a strong implicit message in the fact of the book itself. European science in this arena has noteworthy strengths, and European scientists working on this issue have the will to come together for common purpose and contribute to the wide debate on how alcohol issues should be handled. That's good news.

ALCOHOL RESEARCH IN EUROPE: A VISION FOR THE FUTURE

In its "Conclusions" section this book outlines some bold directions for the future. Several promising specific ideas for research collaboration are identified, but in addition a larger challenge is laid down. The general need for a bolstering of European support for alcohol research is emphasised and the novel suggestion made that a pan-European centre should be established along the lines of NIAAA (America's very influential national agency for alcohol research). In short, the plea in that concluding statement is that however historically diverse our drinking terrains, we should come together to deal with common problems of pervasive European importance. This book argues cogently and with much authority for the need, direct and indirect, to put alcohol research strongly onto the European map. The editor and authors of this volume are to be congratulated on their contribution to science, debate, and the beginnings of important cartography.

CONTRIBUTORS

Dr D. P. Agarwal
Institute of Human Genetics
University of Hamburg
Butenfeld 23
22529 Hamburg
Germany

Dr J. P. Bernard
INSERM
Unité de Recherches de Pathologie
    Digestive
46 Boulevard de la Gaye
F-13009 Marseille, France

Professor Griffith Edwards
National Addiction Centre
Addiction Sciences Building
4 Windsor Walk
London SE5 8AF
United Kingdom

Dr Ramon Estruch
Alcohol Research Unit
Department of Internal Medicine
Hospital Clinic, Villarroel 170
08036 Barcelona
Spain

Dr Joaquim Fernández - Solà
P.O. Manuel Girona 75
Bajos 3A
Barcelona 08034, Spain

Dr Elisabeth M. Higgins
Department of Dermatology
King's College Hospital
Denmark Hill
London SE5 8RS
United Kingdom

Dr C. D. Johnson
INSERM
Unité de Recherches de Pathologie
    Digestive
46 Boulevard de la Gaye
F-13009 Marseille, France

Dr J. Koskinas
Institute of Liver Studies
King's College School of Medicine and
    Dentistry
Denmark Hill
London SE5 8RS
United Kingdom

Dr K. Mann
Associate Professor of Psychiatry
University of Tübingen Medical
    School
Department of Psychiatry
Universität-Nervenklinik
Osianderstrasse 22
72076 Tübingen 1, Germany

Dr T. J. McManus
Department of Genito-Urinary Medicine
King's Healthcare NHS Trust
Denmark Hill
London SE5 8RS
United Kingdom

Dr E. Österberg
Social Research Institute of Alcohol
 Studies
Oy Alko Ab, P.O. Box 350
FIN-00101 Helsinki
Finland

Professor Timothy J. Peters
Department of Clinical Biochemistry
King's College of Medicine and
 Dentistry
Bessemer Road
London SE5 9PJ
United Kingdom

Dr H. Sarles
INSERM U315
Unité de Recherches de Pathologie
 Digestive
46 Boulevard de la Gaye
F-13009 Marseille, Cédex 09
France

Dr D. Sherman
Department of Gastro-Enterology
Queen Elizabeth Hospital
Edgbaston
Birmingham B15 2TH
United Kingdom

Dr J. Simpura
Social Research Institute of Alcohol
 Studies
Oy Alko Ab, P.O. Box 350
FIN-00101 Helsinki
Finland

Dr A. J. Tuyns
International Agency for Research on
 Cancer
150 Cours Albert Thomas
69008 Lyon
France

Dr Alvaro Urbano-Márquez
Muscle Research Group and Alcohol Unit
Internal Medicine Department
Hospital Clinic, Faculty of Medicine
University of Barcelona, Villaroel 170
08036 Barcelona, Spain

Dr P. Weatherburn
Project Sigma
University of Essex
Wivenhoe Conference Centre
Wivenhoe Park
Colchester, Essex C04 3SQ
United Kingdom

Professor Roger Williams
Institute of Liver Studies
King's College School of Medicine and
 Dentistry
Denmark Hill
London SE5 9PJ
United Kingdom

1 Trends in Alcohol Consumption in the EU Countries

Jussi Simpura, Ph.D.

Social Research Institute of Alcohol Studies, PO BOX 350, FIN-00101 Helsinki, Finland

The EU member countries occupy top ranks in the world statistics in alcohol consumption. Large economic interests conflict with the concern about alcohol-related harm in public health. A description of current trends of alcohol consumption levels and patterns shows that a process of homogenization is slowly proceeding in the EU although differences between the countries are still large. Complex explanations are required for the dynamics of aggregate alcohol consumption and, despite the trend towards increasing homogenization, the explanations are different for different countries. Two kinds of proposals for better understanding of the dynamics in the EU are presented. First, a number of issues for improvement of the data bases are discussed. Second, a deeper analysis is called upon on processes that are reformulating the social and political environment of alcohol issue in the EU. Homogenization between countries occurs parallel with fragmentation of everyday life practices within each country, and the relationships between public agencies and citizens are being reshaped in the consumer society. Alcohol consumption and measures to promote or control it appear not only as economic or health policy issues but also as a symbolic battlefield on new social and cultural order. However, the importance of economic interests and health worries should not be overlooked.

1. INTRODUCTION

All indicators of alcohol consumption show unanimously that the EU is the region with highest alcohol consumption and, in many cases, also with highest alcohol-related harm in the world. In the 1993 edition of a compilation of statistics on world alcohol consumption (World Drink Trends 1993, p. 7), the top four countries came from the EU. Among the top 15 countries, there were 10 EU countries. Only Ireland and the United Kingdom belonged to the middle category, occupying the 20th and 21st places in the alcohol consumption statistics. Only recently, the leading position of the EU countries has become challenged, as the somewhat unreliable estimates of alcohol consumption in some ex-socialist countries exceed the present top consumption figures of France, the leading country (see e.g. Strazdins 1994, Subata 1994, and Lehto and Moskalewicz 1994).

Consequently, alcoholic beverages are an important economic issue in the EU. Alcohol could also be an important health policy issue, although this aspect has not gained very much attention within the EU as a whole, until recently. There are signs of an emerging battle around alcohol between alcohol industry and health policy proponents in the EU. Therefore, a discussion on the changing nature of alcohol consumption as a policy issue in the EU is a necessary background for a description of trends in alcohol consumption.

After that background discussion, this paper aims at providing a brief review of statistical material on alcohol consumption, including remarks on specific features of trends in each of the 12 EU countries. Problems related to the quality of data on alcohol consumption will be separately dealt with. The dynamics of changes in alcohol consumption will be discussed. Finally, some proposals for action within the EU will be made, both on issues concerning technical problems in establishing sufficient data bases and on issues of more general political and scientific concern. In the latter point, the parallel but sometimes contradictory processes of homogenization and fragmentation of lifestyles in Europe will be touched, with implications for research as well as public policy.

2. THE ISSUE OF ALCOHOL CONSUMPTION AS A BATTLE FIELD

Until recently, the issue of the level of alcohol consumption has been relatively invisible as a subject of political debate in the EU, with the exception of agricultural policy. Perspectives of health policies have been absent, not to say a word about moral policies and public order. This is contrary to the discussion around alcohol in a number of other developed industrialized western countries, where alcohol-related problems of health and public order have been constant themes in the public debate. Examples of such countries are USA and the Nordic countries, except Denmark. Within the EU, there have been relatively few efforts to provide reviews on the development of alcohol consumption and alcohol-related action in the Community and on the community level (Fahrenkrug (1987) is one of the few examples).

Recently, the situation has changed. Within the EU, the intensification of economic integration and the rise of health and social issues in the community agenda after the Maastricht summit has provoked increasing interest in alcohol issues. Most visibly, international enterprises working in the field of alcohol production and trade have mobilized themselves into an efficient lobby. One of the major goals of that lobby seems to be to prevent the level of alcohol consumption from becoming regarded as an indicator of alcohol-related harm, and consequently, as an instrument of target of preventive health policies (see Alcoholic Beverages and European Society, 1993). The opponent of the industry lobby is most often the WHO Regional Office for Europe. That office has, also recently, launched a new European Alcohol Action Plan (1993; abbreviated later as AAP). The core of that plan is exactly opposite to the views of the alcohol industry lobby. The AAP accepts the idea of the level of alcohol consumption both as a central indicator of alcohol-related harm and as a central target and instrument of preventive policies. Importantly, the European AAP is a direct continuation of alcohol-related views expressed in the worldwide WHO program "Health for all by the year 2000" (see Targets for Health for All, 1985, in particular target 17).

The standpoint of the alcohol industry lobby was neatly stated a few years ago in the foreword to the main statistical source on alcohol consumption (World Drink Trends

1992 foreword by Dr. J.J.M. Verhoek, from the Dutch Commodity Board for the Spirits Industry):

> Everyone knows of countries with a low ranking for alcohol consumption in this book who suffer from more misuse than countries with a higher ranking. There is no correlation between alcohol consumption in a country and alcohol misuse there. People who use this book on that basis are fighting the wrong battle.

This view is repeated, although in a softer formulation, in the recent report by the Amsterdam Group, a main lobbying organization of the alcohol industry (Alcoholic Beverages and European Community, 1993, p. 13):

> However, certain organizations and governments have suggested a number of proposals intended to reduce the total consumption of spirits, beer and wine within Europe as an alternative policy for reducing alcohol abuse. ... The Amsterdam Group is convinced that such a policy will not be successful. There is little reason to expect that measures aimed at lowering total alcohol consumption will reduce alcohol abuse.

The opposite view is condensed in the following quotation from the European Alcohol Action Plan, from the paragraph titled "Strategy" (on p. 12):

> A significant reduction in the health-damaging consumption of alcohol can be achieved through the combination of a population-based approach reducing overall consumption, and a high risk approach targeting high risk behaviors. The population-based approach is needed because; (i), an overall reduction results in less problems at all levels of drinking; (ii), heavy drinking and its problems are particularly sensitive to this approach; (iii), influencing perceptions of reduced levels and patterns has important long-term cultural consequences. An environment in which light drinking is the norm would exert pressure on heavy drinkers to reduce their consumption, thereby potentiating the high risk approach.

An uneven battle may be expected, the industry side being provided with quite superb material resources compared to those of the health promotion proponents. Similarly, within the EU, the alcohol-related expenditure is quite unevenly distributed. It has been estimated that the EU spends almost 2 billion pounds a year subsidizing alcohol production and export — "some 2,000 times more than it spends on alcohol-prevention and education programs" (Leonard Doyle, in The Independent, August 11, 1993). There is a lot of money in the game, and the battle is likely to go on for a long time.

It is beyond the scope of this paper to go into the details of this dispute (see e.g. Wodak (1994) for additional information). Suffice it to say that researchers are also divided in this question. In two subsequent articles in the Journal of the Royal Statistical Society in 1993, it can be read, first, that "some control policies may deter individuals from drinking at high levels, and thus reduce the proportion of deviants and mean consumption, but it is not possible to identify these simply from their effect on average consumption, ..." (Duffy 1993); and second, that "it is not very realistic to deny a connection between per capita consumption, excessive drinking and harm" (Lemmens 1993). In the research field, this dispute goes back to the "single distribution theory" by the Frenchman Ledermann (1956), and the public health perspective on preventing alcohol problems, launched by a prominent research team in the mid-1970's (Bruun *et al.*, 1975; cf. also Edwards *et al.*, 1994). Presently, most researchers admit the complicated nature of the link between mean consumption levels and alcohol-related harm. More detailed research is cumulating on different alcohol-related risks on different consumption levels and for different types of consequences. Still a significant number of researchers would agree with Lemmens (op. cit.) that it indeed is not very realistic to deny the connection between consumption level and alcohol-related harm.

Finally, two new aspects to the battle around alcohol within the EU should be added. First, the prolonged economic depression in many countries threatens the sales of alcoholic beverages. At the same time the competition between alcohol producers is becoming harder, thanks to the abolishment of hindrances for trade in the course of integration. Second, in a number of the countries presently applying for the EU membership, alcohol is an important issue and much of the preventive policies there are based on the idea of regulating aggregate alcohol consumption. Both of these issues make the increasing interest for policy debate around alcohol in the EU more understandable.

3. TRENDS OF ALCOHOL CONSUMPTION IN THE EU

For most of the western industrialized countries, the post-war period until the mid-1970's was a time of continuous growth of alcohol consumption (see e.g. Mäkelä *et al.*, 1981; Single *et al.*, 1981). A notable exception was France where the consumption level was already turned into a decline in the 1960's (see e.g. Sulkunen, 1989). That joint trend was characterized by a double process of homogenization. First, the differences in the level of consumption were diminished as an outcome of the start of a decrease in the countries with high consumption levels, and an increase in countries on low consumption levels. Second, the differences in beverage preferences were also diminished, so that in the time of increasing consumption the relative share of the traditional dominating beverage in each country went slowly down. In absolute terms, however, the consumption volumes of the traditional beverages did not always decrease. The change in drinking took place through a process of addition, rather than by substitution (cf. Mäkelä *et al.*, 1981, p. 9). New beverages and, to some extent new drinking habits, were added to the existing ones. Neither the traditional beverages nor the old habits were replaced by newer ones in the time of increasing alcohol consumption. Of course, the exceptional case of France should be remembered here.

Since the late 1970's, the development is more difficult to characterize in simple terms. The consumption growth was practically stopped in most of the western industrialized countries. Only in Japan, Finland and the former GDR there was a significant increase in the consumption in the late 1980's. Perhaps the United Kingdom should also be joined to this group. At the same time, however, the decline in consumption continued in France, and the other Mediterranean wine countries joined France on a declining path (cf. Pyörälä 1991; see also country reports in Young People and Alcohol in Europe, 1994). The economic depression of the early 1990's has further contributed to stabilization or even decline in aggregate alcohol consumption.

Why did the consumption growth stop in the 1980's? So far, there is no commonly-accepted explanation. The slower pace of overall social change, the problems in economic development, and long-term changes in attitudes and opinion climate, as exemplified by the rise of a health ideology in the U.S. (cf. Room 1991), have been suggested explanations. Of course, the development of consumption in each country contains many details that deviate from this broad overall description although there is a lot of movement in concert in the trends of alcohol consumption in the western industrialized countries. This issue is dealt with in more detail in a number of reviews (see e.g. Sulkunen 1983; Sulkunen 1988; Smart 1990, 1991; Edwards *et al.*, 1994).

Data bases

Before entering a more detailed discussion on the development of alcohol consumption in the EU countries, a few words on the data bases are needed. The standard data base for international comparisons of alcohol consumption levels is the small annual publication called "World Drink Trends", formerly published by the Dutch Distiller's association, covering some 40 countries. Another important publication is the extensive "International Survey on Alcoholic Beverage Taxation and Control Policies", published by The Brewers Association of Canada, with its eight edition from 1989. Besides the consumption figures, this publication gives some background information on factors related to the development of alcohol consumption in some 25 countries. The most detailed compilation of alcohol consumption statistics so far is the "International Statistics on Alcoholic Beverages" (1977), covering the years from 1950 to 1972. It gives information also on the world outside western industrialized countries. Unfortunately, the effort of producing such a world-wide statistics has not been repeated since then. In addition to the publications mentioned above, a number of recent texts contain reviews on trends of alcohol consumption (e.g. Vanston 1990; Moser 1991).

It should be noted that practically all international data sources rely on the same original information from the countries in question. In addition to statistics concerning the volume of alcohol consumption, sales or trade in terms of liters, a number of other sources provide data on the volume of consumption in terms of monetary expenditure on alcoholic beverages (e.g. European Marketing Data, Statistics 1992 and Consumer Europe 1993).

Level of alcohol consumption

Although almost all EU member countries lie on the top of alcohol consumption statistics, there is considerable variation between the countries' consumption levels. This variation has been even larger in the earlier years. Therefore, it hardly makes sense to present a consumption curve for the EU as whole (for such an exercise, see Alcoholic Beverages and European Society, p. 31). In the recent decades, the opposite trends in wine-drinking countries with very high consumption levels, and in other countries with historically much lower consumption levels will get confused with each other within the EU in such a way that an aggregated EU consumption curve is uninformative for any purposes. Suffice it to say that for the EU as a whole the consumption peaked around 1975 at a level of 11 liters of alcohol per capita (according to the data published in "World Drink Trends", 1992 edition). In 1990, the all-EU mean consumption was 9.8 liters per capita. The respective figure thirty years earlier, in 1960, was almost the same, or 9.2 liters. The confusing nature of these figures is evident when one remembers that the rise by mid-1970 took place solely in non-wine-drinking northern EU countries, whereas the decline since 1980 is dominated by the Mediterranean wine-drinking countries.

For a better understanding of alcohol consumption trends, a separate presentation for each country is indispensable (see Figure 1.1). The available data point out remarkably different trends in different EU countries over the post-war period. For most of the northern EU countries, a strong upward trend was indeed visible until the late 1970's. France is distinguished with its already downward trend in the 1960's. The other Mediterranean wine countries joined that trend later, beginning with Spain in the early 1970's, Italy a little later and Portugal in most recent years. The information on Greece is mostly lacking or unreliable. Germany, after having recovered from the years of reconstruction, showed stabilized consumption level earlier than many other countries. Luxembourg is a special case with its intensive contacts with neighboring countries and high foreign population.

There is a lot of homogenization in consumption levels between the EU countries. In 1960, for instance, the difference between France and Britain was over 13 liters alcohol per capita. Today, that difference is only 4.5 liters. On the other hand, the difference between Britain and Morocco, for instance, was only 4 liters in 1960 and has increased to

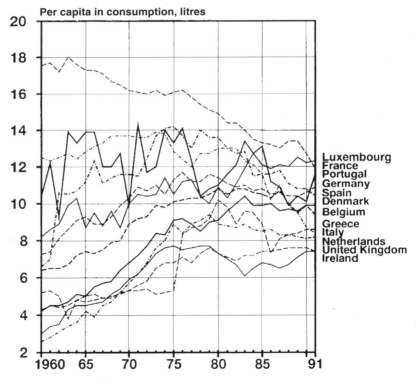

Source: World Drink Trends 1993

Figure 1.1   Trends of aggregate alcohol consumption in the EU countries, 1960–1991.

7 liters by 1990. Europe has come closer to Britain, or Britain has gained some distance to Northern Africa, as far as drinking patterns are concerned.

Beverage preferences

The EU countries, understandably, also hold top positions on consumption statistics by beverage type (see Table 1.1). For wine, the top four positions belong to EU countries,

Table 1.1 The positions of the EU countries (italics for in the top ten) in the consumption of beer, wine and spirits in 1991 (the number of countries in the statistics for each beverage type between parentheses; Source: World Drink Trends, 1993)

	Position	Country	Liters of beverage p.c.
Beer (48)	1	*Germany*	143
	2	Czechoslovakia	135
	3	Denmark	126
	4	Austria	124
	5	*Ireland*	123
	6	*Luxembourg*	116
	7	*Belgium*	111
	8	New Zealand	110
	9	Hungary	107
	10	*United Kingdom*	106
	...		
	12	Netherlands	89
	...		
	16	Spain	71
	...		
	18	Portugal	67
	...		
	31	France	41
	32	Greece	40
	...		
	38	Italy	23
Wine (46)	1	*France*	67
	2	*Portugal*	62
	3	*Luxembourg*	60
	4	*Italy*	57
	5	Argentina	52
	6	Switzerland	49
	7	*Spain*	34
	8	Austria	34
	9	*Greece*	32
	10	Hungary	30
	...		
	13	Germany	25
	14	Belgium	25
	...		
	16	Denmark	22
	...		
	20	Netherlands	15
	...		
	25	United Kingdom	12
	...		
	33	Ireland	5

Table 1.1   (*Continued*)

	Position	Country	Liters of beverage p.c.
Spirits (40)	1	Poland	4.5
	2	Hungary	3.4
	3	Cyprus	3.3
	4	Czechoslovakia	3.3
	5	Bulgaria	2.8
	6	*Germany*	2.7
	7	*Spain*	2.7
	8	*Greece*	2.7
	9	Finland	2.6
	10	*France*	2.5
	...		
	14	Netherlands	2.0
	...		
	20	Ireland	1.7
	...		
	22	United Kingdom	1.6
	...		
	27	Luxembourg	1.6
	...		
	29	Denmark	1.3
	...		
	31	Belgium	1.2
	...		
	33	Italy	1.0
	...		
	36	Portugal	0.8

and among the top ten there are altogether six EU countries. For beer, the situation is very similar. The dominance of the EU countries in wine and beer consumption is well-known in the public debate. Less attention has been paid to the fact that in consumption of distilled spirits there are four EU countries in the top ten. The former GDR would have had the highest position in the spirits consumption in 1989 and 1990. Thus, for all beverage types, the area with highest consumption in the world is to be found within the EU.

One way of describing changes in beverage preferences is to use so called triangle diagrams (Figure 1.2). In that diagram, the position of each country is determined by the distribution of the country's aggregate alcohol consumption into beer, wine and spirits, in terms of liters of alcohol. In the diagram, countries where more than 50 percent of total alcohol consumption is drunk as beer will be located in the subtriangle on the top. Respectively, countries where the share of wine exceeds 50 percent are located in the bottom left triangle, and countries where beer dominates lie in the bottom right triangle. In the fourth triangle in the middle, none of the beverage types has a share over 50 percent.

The triangle is useful in illustrating changes in beverage preferences. In Figure 1.2, all EU countries except Greece are included, and information from both 1970 and 1990 has been used. The short lines, or arrows, beginning from the dot at the symbol of the country indicate the change in beverage preferences between 1970 and 1990. The interpretation of the figure is straightforward. Wine countries in the bottom left triangle have moved towards the centre and in direction of increasing popularity of beer. This is particularly true for Spain and Portugal, but to a much less extent for France and Italy. Respectively, the beer countries in the top triangle have moved towards the wine corner. Ireland, however, has stayed on its own. The two countries in the more neutral area in 1970 were Luxembourg and Netherlands. The former has moved towards the increasing popularity of wine, whereas in the latter both beer and wines have gained in popularity. It should be remembered that the arrows are based on information for two years only, and thus do not describe movements between 1970 to 1990 in any detail. The whole truth on these movements is much more complicated than that depicted in Figure 1.2.

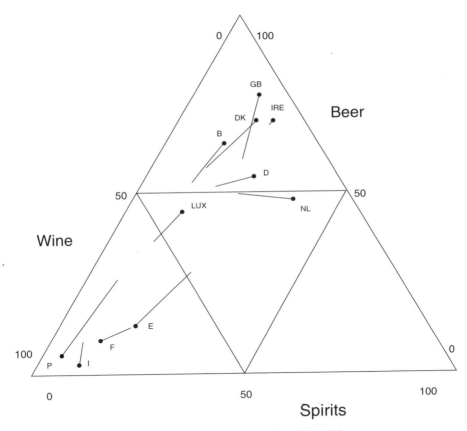

Figure 1.2 Changes in beverage preferences in the EU countries, 1970–1990.

A country's location is determined by the distribution of alcohol consumption into beer, wine and spirits. In the subtriangle on the top, the share of beer exceeds 50 percent. Respectively, the share of wine is over 50 percent in the bottom left triangle, and the share of spirits exceeds 50 percent in the bottom right triangle. In the central triangle, none of the beverages has a share over 50 percent. The change in each country is indicated by an arrow, starting from a dot denoting the situation in 1970. The other end of the arrow shows the location in 1990. The years between have not been shown.

If one is to speculate about the further homogenization of beverage preferences in the EU countries, the information in Figure 1.2 would suggest that there is a point of convergence somewhere in the vicinity of the location of Luxembourg in the year 1970. That is, over 40 percent of the consumption would be beer, a little smaller share would be given to wine, and less than 20 percent would be left for spirits. This is, however, a highly speculative forecast. As is evident from figure 1.2, many of the EU countries would have a long way to go towards that point of convergence. It is unlikely, although not impossible, that the changes in the next twenty years would be very much larger than in the last 20 years depicted in Figure 1.2. In that case, there would still be relatively large differences between the EU countries 20 years from now.

Long waves and short-term fluctuations

It would be fascinating to forecast that the post-war trend of homogenization of consumption levels and beverage preferences would continue for a long time in the future. There has been a lot of discussion of really long historical waves in alcohol consumption. Room (1991, 151) suggests that industrialized countries have undergone during the last two centuries long waves of alcohol consumption with the periodicity of approximately three generations, or some 70 years. It is a matter of further research to find out whether the 1980's are a turning point in the long wave of increasing alcohol consumption in the western industrialized world. To talk about a long wave in terms of consumption levels might seem ungrounded in the EU as the wine countries certainly have experienced a development different from most other countries. Also, the role of the process of homogenization in the suggested long waves awaits further discussion.

It is undeniable that each country is undergoing long-term historical changes that have an effect on alcohol consumption and drinking patterns. The post-war urbanization in Western Europe has eroded rural life-forms in many countries. The variation of structure with time is different in urban waged labour compared with subsistence farming. In the modern or even post-modern consumer societies, the way of life does not much resemble the patterns in traditional industrial communities. Housing, family relations and social networks in the EU countries are today quite different from those some 30 years ago. Items that are sometimes called "the culture" or "the consciousness" of people are changing all the time. The meaning and interpretation given to alcoholic beverages, their uses and even consequences of drinking will also vary with time. It has been suggested that such cultural changes often occur on the time scale of generations rather than in shorter periods (cf. Sulkunen 1983).

The effect of historical and generational changes on alcohol consumption may be different in different countries. In many wine-drinking countries, the habit of consuming daily large amounts of wine, predominantly at meals and as a part of nutrition, has been most strongly associated with rural life-forms. In some other countries, rural life-forms may have been characterized by a very moderate consumption of alcoholic beverages. The process of urbanization, then, may have led to quite opposite effects on alcohol consumption in different countries. Basically the same processes may reduce consumption growth in one country but increase drinking in some other country.

In addition to long-term historical waves and medium-term generational changes, there are also short-term fluctuations that may influence the level of alcohol consumption.

Typical examples of such variation are economic conjectures. Changes in purchasing power are reflected in alcohol consumption in all developed countries, and this is true for the EU of early 1990's. Another type of short-term fluctuation arises from changes in political and institutional environment. In Denmark, joining the EU in 1972 led to a marked increase in wine consumption, despite the economic depression in the following few years (see Thorsen 1990, 1993). It is likely that deepening integration within the EU will have numerous short-term and medium-term effects on the level of alcohol consumption in most of the member countries. Harmonization of the taxation of alcoholic beverages, changes in regulation of border trade, etc. all will influence the relative prices and availability of alcoholic beverages and will be reflected in consumption levels (cf. Tigerstedt (ed.) 1990).

4. SPECIFIC REMARKS ON EACH OF THE EU MEMBER COUNTRIES

The above discussion already shows that it is insufficient to treat all the EU countries as a supposedly homogeneous group. In each country, there are some specific features in the development of alcohol consumption, both in long-term effects and in short-term fluctuations. The notes below are not a systematic analysis but serve as examples of factors to be considered. Besides the processes of change, some problems related to the reliability of the consumption data in each country will be touched. Figure 1.1 should be used as the general description of the development of alcohol consumption in each country.

Belgium

Although the level of alcohol consumption has been relatively stable in Belgium since the early 1970's, there has been a remarkable change in beverage preferences. This is indicated by a sharp drop in the share of distilled spirits since the mid-1980's. The reports available do not provide much explanation for this development. The drop in the consumption of spirits is partly compensated by increasing wine consumption. There is a long-term trend of increasing wine-drinking in the country, dating back to the 1960's. A question worth considering in Belgium is the share of foreign citizens, both residents and tourists, in the total alcohol consumption. Another issue is the border trade in alcoholic beverages. Neither of these questions have been discussed in the standard references on alcohol consumption in Belgium.

Denmark

In Denmark, much of recent research literature is available on the long-term development of alcohol consumption and consequences of drinking (see in particular Thorsen 1990 and 1993). Economic changes and the joining of the EU in 1972 are reflected in the development of alcohol consumption. A rapid rise in wine consumption and a slower long-term trend of increasing beer-drinking resulted in a significant growth by the early 1980's. After that, there has been a very stable period. The issue of unregistered alcohol consumption is important in Denmark. It has been estimated that as much as 20 to

25 percent of alcohol consumption is the border trade between Denmark and Germany (cf. Bygvrå 1990). Home production is also an important part of the supply of alcohol. Along with the new EU regulations on alcohol imports by private EU citizens since 1993, the volume of border trade has forced the Danish government to reduce the taxation on beer several times. Border trade between Denmark and Sweden should also be considered as a factor requiring correction in the consumption statistics.

France

In France, the general trend of a long-term decrease in wine consumption has been the subject of several studies (e.g. Sulkunen 1988, 1989). The major explanation for that development lies in the modernization of life-styles, spreading from the centre to the periphery. Traditional wine-drinking is disappearing from the modern life-form. As a technical issue concerning French statistics on alcohol consumption, the volume of home production seems to be a marginal element. By the mid-1980's, unregistered distillation was estimated at some 5 percent of the consumption of spirits (Haut Comitée ..., cited in the International Survey, 1989, p. 137). No estimates of unregistered wine consumption were presented.

Germany

In the former Federal Republic of Germany, the level of alcohol consumption was relatively stable in the 1970's and 1980's. The changes were quite different in the former German Democratic Republic. The former GDR showed a consistent growth in alcohol use all through the 1970's and 1980's (cf. e.g. Winter 1990). Although the data on the GDR may be unreliable, the country was evidently one of the few industrialized countries with a growth of alcohol consumption in the late 1980's. Already before the reunification, there were large differences in beverage preferences between the northern Germany and the rest of the country. Recent reports on the eastern regions indicate a higher level of alcohol consumption than elsewhere in Germany (Junge 1993; see also Herbst *et al.*, 1993). The eastern "Neue Bundesländer" have brought a strong element of spirits drinking into the German spectrum of alcoholic beverages, thereby strengthening the distinctions between Schnapps regions, beer drinking and the wine-using areas in Germany.

Greece

The statistical material on alcohol consumption in Greece has been quite limited and often regarded as unreliable (cf. World Drink Trends 1993, p. 7). Therefore, it is difficult to make any comment on the trends of alcohol consumption in this country. Additional problems to the reliability of the statistics may be caused by the unknown extent of home production and the presumably significant consumption by the millions of foreign tourists. A recent source (the country report on Greece in "Young People and Alcohol in Europe", 1994, pp. 361–371), dares to arrive at a conclusion that the level of consumption in Greece has been fairly stable since the 1960s. The structure of consumptions has, however, changed in favor of beer at the expense of wines. The same source repeats (ibid. p. 371) the well-known fact that alcohol problems are of little concern in Greece as a health or public policy issue. The standard explanation for this is that drinking is so deeply integrated in everyday life that informal control has been sufficient to prevent excessive problems. Of course, the economic interests of local wine industries may also have discouraged health policy initiatives in Greece.

Ireland

The trend of alcohol consumption in Ireland is somewhat different from the most general patterns among the EU countries. A lengthy period of increasing consumption was stopped by a deep economic recession in the late 1970's, and the consumption trend turned downward after a peak of a few years. Indeed, economic factors have been presented as the major factor underlying the turn in the trend (cf. Walsh l'1987). There are some doubts on the reliability of the Irish consumption data in the leading statistical source (World Drink Trends, 1993), but the nature of these doubts is not clarified there.

Italy

The decline in alcohol consumption in Italy since the mid-1970's is even more spectacular than the decline in France. Similar processes of modernization as those referred to in France are involved here. The generational gap, with young people turning away from wine, has been reported to be a significant factor (Rossi 1992; see also Pyörälä 1990). Recent survey results show that a decline in consumption involves all beverage types, but wine consumption has been hit hardest (Gli italiani e l'alcool, 1994, p. 31). The results also show that the trend in reduction in alcohol consumption is highest among working-class males, but is also significant in other male groups (Gli italiani e l'alcool 1994, p. 30). As a technical detail, the concerns over home production and tourist consumption as confounding factors behind the consumption statistics should be repeated here.

Luxembourg

In some earlier editions of the world alcohol consumption statistics, Luxembourg reached unusually high consumption figures for the early 1980's. This peak was corrected in later editions. The explanation for such fluctuation is the extensive border trade in Luxembourg, in particular with wine. In the 1992 edition of the "World Drink Trends", a footnote states that "national sales are heavily influenced by tourist and cross-border consumers". It is therefore difficult to say anything definite about the trends of alcohol consumption in Luxembourg.

The Netherlands

The Netherlands experienced a very rapid growth of alcohol consumption in the 1960's, and the growth has continued at a lower pace until 1980 (cf. de Lint 1981; Knibbe *et al.*, 1985). Thereafter, the consumption has become stabilized and changed to a slow decline by the end of the 1980's. The standard explanations of modernization and generational shifts have been proposed here (cf. Knibbe *et al.*, 1985). An interesting feature in the

Netherlands has been the rapid rise of consumption of low-alcoholic and non-alcoholic beers since the mid-1980's. It has been estimated that some 5 to 10 percent of all beer consumed is low-alcoholic (cf. Nachrichten für Aussenhandel, May 19, 1992). More recent information indicates, however, that the boom of non-alcoholic and low-alcoholic beverages may be slowing down. Similar growth of consumption of low-alcoholic beverages has been reported in some other countries but the phenomenon is probably most visible in the Netherlands.

Portugal

Portugal has relatively late joined the declining trend of alcohol consumption found in other wine-drinking countries (cf. Pyörälä 1990). In Portugal, the declining wine consumption is strongly paralleled, although not compensated, by increasing beer drinking. Again, the consumption of domestic products and the amounts consumed by increasing numbers of tourists might require further checks of the data. The 1989 edition of the International Survey by The Brewers' Association of Canada (p. 302) reminds the reader that in Portugal "... practically all farmers have small vineyards and produce wine for their own use". Similarly, "without the tourist industry consumption of alcoholic beverages would probably be 10 per cent lower than the figures shown in official statistics" (p. 303).

Spain

The trends of alcohol consumption in Spain have been relatively well-reported in a number of studies (e.g. Pyörälä 1990; Alvarez *et al.*, 1991; Gili *et al.*, 1991). Again, the standard explanations for changes in living conditions and resulting generational shifts have been reported as underlying factors for the decline of wine and the rise of beer usage. A study on the drinking patterns of young adults in Spain (Pyörälä 1991) shows that abandoning wine-drinking at home meals is commonplace among young Spanish people. The traditional pattern is becoming replaced by a leisure-type drinking with peers and with intoxication as a recognized element of drinking. The new pattern may lead to lower overall alcohol consumption compared to the traditional ones. In Spain, as in other Mediterranean wine countries, domestic production of wine for domestic use is an error factor in consumption statistics. The tens of millions of foreign tourists make another problem. A few years ago it was estimated that as much as 25 percent of the consumption of distilled spirits in Spain is drunk by foreign tourists ("speculation by Spanish distillers", quoted in the International Survey, ..., 1989, p. 314).

United Kingdom

In Britain, the 1980's was a period of relatively stable alcohol consumption after an increase in the 1970's. No special effects due to fluctuation of economic status can be seen in the trends of alcohol consumption. In the pattern of consumption there is a remarkable shift from beer in favour of wine. However, beer has kept its dominating position. British sources (e.g. Duffy 1991, Harding 1991) do not contain any references to unregistered consumption or extensive home production of alcoholic beverages. From the beginning of 1993, however, the British have taken advantage of the more liberal cross-border trade rules of the EU, and tourist imports of alcohol from France have grown to an unknown extent.

5. ON THE DYNAMICS OF CHANGES IN ALCOHOL CONSUMPTION

This brief review, country by country, supports the view that there are multiple factors affecting the volume of alcohol consumption, and these factors operate on variable time horizons. Long-term historical waves, generational shifts and short-term fluctuations are already discussed above. These three levels of change are certainly intermingle. In the EU context, for instance, one has to regard the integration itself as a historical process influencing through various channels a short-term perspective. Clearly, some of the changes in the level of alcohol consumption and in beverage preferences can be attributed to the EU integration. Increase of wine consumption in Denmark at the mid-1970's and in general the slowly but steadily strengthening popularity of wine in the northern EU member countries are good examples. Another issue related to the EU is the process of harmonizing alcohol taxes, producing price changes and thereby consumption effects.

Generational shifts are most visible in Spain and Italy, and these shifts cannot necessarily be connected with the ongoing integration. Rather, they are linked with deeper processes of modernization operating through cultural patterns. A pattern that may look modern in one society can be regarded as a remnant from old times in another. Drinking wine at meals serves here as a good example. It appears as a slowly decreasing pattern in the Mediterranean wine countries whereas in the northern EU countries that pattern is becoming stronger (cf. Hupkens *et al.*, 1993). In both directions, this shift seems to be generational in many countries, the young and the well-educated being the avant-garde in adopting new habits. Of course, integration effects may have supported these cultural changes. One needs not worry about the disappearance of national cultural identities, as those processes are slow. For instance, the British drink most of their wine outside meals, quite contrary to the prevailing patterns in Mediterranean countries (see Hupkens *et al.*, 1993).

Three additional factors should be mentioned. In many EU countries, medium-term fluctuations in alcohol consumption have been related to general economic developments. In some cases, which are admittedly rare within the EU, public policy measures may have had an impact on consumption levels. Of course, much of the integration is produced by public policy measures, although not specifically targeted to the level of alcohol consumption. The third factor here is the attitudinal and ideological change. In the EU countries there is so far no parallel to the health ideology so prominent in the U.S.A. A European variant of such an ideology cannot be excluded from European scenarios, although the impact of healthy lifestyles on alcohol consumption is not necessarily the same in Europe as in America.

Changes in alcohol consumption often appear to take place collectively. They seem to penetrate the whole population, at least in the course of time (cf. Skog 1985). Through interaction in various social networks, the changes originating in smaller groups may spread over larger numbers of people. The population, then, seems to move in concert over the distribution of consumption. In such a way, the phenomenon called "peer drinking" is an essential factor in the dynamics of alcohol consumption, not only among adolescents, but also, and more importantly, among the adult population. This view has been criticized for being too simplistic, and some evidence has been presented on changes that go to opposite directions in different subgroups of population (e.g. Duffy 1991, 1993). Thus, the qualitative changes in drinking patterns seems to spread unevenly, as is the case in the modernization of Mediterranean drinking patterns. The question of collectivity of changes in drinking requires more research in the EU countries, in order to better understand both the quantitative and qualitative dynamics behind changes in consumption levels.

There are a number of differences in drinking trends between the EU countries. The discussion above suggests that these differences are mostly outcomes of cultural, social and political processes. The effects are often indistinguishable and may go in opposite directions in different countries. A good example is the urban vs. rural distinction. In wine countries, heaviest wine drinking and thus heaviest alcohol consumption in general is related to rural and even backward ways of life, whereas the modern urban dwellers have a stronger tendency to reduce their drinking. In some northern EU countries, rural life is connected with more restricted alcohol consumption, but the modern urban lifestyle fosters heavy drinking. Genetic factors are sometimes suggested as an additional explanation of different alcohol consumption trends in different countries. Although genetics certainly play a role in individual differences in experiencing alcohol problems, there is little evidence that the genetic explanation could be extended to concern population differences in alcohol consumption trends.

6. PROBLEMS OF DETERMINING THE LEVEL OF ALCOHOL CONSUMPTION IN THE EU COUNTRIES

The country by country review also revealed a number of technical problems in determining the actual consumption level in each country. A list of problematic issues will serve as a summary here (see e.g. International Statistics for a more extensive discussion, 1977). These problems are becoming more openly discussed in the international statistics. In the 1993 Edition of "World Drink Trends", the summary table on aggregate alcohol consumption is, for the first time, provided with a three-point evaluation of the reliability of data for each country.

What is an alcoholic beverage?

The EU norms and standards provide a league of exact definitions for various categories of alcoholic beverages. A problem arises, however, at the lower end of the alcohol content scale, with low-alcoholic beverages. It is a matter of convention to what extent such beverages are included in national and international statistics. The question on how alcoholic beverages are defined is important both from the commercial and public health perspectives, as low-alcoholic beverages are an increasing part of market and consumption.

Consumption vs. sales vs. production

A pertinent problem in international statistics has been the distinction between data on production, sales and consumption. Evidently, this problem is diminishing within the EU with better standardization of industry and trade statistics. On the other hand, the longer the integration goes on, the more difficult it may become to trace the products from the site of production to the site of consumption. A recent example of this kind of problem comes from outside the EU. In Poland, the official statistics show a decline in alcohol consumption in the late 1980's. However, only domestic production is included in the statistics, whereas the huge and uncontrolled import is completely omitted (see Wald *et al.*, 1993).

Per capita consumption and demographic structures

It is a standard procedure in comparing counties to calculate per capita consumptions for the whole population. This is a problem in two cases. In the first case, countries may have very different shares of population in the most active drinking age. Large numbers of very old or very young citizens may cause problems in determining the "true" alcohol consumption levels for comparison. One solution here is to calculate the figures for some specific age bracket, such as those over 15 years of age. However, a second problem may arise. In some countries, children and young people hardly drink at all, whereas in others drinking of diluted alcoholic beverage may be a common practice among some groups of children. For instance, a report from Spain (quoted by Quiros Corujo and Riesgo Gonzales, 1985) estimated that in a certain region the average consumption for the age group 4 to 14 years was 4 liters alcohol per capita each year. Similar problems will arise if differences in demographic structures are corrected by excluding some of the oldest age groups.

Consumption by foreigners and consumption abroad

The consumption of alcohol by foreign tourists has a considerable share of aggregate consumption in may EU countries. The resulting error in consumption statistics is seldom completely compensated for by the consumption abroad by the country's own citizens. Specific studies and statistics on travel and tourism would help to estimate the extent of this part of consumption.

The unregistered consumption: home production, smuggling, tourist imports

Various forms of home production may play an important role in alcohol consumption. This issue is often mentioned in Mediterranean countries but seldom in other EU countries. The extent of smuggling within the EU is also seldom discussed in this context. The legal imports by tourists and other travellers evidently play an important role in the alcohol consumption in some countries (e.g. Luxembourg and Denmark). Most of the estimates of unregistered consumption must be regarded as "guesstimates" (see e.g. Hannibal 1993). There are, however, serious efforts to develop better methods of estimating this "dark figure" of alcohol consumption (see e.g. Nordlund 1992).

7. PROPOSALS FOR IMPROVING DATA BASES ON CHANGES IN AGGREGATE ALCOHOL CONSUMPTION WITHIN THE EU

This review has listed a number of areas where administrative cooperation and joint research efforts would be useful within the EU, in order to provide better data on trends in alcohol consumption. The work done so far by industrial organizations, official statistics organizations and researchers has been most valuable, and the proposals here would be best realized by some kind of collaboration between the existing bodies, both private and public. Understandably, the fact that the discussants around alcohol consumption are divided into opposite lobbies may distort any form of collaboration. Therefore, initiatives from EU bodies would be crucial in supporting the efforts proposed here.

Improving the reliability of alcohol consumption statistics

The numerous problems on consumption statistics certainly indicate a need for research and technical collaboration. Both national and international bodies should be involved. Each of the problems mentioned above would serve as a specific issue of collaboration. Statistical organizations within the EU with their extensive experience and with their presumably neutral position might have a strong role in such efforts.

Completing consumption statistics by information from comparable alcohol consumption surveys

An indispensable part of the data base for describing and understanding the trends in alcohol consumption would be population surveys of drinking patterns. In the above discussion, a number of issues could be at least partly illuminated by survey results. So far, there are very few attempts to compare drinking habit surveys of all the EU countries (Eurobarometer from 1988 is one of these; see Hupkens *et al.*, 1993 for results). National general population surveys are available for most of the EU countries (e.g. Estudio ..., 1984 from Spain; Simon and Wiblishauser 1993 from Germany; Sabroe 1993 from Denmark; Goddard and Ikin 1988 from Britain; Aigrain *et al.*, 1991 and Balmes *et al.*, 1988 from France; Knibbe and Swinkels 1992 from the Netherlands, etc.). These studies are, however, very different in scope and methodology, which makes it difficult to use them in secondary comparative analyses (for attempts see e.g. Simpura *et al.*, 1995, Simpura 1995). In Europe, informal groups of involved researchers have made a few efforts to set foundations for a better international comparability between studies on drinking patterns and alcohol consumption, but so far the efforts have been unsuccessful. The efforts will most likely continue, as the extending and deepening integration raises more interest in comparative European studies. Various EU bodies could have an active role in supporting these attempts.

8. CONCLUSION

To conclude, the complexity of the dynamics behind the trends in alcohol consumption makes it necessary to extend the discussion beyond the mere consumption figures. The intermingled processes operating over different time ranges should all be simultaneously considered.

In 1995 it appears that the homogenization of consumption levels and beverage preferences within the EU will continue and will become strengthened by the intensification of integration in Europe. The worldwide experience of the post-war history of alcohol consumption indicates that large changes are possible in any direction. Therefore, it is not automatically true that alcohol consumption in the EU countries will converge toward the level of 10 liters. After one generation, the situation can be quite different, in particular as uncertainty in the world as a whole is increasing.

Presently, the level of alcohol consumption is an important symbolic issue in the battle between opposite alcohol lobbies within the EU. But the importance of trends of alcohol consumption is not limited to the symbolic level. The huge economic interests of alcohol production and trade cannot be denied. At the same time, it seems that the importance of consumption levels as an indicator of, and instrument for, preventing alcohol problems is becoming more openly discussed. Whatever the outcome of the battle around alcohol in the EU will be, the issue of alcohol consumption has come there to stay on the agenda. Maybe the battle will be solved by arriving at a reformulation of the goals of the prevention of alcohol problems. "Harm reduction" would be a good candidate for the title of an European agenda, with the focus on minimizing harmful consequences of drinking with a strategy that would contain not only control consumption levels but also target action on specific alcohol-related risks.

9. PROPOSALS FOR FURTHER RESEARCH

Section 7 above contains a number of technical proposals to facilitate comparisons between the EU countries. Another direction for future action and research is to consider the dynamics of alcohol consumption and drinking patterns in a broader social, cultural, economic and political context in Europe. Much of the scientific discussion concerning the dynamics of alcohol consumption comes from outside the EU countries. Given the importance of EU as the leading alcohol producer and consumer in the world, it is worthwhile to start efforts to understand these dynamics within the EU. There is certainly space for different approaches, ranging from econometric to politological and cultural studies. It is very likely that any single standard approach would be insufficient for grasping the complexity of these phenomena.

Intensifying research on the link between alcohol consumption levels and alcohol-related harm is an essential component in setting the agenda for the public debate around alcohol. Although some participants in the debate deny the existence of the link between consumption level and the prevalence of harm on population level, the need for compiled EU data on the consequences of drinking is evident for all partners. A proposal from the EU in that direction would certainly make it possible to recruit the best available experts to the work.

As an example of research proposals in this field, the question of life histories of drinkers in general and problem drinkers in particular is a much-disputed but little studied issue. It is not very well known to what extent, how permanently and how consciously heavy drinkers actually manage to reduce or otherwise control their drinking over the lifetime. Besides the implications of such research for prevention of problem drinking on the individual level, this question is also related to the interpretation of changes in consumption levels in various populations. It was suggested above that alcohol consumption typically changes over the time-scale of generations, and even longer waves may be involved. This would imply, among other things, that changes in the drinking patterns among the present adult population are less important than those occurring in the rising new generation. This is of course a contradictory statement, as many studies show that changes in alcohol consumption patterns mostly take place in all population segments and not only in the younger generation.

The next question, then, would be about the changes that influence the formation of new generational patterns and attitudes towards alcohol. Both the proponents of controlling consumption and the advocates of alcohol education find ammunition here. For the former, the undeniable importance of access to alcohol as a shape-giver to later drinking patterns is important. For the latter, the new generation is always the ideal target of alcohol education, not least because of the subordinate position of young people. However, in a broader perspective of the social change in Europe, the question should be formulated in more general terms. This reformulation should begin with considerations of what is happening in the social and political life in Europe. The common way of speaking about Europe as a whole already creates a bias of uniformity, supported by the slogans of integration, homogenization, convergence and harmonization.

The other side of the mirror looks quite different. Prominent social scientists stress the processes of fragmentation of social structures in everyday life, disappearance of the ties of tradition, the loss of cohesion as presented in the institutional basis of industrial society etc. (see e.g. Beck, 1994; Giddens, 1994). Disintegration and destructuration are proceeding parallel with the visible processes of political and economic integration. The late modern world is in itself challenging the public intervention of any kind in private lives. The heralds of the new Europe, sometimes called the new middle classes, may prove to be particularly reluctant to approve of public interventions in their drinking, be it control or education (cf. Sulkunen, 1994). The battle between alcohol lobbies, fought within the framework of public institutions and nation-states, looks different from the perspective of the postmodern world. The premises of prevention as well as those of marketing may be radically changing, irrespective of political decisions.

References

Aigrain, P., Boulet, D., Lambert, J.L. and Laporte, J.P. (1991). La consommation du vin en France: evolutions tendancielles et diversite des comportements. *Revue de l'Economie Meridionale*, **39** (3 and 4):19–52.
Alcoholic beverages and the European society (1993). A report from the Amsterdam Group. Amsterdam.
Balmés, J.-L., Boulet, D. and Picheral, H. (1989). Approche des processus d'alcoolisation: L'exemple du Languedoc-Roussillon. *Journal d'Alcoologie* 2:99–113.
Beck (1994). The reinvention of politics: towards a theory of reflexive modernization. pp. 1–55 in: Beck, U., Giddens, A. and Lash, S. *Reflexive Modernization*. Polity Press, Cambridge.
Bruun, Kettil *et al.* (1975). *Alcohol Control Policies in Public Health Perspective*. WHO and FFAS, Helsinki.
Bygvrå, Suzzane (1990). Border shopping between Denmark and West Germany. *Contemporary Drug Problems* **17** (4):595–610.
Consumer Europe (1993). Euromonitor. London.
de Lint, J. (1981). The influence of much increased alcohol consumption on mortality rates: the Netherlands between 1950 and 1975. *British Journal of Addiction*, **76**:77–83.
Duffy, J.C. (1991). *Trends in alcohol consumption patterns*. NTC Publication Ltd, Henley-on-Thames.
Duffy, J.C. (1993). Alcohol consumption and control policy. *Journal of Royal Statistical Society*, A:**156**, part 2: 225–230.

Edwards, G., Anderson, P., Babor, T.F., Casswell, S., Ferrence, R., Giesbrech, N. *et al.* (1994). *Alcohol Policy and The Public Good*. Oxford University Press, Oxford.

Estudio de los habitos de consumo de alcohol de la poblacion adulta espanola (1904). Ministerio de Sanidad y Consumo, Madris, Spain.

European Alcohol Action Plan (1993). Alcohol, Drugs and Tobacco Unit Lifestyles and Health Department, Regional Office for Europe, World Health Organization, Copenhagen, Denmark.

European Marketing Data and Statistics (1992). Euromonitor, London.

Fahrenkrug, Hermann (1987). *Gesundheitspolitische Initiativen zur Alkoholproblematik in den Mitgliedstaaten der europäischen Gemeinschaften*. Gesomed, Freiburg, Germany.

Giddens, Anthony: Living in a post-traditional society. Pp. 56–110 in: Beck, U., Giddens, A. and Lash, S. *Reflexive Modernization*. Polity Press, Cambridge, UK.

Gili, M., Giner, J., Lacalle, J.R., Franco, D., Perea, E. and Dieguez, J. (1989). Patterns of consumption of alcohol in Seville, Spain. Results of a general population survey. *British Journal of Addiction* **84**:277–285.

Gli Italiani e l'Alcool (1994). Consumi, tendenze ed attegiamenti. Osservatorio Permanente sui Giovane e l'Alcool. Roma, Italy.

Goddard, Eileen and Ikin, Clare (1988). *Drinking in England and Wales* in 1987. HMSO, London, UK.

Hannibal, J. Alcohol control policy: Sweden with examples from Finland and Norway. Annex to the Report by the Amsterdam Group, "*Alcoholic Beverages and the European Society*", op. cit., 1993.

Harding, R.J. Consommation d'alcool au Royayme-Uni/Alcohol consumption in the United Kingdom (1991). *Bulletin de l'O.I.V.*, **64**, 725–726:555–574.

Herbst, K., Schumann, J. and Wiblishauser, P.M. (1993). Repräsentativerhebung zum Konsum and Mißbrauch von Illegalen Drogen, alkoholischen Getränken, Medikamenten und Tabakwaren. IFT Institut für Therapieforschung. München.

Holder, H.D. and Edwards, G. (1995). *Alcohol and Public Policy. Evidence and Issues*. Oxford University Press, Oxford.

Hupkens, L.H., Knibbe, R.A. and Drop, M.J. (1993). Alcohol consumption in the European Community: uniformity and diversity in national drinking patterns. *Addiction* **88**:1391–1404.

International Statistics on Alcoholic Beverages (1977). Production, Trade and Consumption 1950–1972. FFAS, Helsinki.

International Survey. Alcoholic Beverage Taxation and Control Policies (1992). Brewers' Association of Canada, Ottawa 8th edition.

Junge, D. (1993). Alkohol In: *Jahrbuch Sucht '94*. Deutsche Hauptstelle gegen die Suchtgefahren. Geestahackt.

Knibbe, Drop, M.J., van Reek, J. and Saenger, G. (1985). The development of alcohol consumption in the Netherlands: 1958–1991. *British Journal of Addiction*.

Knibbe R.R.A. and Lemmens, P.H. (1987). Korrelate des Alkoholkonsums in der Schweiz, Deutschland und den Niederlanden. *Drogalkohol* **11**.27–41.

Knibbe, R. and Swinkels, H. (1992). Alcoholgebruik in Nederland: een analyse van gegevens uit de CBS-gesondheidsenquete 1989. *Tijdschrift voor alcohol en drugs* **18(3)**:124–138.

Ledermann, (1956). Alcool, alcoolisme, alcoolisation. Vol I and II. Presses Universitaires de France, Paris.

Lehto J., and Moskalewicz, J. (1994). Alcohol Policy During Extensive Socio-Economic Change. WHO Regional Office for Europe, Copenhagen.

Lemmens, P.H.H.M. (1993). Regurality in the distribution of alcohol consumption. *Journal of Royal Statistical Society* A:**156**, part **2**:231–235.

Mäkelä, K., Room, R., Single, E., Sulkunen, P, Walsh, B. *et al.* (1981). Alcohol, Society and the State 1. A comparative study of alcohol control. Addiction Research Foundation, Toronto.

Moser, J. (1992). *Alcohol problems, policies and programs in Europe*. WHO, Regional Office for Europe, Copenhagen.

Nordlund, S. (1992). Metoder og metodproblemer ved estimering av alkoholforbruk. National Institute for Alcohol and Drug Research, Reports Nr. 3/92, Oslo.

Pequignot, G., Crosignani, R.P., Terracini, B., Ascunce, N., Zubiri, A., Raymond, L. *et al.* (1988). A comparative study of smoking, drinking and dietary habits in population samples in France, Italy, Spain and Switzerland. III. Consumption of alcohol. *Revue d'Epidemiologie et de Sante Publique*, **36**:177–185.

Quirós C.P. and R. Gonzales, Gonzalo (1987). Habit modifications in alcohol consumption in Spain. pp. 33–34 in: Paakkanen, Pirjo and Sulkunen, Pekka (eds.): *Cultural Studies on Drinking and Drinking Problems*. Report on a Conference. Reports from the Social Research Institute of Alcohol Studies, No 176.

Pyörälä, E. (1990). Trends in alcohol consumption in Spain, Portugal, France and Italy from the 1950's until the 1980's. British Journal of Addiction, **85**:469–477.

Pyörälä, E. (1991). *Nuorten aikuisten juomakulttuuri Suomessa ja Espanjassa* (Drinking culture among young adults in Finland and Spain). Reports from the Social Research Institute of Alcohol Studies, No 183, Helsinki.

Reader's Digest Eurodata (1991). A Consumer Survey of 17 European Countries. The Reader's Digest Association Ltd., London.

Room, R. (1991). Cultural changes in drinking and trends in alcohol problems indicators: Recent U.S. experience. Pp. 149–163 in: Clark, W. and Hilton, M. (eds): *Alcohol in America*. SUNY, New York.

Rossi, R. (1992). Alcool: consume e politiche in Europa. Edizioni Otet, Roma 1992.

Sabroe, Knud-Erik: Udviklingtendenser in alkoholforbrug 1988–1990 (Trends in the use of alcohol 1988–1990). Pp. 143–169 in Petersen, E. *et al*: *De trivsomme og arbejdsomme danskere*. University of Aarhus, Institute of Psychology, Aarhus.

Simon, R. and Wiblishauser, P.M. (1993). Ergebnisse der Repräsentativerhebung 1990 zum Konsum und Missbrauch von illegalen Drogen, alkoholischen Getränken, Medikamenten and Tabakwaren. *Sucht* **3**:177–180.

Simpura, J. (1995). Trends in alcohol consumption and drinking patterns: lessons from worldwide development. Pp. 9–37 in Holder, Harold and Edwards, Griffith (eds): Alcohol and Public Policy. Evidence and Issues. Oxford University Press, Oxford.

Simpura, J. Paakkanen, Pirjo, Mustonen, Heli (1995): New beverages, new drinking contexts? *Addiction*, in press.

Single, E., Morgan, P. and de Lint, J. (eds) (1981). *Alcohol, Society and the State 2*: The Social History of Control Policy in Seven Countries. Addiction Research Foundation, Toronto.

Skög, O. (1985). The collectivity of drinking cultures. British Journal of Addiciton, **80**:83–99.

Smart R.G. (1989). Is the postwar drinking binge ending? Cross-national trends in per capita alcohol consumption. *British Journal of Addition*, **84**:743–748.

Smart, R.G. (1991). World trends in alcohol consumption. *World Health Forum*, **12**:99–103.

Strazdins, J. (1994). Opportunities for an effective alcohol policy in Latvia. Paper presented at the Baltic Meeting on Alcohol Policy, organized by the WHO Regional Office for Europe, Riga, Latvia, August 31 to September 2, 1994.

Subata, E. (1994). Trends in alcohol consumption and alcohol–related problems in Lithuania. Paper presented at the Baltic Meeting on Alcohol Policy, organized by the WHO Regional Office for Europe, Riga, Latvia, August 31 to September 2, 1994.

Sulkunenv, P. (1993). Alcohol consumption and the transformation of living conditions. A comparative study. Pp. 247–297 in: R.J. Gibbins *et al*. (eds.) *Research Advances in Alcohol and Drug Problems*, Vol. **8**, Plenum, New York.

Sulkunen, P. (1989). Drinking in France 1965–1979. An analysis of household consumption data. *British Journal of Addiction*, **84**:61–72.

Sulkunen, P. (1992). *The European New Middle Class*. Individuality and Tribalism in Mass Society. Avebury, Aldershot.

Sulkunen, P. (1994). The conservative mind. Why does the now middle class hate alcohol control? *Addiction Research*, **1**(4):295–308.

Targets for health for all. Target in support of the European strategy for the health for all, WHO, Copenhagen 1985

Thorsen, T. (1988). Danskerne drikker mere end som så. *A and N-Debatt*, **33**:16–21.

Thorsen, T. (1990). Hundrede års alkoholmisbrug. Sundhetsstyrelsen, Copenhagen.

Thorsen, T. (1993). Dansk alkoholpolitik efter 1950. Forlaget Socpol, Hotle.

Tigerstedt, C. (ed) (1990): EG, alkohol och Norden (1990). (ed. by Christoffer Tigerstedt). NAD-*publikation* 19, The Nordic council for alcohol and drug research, Helsinki (Parts of this report are published in English in *Contemporary Drug Issues*, Winter 1990).

Vanston, N. (1991). Patterns and trends in alcohol consumption. A statistical survey. Pp. 333–46 in: Expert meeting on the negative social consequences of alcohol use. Oslo 27.–31. August 1990. Norwegian Ministry of Health and Social Affairs, in collaboration with the UN Office at Vienna Center for Social Development and Humanitarian Affairs, Oslo.

Wald, I., Markiewicz, A., Moravski, J., Moskalewicz, J., Sieroslawski, J., Swiątkiewicz, G. (1993). Alcohol *policy in the light of social changes. Pp. 88–94 in: Greenfield, T.K. and Zimmerman, Robert: Experiences with Community Action Projects: New Research in the Prevention of Alcohol and Other Drug Problems.* CSAP Monograph 14, DHHS, Rockville.

Walsh, B. (1987). Alcohol and Ireland. *British Journal of Addiction*, **82**:118–120.

Winter, E. (1991). Alkoholismus im Sozialismus der Deutschen Demokratischen Republic — Versuch eines Ruckblickes. *Sucht* **37**:71–85.

Wodak, A. (1994). Just say "no" to alcohol abuse and misuse. *Addiction* **89**:787–789.

World Drink Trends 1992. NTC Publications Ltd., Henley-on-Thames, 1992.

World Drink Trends 1993. NTC Publications Ltd., Henley-on-Thames, 1993.

Young People and Alcohol in Europe (1994). A tool for monitoring consumption and institutional action policies. Edizioni Otet, Roma.

2 Racial/Ethnic and Gender Differences in Alcohol Use and Misuse

Dharam P. Agarwal, Ph.D

Institute of Human Genetics, University of Hamburg, Butenfeld 32, 22529 Hamburg, Germany

This chapter gives an overview of the putative role of racial/ethnic and gender factors in alcohol use and misuse. Although the use of alcoholic beverages is found in virtually all societies, certain socio-economic, cultural, biobehavioural factors and ethnic/gender differences are among the strongest determinants of drinking pattern in a society. There is a considerable variation in the proportion of drinkers in a given population when divided by ethnicity, gender, age, religious affiliation and socio-economic status. The legacy of alcoholism among certain ethnic groups suggests that genetic factors can increase an individual's vulnerability for this disease. Although some of the putative environmental factors remain obscure in their nature, there is a strong evidence that there is a crucial interplay of nature and nurture, heredity and environment, and biology and culture in the development of alcoholism across ethnic groups and gender. Following the overview, proposals are made for future research.

INTRODUCTION

The distribution of drinking patterns in specific racial and ethnic groups is of great interest from the public health perspective. The "governing images" of alcohol problems differ considerably from one society to another, and they shift over time in a particular society or culture. Past epidemiological studies clearly indicate that race and gender differences in drinking pattern may play an important role in the development of medical conditions associated with alcohol misuse. Thus there is a considerable variation in the proportion of drinkers in a given population when divided by ethnicity, gender, age, religious affiliation and socio-economic status.

The legacy of alcoholism among certain ethnic groups suggests that genetic factors can increase an individual's vulnerability for this disease. Different underlying genetic factors may thus be responsible for the development of such disorders as FAS, cirrhosis and Wernicke-Korsakoff's syndrome in people exposed to high levels of alcohol use. On the other hand, individuals within certain ethnic groups have protective genetic factors that make them very sensitive to alcohol actions thereby acting as a deterrent to alcohol misuse. A better understanding of the contribution of these variables in drinking patterns may help to reduce the alcohol-related problems.

This report will focus on two main aspects of alcohol use and misuse: racial/ethnic differences in prevalence of alcohol-related morbidity and mortality, and gender difference in individual vulnerability to medical consequences of alcohol misuse. The aggregate data gathered from various sources have been used in the present report to elucidate possible interethnic and intergender relationships concerning alcohol metabolism, initial sensitivity reactions to alcohol drinking, alcohol drinking profile, and alcoholism.

FACTORS AFFECTING DRINKING BEHAVIOUR

Racial/Ethnic Perspectives

Interethnic differences in alcohol misuse is of great public health interest (Blane, 1993). However, an important problem is the recognition of genetically distinct subgroups within a population. Geneticists recognize five human races including Bushmen and Australian aborigines. The three larger races are the Caucasoids, Mongoloids, and Negroids. Each of the larger races consists of subgroups which do not always represent distinct and uniform groups; rather they represent populations with racial admixtures differing in geography, culture, lifestyle, and social and religious norms. Ethnicity on the other hand, may include different groups such as race, national heritage, religion, bureaucratic category, and special population.

Although the use of alcoholic beverages is found in virtually all societies, certain socio-economic, cultural, biobehavioural factors and ethnic/gender differences are among the strongest determinants of drinking pattern in a society (deLint, 1976). In particular, studies accrued in recent years clearly hint to a greater involvement of racial/ethnic factors in the evolution of alcohol use and misuse (Reed, 1985; Akutsu *et al.*, 1989; Agarwal and Goedde, 1990; Blane, 1993). Though restrictions on the accessibility of alcohol have a major impact on the lowering of the aggregate level of alcohol intake in a community, among immigrant populations, indigenous cultural styles and assimilation and acculturation to the so-called western societies have made a powerful impact on alcohol use. Thus the reported ethnic variations in alcohol use have a meaning only in regions where alcohol is freely available without widespread religious, moral, or economic restrictions.

Per Capita Alcohol Consumption in Different Population Subgroups

Yearly per capita consumption of alcohol in terms of absolute alcohol in liters in various population subgroups is displayed in Figure 2.1. The data have been compiled from the available survey reports of the past 10 years and indicate a secular trend only.

European as well as North American Caucasoids and Chileans show the highest per capita alcohol consumption followed by the Australian Aborigines, Brazilian Indios and partly by Papua New Guineans. Mexican Hispanics, South African Negroids, Japanese, Koreans, Chinese and Thais have an intermediate level of per capita consumption while Malays shows the lowest alcohol consumption.

Per Capita Alcohol Consumption

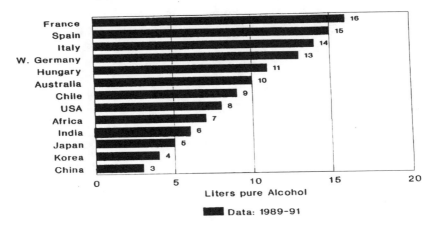

Figure 2.1 Approximate per capita consumption of alcohol (in terms of pure alcohol in liters) in various countries.

Alcohol Drinking Pattern, Alcohol Morbidity and Mortality Rate

Alcohol drinking pattern in different populations is usually estimated on the basis of quantity-frequency-variability classification. The populations are broadly divided into abstainers and drinkers. The drinking group is further divided into heavy, moderate/light, and infrequent drinkers. While it is quite difficult to classify different populations on the basis of any single criterium set for drinkers and nondrinkers, the available data (Table 2.1) do hint to a general pattern of drinking habits in these populations. Whereas the number of abstainers and infrequent drinkers is significantly high in the Mongoloids and Mexicans, the proportion of heavy and moderate drinkers is relatively higher in the Caucasoids, Australian Aborigines, Chileans, Filipinos and U.S. Blacks. The alcoholism rate, as percentage of the total population, and the alcohol-related mortality rate (per 100.000 persons) are compiled in Table 2.2. These data have been gathered from sources such as WHO reports and public health authorities, as well as through personal communications from scientist colleagues (Agarwal and Goedde, 1992). The cross-national pattern of alcohol-related morbidity is found to be very similar with about 3 to 5% alcoholism rate in most of the countries representing different racial and ethnic groups. However, the alcohol-related mortality rate (in terms of deaths from cirrhosis) varies considerably from country to country. The figures range from as low as between 3 to 6% in Thailand, Filipines and China, and as high as between 8 to 36% in Finland, Sweden, Mexico, Japan, Hungary, Germany, and Chile. For the Caucasoid populations living in Europe, North America, Australia, and Chile the average per capita yearly consumption ranges between 5 to 20 liters. These figures are considerably higher than the corresponding figures in the other populations except for Native Americans and Latin Americans (Hispanics). In most

Table 2.1 Alcohol drinking pattern in different populations* (Agarwal and Goedde, 1992)

Population	Drinkers (%)			Abstainers (%)
	Heavy	*Moderate*	*Infrequent*	
Caucasoids				
North Americans	21	46	22	11
Germans	16–47	32–53	9–16	6
Finns	12–18	48	0	25
Hungarians	20	30	30	20
Asian Indians	0–4	9–16	54–80	0–37
Australians	2–14	23–37	27–63	12–22
Mongoloids				
Chinese (Singapore)	3–6	8–10	50–86	0–36
Chinese (USA)	14	55	10	22
Japanese	31	29	25	14
Japanese (USA)	29	39	16	17
Koreans (USA)	26	28	1	45
Filipinos (USA)	29	37	16	17
Malays	1	0	0	99
Negroids				
US Blacks	13–22	38–71	0–24	0–16
Other populations				
Mexican Americans	7–18	26–42	0–12	27–60
Brazilian Indians	7	17	56	22
Chileans	20–25			
Papua New Guineans	9	47	16	22
Australian				
Aborigines	53	31	6	10

* = in most cases the data refer to male population age 15 and above

European countries, the U.S. and Chile, the aggregate alcohol consumption is relatively higher compared to other parts of the world except the Latin American countries. In the Scandinavian countries, particularly in Finland the per capita alcohol consumption has grown in recent years after a long stable period due to an increase in the availability of alcohol beverages and better economic conditions (Rahkonen and Ahlström, 1989).

Chinese cultural values stress moderate and infrequent drinking in that intoxication is permissible only at certain social situations such as wedding, banquets and family association meetings (Lee, 1987; Yeh *et al.*, 1989; Hughes *et al.*, 1990). On the contrary, drinking of alcohol has spread rapidly through the Japanese society during the past 20 years when Japan achieved her postwar reconstruction (Kono *et al.*, 1977; Saito, 1978). The spread of alcohol and alcoholic beverages has resulted in an increase in the drinking population, an increase in alcohol consumption, diversification of occasions for drinking and diversification of alcoholic drinks (Kono *et al.*, 1977; Suwaki and Ohara, 1985). The smallest consumption of alcohol is found in the Malay population in comparison with those of the other ethnic groups investigated (Hong and Isralowitz, 1989). For the Malay community, the Islamic religion acts as a deterrent to drinking alcohol because it counsels moderation (Armstrong, 1986).

Table 2.2   Alcoholism rate and alcohol-related mortality in different countries (Agarwal and Goedde, 1992)

Country	Alcoholism rate (%)	Alcohol-related mortality rate*
Germany	3–5	26.9–27.7
Sweden	2.4–3.6	8.0–12.2
Finland	4	4.3–8.2
Hungary	2.5–5	13.0–23.1
India	4.2	n.d.
Australia	5	7.7–8.3
China	3.4	6.4
Japan	3.7	13.4–24.3
Korea	9.9	n.d.
Thailand	n.d.	3.2–5.5
Filipines	n.d	4.1
Africa	**	13.8
Mexico	**	19.3
Brazil	3–12	n.d.
Papua New Guinea	**	**
Chile	5–13	35.7
Australia (Aborigines)	1.6	**

n.d. = no data available.
*   = deaths from alcoholic cirrhosis (per 100.00 persons).
**   = although exact data are not available, the reported epidemiological studies show a high rate of
       alcoholism and alcohol-related cirrhosis among these communities.

The Australian Aborigines comprise the population group with the highest percentage of heavy drinkers. Aborigines were noted to consume more alcohol and drink more often than non-Aborigines (Kamien, 1975; Thomson, 1984; Marshall *et al.*, 1985; Marshall, 1988). In Papua New Guinea drunkenness is widely accepted as an excuse for untoward behaviour, and the purchase and consumption of alcohol symbolizes participation in a sophisticated, modern, emergent Melanesian lifestyle (Marshall *et al.*, 1985). Papua New Guineans possessed a number of recreational drugs before alcoholic beverages came on the scene. Even though alcoholic beverages are easier to obtain all the time in Papua New Guinea, the great majority of the country's citizens still do not drink. When Papua New Guineans gather to drink, they do so with the intent of continuing until all available alcohol is gone, at which point they will go to search for more.

Among Mexican Americans both abstention and drinking are effected by a number of sociodemographic characteristics (Gilbert, 1989). Drinking decreases with age (Caetano, 1989; Christian *et al.*, 1989), and the alcohol consumption varies with education and income levels. Abstainers tend to be older with lower income and education, while drinkers tend to have the opposite characteristics (Caetano, 1989; Christian *et al.*, 1989; Gilbert, 1989). Alcoholism and alcohol-related problems are endemic in Chile, representing one of the most important Public Health problems of the country (Téllez, 1984). In Brazil the per capita consumption of alcohol is on a level which is comparable with that of the Caucasoids with the exception of the Scandinavians. The consumption of alcohol beverages is a widespread behaviour among the adolescent population in Sao Paulo, i.e. students from a low socioeconomic level and aging from 9 to 18 years (Carlini *et al.*, 1986). Nearly the same proportion of excessive regular drinkers is found in all the age groups.

Among the Asian-American groups, Koreans have the highest percentage of abstainers. The Koreans are likely to be one of the extremes, either abstainers or heavy drinkers (Lubben *et al.*, 1989). Heavy drinking among Japanese- and Korean-Americans is as prevalent as it is among men in the general U.S. population (Chi *et al.*, 1988; 1989). Data about Filipino Americans living in Los Angeles show that their drinking behaviour appears more comparable to the Western pattern (Herd, 1989; Lubben *et al.*, 1987).

Although in the U.S. black men, a greater proportion of lifelong abstinence is reported than in North Americans, the proportion of those black men reported to be heavy drinkers is only slightly lower than among whites (Herd, 1989). At the aggregate level both black and white men (North Americans) appear to have similar drinking patterns (Klatsky *et al.*, 1983). The per capita alcohol consumption of South Africans is relatively low; they evaluate both drinking and drunkenness in general negatively, although a substantial proportion accepts both in certain situations, particularly when the situation concerned is of a non-work nature (Rocha-Silva, 1988).

More recent epidemiological studies (Buchholz, 1992) further support the notion that there are ethnic differences in patterns of alcohol use and alcoholism prevalence, particularly across the racial and ethnic groups (African Americans, Hispanic Americans and Asian Americans as well as Pacific Islanders) living in the United States.

GENDER DIFFERENCE IN ALCOHOL INTAKE AND ALCOHOLISM

Most research on alcoholism has focused on men, largely because men are more likely than women to drink at all, and are particularly more likely to drink frequently and heavily (Gomberg, 1993). Even if gender difference in body weight and water content are taken into account, male predominance in heavy drinking persists (Dawson and Archer, 1992; Midanik and Room, 1992). Estimates from the Epidemiological Catchment Area (ECA) study (Helzer *et al.*, 1991) indicate that lifetime alcoholism prevalence rate was much higher for men (23.8 percent) than for women (4.6 percent). Patterns of 1-year prevalence were generally similar to those observed for lifetime prevalence. Male-to-female ratio increased with age; the ratio was lowest for the youngest age group and highest for the oldest age group. Taken together, these studies suggest that alcoholism is more common among men than among women, but the gender gap in alcoholism rates is closing rapidly as social attitudes surrounding drinking are changing. This is evident from a decreasing male-to-female ratio for alcohol misuse among younger age groups.

Basis of Gender Difference in Alcohol Actions

It is no secret that men and women respond differently to alcohol. Women are quicker to get giddy, and they stay drunk longer than men matching them drink for drink. The unique gender-related difference in alcohol drinking behaviour has been attributed to gross anatomical differences: on average, women are smaller than men, thus alcohol gets into body tissues more rapidly; they carry proportionately more fat and less water in their bodies resulting in higher cellular concentration of alcohol. Recent studies indicate that in women a relatively lower level of alcohol dehydrogenase (ADH), a primary enzyme in alcohol metabolism, in the gastric mucosa results in decreased gastric metabolism of alcohol and therefore higher peak blood alcohol levels are achieved in women than in men after ingesting similar quantities of alcohol (Frezza *et al.*, 1990; Seitz *et al.*, 1993). Moreover, alcoholic women showed almost no ADH activity at all, loosing all gastric protection. This lack of protection may help explain why alcoholic women suffer more heavily from liver damage than do alcoholic men.

Women may be more vulnerable to alcoholic cirrhosis for another reason. A sex difference in rates of alcohol elimination has been reported (Mishra *et al.*, 1989). The average rate of alcohol elimination was found to be significantly greater in women when compared with their male siblings. Thus higher alcohol elimination rate may lead to increased susceptibility to alcohol-related liver disease in women. Indeed, a disproportionate number of deaths from alcoholic liver disease in women compared with men (Mezey *et al.*, 1988) provides a clear evidence for a gender-specific difference in alcohol-related end organ damage.

These findings intensify earlier warnings that women are at higher risks for alcohol misuse related consequences. What is moderate drinking for men is not moderate drinking for women. This warning is of special significance in alcohol dependent women while pregnant. The injury caused by alcohol to the developing fetus leads to the birth defect known as "fetal alcohol syndrome" (FAS). This congenital disorder is characterized by a distinct cluster of symptoms including permanent physical abnormalities and mental retardation.

Genetic Contribution to Gender Differences

Conventionally, it is believed that social and psychological forces are far stronger among women than genetics in the steps leading to alcoholism. However, in a recent study, genetics has been shown to be an important determinant of vulnerability to alcoholism (Kendler *et al.*, 1992). The authors have investigated 1,080 adult pairs of female twins for their alcohol-related behaviour. The study revealed that at every level of alcoholism, identical twins were significantly more likely than fraternal twins to have similar histories of alcoholism. These results support an earlier finding from a Swedish study of women who had been adopted (Cloninger *et al.*, 1981). They had found a pattern of genetic transmission of alcoholism from mothers to daughters.

GENETIC DETERMINANTS OF ALCOHOL MISUSE AND ALCOHOLISM

In the last quarter century, biomedical, psychiatric and epidemiological research has increasingly supported the presence of a genetic influence in the development of alcoholism (for recent reviews on genetics and alcoholism, see Agarwal and Goedde, 1987; Goedde and Agarwal, 1989; Agarwal and Goedde, 1990, 1992; Couzigou *et al.*, 1993). However, still very few studies give specific findings indicating a basic genetic contribution to the disease alcoholism. Genes have long been suspected to play a role in the etiology of alcoholism. The phenomenon that "alcoholism runs in families" has been described by ancient Greek scholars. The current evidence strongly suggests that alcoholism may be a genetically influenced complex multifactorial disorder (Dinwiddie and Cloninger, 1989, Agarwal and Goedde, 1990). Among the most common strategies employed thus far to identify hereditary factors in alcoholism are: 1) family studies (family system variables, drinking behaviour, drinking history); 2) twin studies (alcohol metabolism, pattern of alcohol use and misuse); 3) adoption studies (biological parents vs foster parents) and 4) high risk groups (identification of biological markers of vulnerability to alcoholism).

Family Studies

Studies for the past many years have constantly shown a higher frequency of alcoholism and related disorders among the biological relatives of alcoholics. Family investigations of alcoholic probands have yielded consistently higher rates of alcoholism than would be expected in the general population regardless of the nationality of the sample (Goodwin 1987). A review of 29 family studies covering 6251 alcoholics and 4083 nonalcoholics clearly showed that regardless of the nature of the population of nonalcoholics studied, an alcoholic is more likely to have a mother, father or a distant relative who is an alcoholic (Cotton, 1979). When lifetime prevalence of alcoholism in relatives of alcoholics was compared to that in the general population, a 4-fold increased risk in first-degree relatives and a 2-fold increased risk in second-degree relatives was observed. More recent studies have reported that on average the risk for developing alcoholism is seven times greater among first-degree relatives of alcoholics than among controls (Cloninger, 1987; Merikangas, 1990).

Male relatives of male alcoholics appear to be at particular risk for the disease. However, possible mechanism(s) mediating between alcoholism and family history of alcoholism, remain obscure as the potential role of family environment in the aggregation of alcoholism in families is difficult to assess. Higher family incidence of alcohol use and misuse does not necessarily reflect a genetic determination of alcoholism. Besides family traditions and cultural habits, there are within-family environmental effects like parental loss, birth order and the gender of the immediately elder sibling which may influence an individual's drinking behaviour. Heritable familial attributes as well as similarities in the social environment of family members also appear to play a role in familial transmission of alcoholism. Recent studies support the conclusion that family systems (family reactivity patterns, ethnic family styles, gender of the alcoholic spouse, and stages of alcoholism) are an important variable in the genesis, consequences and treatment of alcoholism (Kaufmann, 1984).

Recent family studies further emphasize fundamental differences in the concept of the two major research paradigms currently used in genetic studies in alcoholism. One model views alcoholism as a discrete disease entity with a unitary cause, whereas the other paradigm considers alcoholism as a multi level disorder with many steps between the genotype and phenotype (Cloninger, 1987).

Twin Studies

While most classical twin studies applied to the problem of alcoholism indicate a modest genetic predisposition, the recently available data on twin studies do not always provide a conclusive evidence for a genetic role in alcoholism (Gurling and Murray, 1987). More recent twin studies indicate a modest to strong genetic predisposition (Merikangas 1990; Marshall and Murray, 1991; McGue *et al.*, 1992). In a recent study conducted by Pickens *et al.* (1991), significant differences in concordance rate were found between the male MZ and DZ twins for alcohol misuse (74% vs 58%), and for alcohol dependence (59% vs 36%). For the female twin pairs, differences in concordance rates were found for alcohol dependence (25% vs 5%). In another recent study, Kendler *et al.* (1992) found a significantly higher concordance rate for alcoholism in female MZ than in DZ twins (26.2% vs 11.9%). The authors estimated that genetic influences account for 50 to 61 percent of the risk for alcoholism in women. These reports strongly support the hypothesis that genetic factors play a major role in the etiology of alcoholism in women.

Adoption Studies

Extensive adoption studies conducted in Denmark and Sweden have provided substantial evidence that alcoholism is genetically influenced, and that there are distinct patterns of alcoholism with different genetic and environmental causes (Devor and Cloninger, 1989). When the adopted away sons of an alcoholic parent were compared to their siblings raised by the alcoholic biological parent, a remarkably similar rate of alcoholism was noted in both groups. However, similar studies conducted for female adoptees did not replicate the findings of those in males. Subsequent adoption studies from other countries have clearly shown that children born to alcoholic parents but adopted away during infancy were at greater risk for alcoholism than adopted-away children born to nonalcoholic parents (Merikangas, 1990).

The findings regarding female alcoholism are more equivocal (Bohman *et al.*, 1981). In general, heavy drinking was far less frequent in women than in men. Of those women who did drink heavily, an unusually high percentage became alcoholic. Daughters of alcoholics raised by their alcoholic parents had more depression problems than the controls, but this was not true of daughters raised by nonalcoholic foster parents. This suggests that in women environmental influences may be more important in producing depression than in producing alcoholism. In a recent analysis of 913 adopted women in Sweden (Gilligan *et al.*, 1988), it was found that although having a biological parent with alcoholism increased the risk of alcohol misuse in the daughter, the alcoholic fathers who had an excess of alcohol-misusing daughters themselves had mild misuse. Alcoholic mothers of alcohol-misusing daughters had a low occupational status and also had a low criminality record.

Clinical Subtypes of Alcoholics

Adoption studies have also helped to characterize clinical subtypes of alcoholics who differ in their patterns of inheritance. At least three distinct genetic subtypes of alcohol misusers with characteristic clinical features and heterogeneous genetic and environmental backgrounds have been identified (Dinwiddie and Cloninger, 1989; Cadoret and Wesner, 1990; Hill, 1992). Data from a large adoptee sample in Sweden demonstrated, for the first time, the existence of two forms of inherited vulnerability to alcoholism, type I and type II (Cloninger *et al.*, 1981).

Type I alcoholism is the more common form (75%), is less severe (mild) and affects both men and women. The genetic contribution comes from either the biological father or the mother (or both), but is sensitive to environmental factors for its expression. It is associated with adult-onset alcoholism in either biological parent. Furthermore, it is considered to be "milieu limited" as postnatal environment affects its occurrence and severity in genetically susceptible offspring. They start chronic drinking usually well after the age of 25, rarely have trouble with the law, and often successfully become abstinent. Their children are only twice as likely to have trouble with alcohol compared with the general population.

In contrast, type II alcoholism is characterized by severe type of susceptibility that is more influenced by genetics than environment. This form is limited to males with an early onset associated with aggressive behaviour and antisocial personality. Biological fathers of these individuals also have similar features. The alcoholics in this group (25% of the total) tend to drink heavily before the age of 25, have bad work and police records and meet with little success with treatment programs. Drinking is a habit these alcoholics seem to pick up on their own with little encouragement from friends or other influences. Alcoholism surfaced nine times as often as in the general population when the sons of men with this form of alcoholism were followed-up. This form is called "male limited".

Recently, a third type of alcoholism has been proposed (Hill, 1992). Like type II alcoholism, it is significantly influenced by genetic factors, but it is not associated with antisocial behaviour.

Although adoption and twin studies have proven useful in answering the question of nature versus nurture, the mode of inheritance of alcoholism is still an unresolved matter. None of the evidence hitherto put forward suggests that susceptibility to alcoholism is inherited via a simple Mendelian dominant, recessive or sex-linked transmission. Even if the inheritance of certain biological factors involved in alcoholism is assumed to be Mendelian, the effect of these factors on the development of complex disorders may still not fit a simple genetic model. The observed transmission of the liability of risk for alcoholism does not fit a single autosomal or sex-linked gene as the first- and second-degree relatives of alcoholics are about equally at risk to become alcoholic and the sex of the proband does not influence the degree of risk in relatives (Cloninger, 1990).

There are, however, serious limitations of the generalizability of the findings implicating genetic factors in the development of alcoholism. According to Fillmore (1990), a genetic hypothesis would deflect attention away from consideration of the more important psycho-social issues related to alcohol use and misuse. Of course, implementation of scientific findings in terms of social policy requires great caution in evaluation and interpretation of the data, especially in view of the involvement of powerful environment variables confounding the development and outcome of alcohol problems.

THE IMPORTANCE OF ENVIRONMENTAL FACTORS IN ALCOHOL DRINKING AND ITS OUTCOMES

The influence of alcohol can be understood in terms of the interaction of the agent (alcohol), the host (the individual who ingests it), and the environment (encompassing ecological, social, and cultural variables). Environmental influences such as moral and religious instructions, exposure to alcoholic beverages, drinking patterns of the family and peer groups, the age, gender, diet, health, life style, behaviour, culture and social traditions must be taken into consideration. Certain socio-economic components such as the availability of alcohol and the price are among the major determinants of alcohol-seeking behaviour in a society. Peer pressure and attitudes to drinking and drunkenness influence directly or indirectly the decision to drink and even to drink to excess occasionally. Moreover, drinking norms in a given society significantly influence the actual drinking behaviour of an individual.

Gene-Environment Interactions

While discussing the role of genetic factors in alcohol use and alcoholism, complex genetic-environmental interactions have to be taken into account. Several different genetic and environmental factors may participate in generating a heterogeneous clinical picture of the disease alcoholism. Certain environmental factors may be playing a greater role in determining the "alcoholic phenotype" in a polygenic multifactorial disorder like alcoholism as they may modulate to different extends the multiple gene loci involved (Vesell, 1989). Therefore, it may not be correct to separate "genes" and "environment" to elucidate their relative contribution. Rather, both genes and environment may participate simultaneously, interacting dynamically to influence the "alcoholic phenotype".

As mentioned before, for recognition and separation of genetic and environmental factors, the age, diet, health, lifestyle, behaviour, culture as well as religious and social traditions have to be considered for their contribution towards drinking practices and increased risk against alcoholism (Heath, 1989). One approach towards this goal is therefore the prospective and retrospective longitudinal study of individuals separated from their alcoholic biological relatives soon after birth and raised by nonalcoholic adoptive parents (see above). The combined twin and adoption studies have clearly demonstrated an important role of genetic and environmental interactions in the development of alcoholism. What we learned from adoption studies is not that nature was important or nurture was important but that both are important.

Cross-fostering studies have shown that both genetic and environmental variables play a significant role in the development of "milieu-limited" (mild alcohol misuse) alcoholism, and the risk was increased four-fold when both genetic and environmental factors were combined (Cloninger *et al.*, 1981). For the moderate alcohol misuser, environmental factors played no significant role. The genetic vulnerability to alcohol use could be extensively modified by environmental factors depending upon postnatal experience. In contrast, the expression of "male-limited" (severe alcohol misuse) form was not significantly modified by environmental forces.

A key role of environmental factors has been also evident in some heritable forms of alcoholism associated with antisocial personality, impulsiveness, sensation-seeking behaviour and extreme emotional volatility (Hesselbrock *et al.*, 1985; Cloninger, 1987; Tarter *et al.*, 1989; 1990). To study the gene-environment interaction, particularly the effect of socio-cultural influences on heritable susceptibility factors, Cloninger *et al.* (1988) examined the relationship between increasing average alcohol consumption in the general population (USA and Sweden) and the risk of heavy drinking or alcohol misuse in the relatives of alcoholics. The rational behind this study was that if there were fundamental differences between familial and non-familial alcoholism, then an increase in average alcohol consumption would lead to an increase in sporadic cases only and no change in the inheritance of familial alcoholism. On the other hand, if the risk of alcoholism was influenced by the interaction of socio-cultural influences and heritable susceptibility factors shared by biological relatives, then increasing average alcohol consumption would lead to both an increase in sporadic cases and a marked exponential increase in the proportion of relatives who misuse alcohol. The results of this study indicate that both social and temporal trends in the use of alcohol markedly influence the inheritance profile of alcohol misuse. The study emphasize the need to distinguish between variables that influence exposure to heavy drinking and variables related to susceptibility to various social and medical outcomes of alcohol misuse in the context of various exposure patterns.

HOW BIOLOGICAL FACTORS MODIFY ALCOHOL DRINKING HABITS

Recent studies have focused on the role of biological factors such as genetic variation in alcohol metabolizing enzymes to be responsible for the inter-ethnic differences in alcohol elimination rate, alcohol-induced skin flush, and alcohol use and misuse (Agarwal and Goedde, 1989; Goedde and Agarwal, 1989; Agarwal and Goedde, 1990). Humans possess varying sets of enzymes involved in the metabolism of alcohol. Both alcohol dehydrogenase (ADH) and aldehyde dehydrogenase (ALDH) exhibit genetic polymorphisms, and the variant isozymes have varied distributions in human populations (Goedde *et al.*, 1992).

An intense alcohol-related flushing reaction — an unpleasant response to small amounts of alcohol — is commonly observed in large percentages of Asian populations. Ethnic differences in sensitivity to alcohol (flushing response and intoxication) are well recognized, and may account for the observed racial and ethnic variations in alcohol metabolism, prevalence of alcoholism, and alcohol-related mortality (Agarwal and Goedde, 1992). Dysphoric reactions to alcohol, producing uncomfortable symptoms, are believed to be due to a buildup of acetaldehyde associated with a deficiency or absence of ALDH2 activity (Goedde *et al.*, 1979; Harada *et al.*, 1985; Agarwal and Goedde, 1987; Goedde and Agarwal, 1989).

Quantity-frequency-variability classification of the ethnic groups indicates an apparent difference between Mongoloids and Caucasoids; the percentage of heavy and moderate drinkers being higher among Caucasoids, with the percentage of abstainers and infrequent drinkers being higher among the Chinese, Japanese, and other Orientals. The alcoholism rate is also found to be lower among Japanese, Chinese, and other Orientals as compared to Caucasoid populations living in the Western society. A markedly low incidence of ALDH2 isozyme abnormality has previously been observed in alcoholics compared to psychiatric patients, drug dependents and healthy controls in Japan, China, Korea, and Taiwan (Goedde and Agarwal, 1989; Agarwal and Goedde, 1990; Yeh *et al.*, 1989; Yamashita *et al.*, 1990). Moreover, a significantly fewer number of patients with alcoholic liver disease possess the ALDH2 deficiency gene (Shibuya and Yoshida, 1988).

All these findings imply that subjects with a "normal" ALDH2 enzyme form are at greater risk from developing alcohol-related organ damage than those with an "abnormal" isozyme form. Thus, ALDH2 deficient individuals drink less, have the tendency not to become habitual drinkers, suffer less from liver disease, and rarely become alcoholics. However, very little is known about the incidence of this "Oriental type" of facial flushing and related symptoms among non-Mongoloid populations. A frequency of about 4 to 12% incidence of alcohol sensitivity was reported among North American Caucasoids (Wolff, 1973). A similar percentage of Germans and Hungarians have been found to respond to alcohol drinking with adverse reactions (Agarwal *et al.*, 1995). Since ALDH2 isozyme abnormality has not been detected in Caucasoids as yet, the basis of this "Caucasoid type" of flushing remains to be explained. Recently, a decreased erythrocyte ALDH activity was suggested to be the major cause of alcohol-induced facial flushing among Caucasians (Yoshida *et al.*, 1989).

SOCIAL AND CULTURAL VARIABLES

While the most important determinant of an individuals drinking problems is a positive family history of alcoholism, a particular profession or occupation may also be determinative in an individual's liability to alcoholism. High rates of alcoholism are usually noted among various occupational groups such as military, police, fire-control, mariners, brewers, etc. Social, ethnic, and cultural factors are some of the strongest determinants of drinking patterns in a society. It has been long suspected that the influence of national and ethnic origin may account for a major part of the variance observed in comparative studies of alcoholism rates within different populations. Certain features of social structure and organization constitute environmental factors that interact with genetic and biomedical factors in shaping how, when, with whom, and for what reason people drink (Heath, 1989). Religions constitute environmental factors that influence individuals and groups in various ways: it can favour drinking or it can preach abstinence. Education, on the other hand, can influence norms, attitudes, and values toward drinking at the individual or group level.

A marked difference in the extent of alcoholism and related problems among Israeli Jews of the three major ethnic communities, Ashkenazi, Sephardi and Oriental has been reported (Snyder *et al.* 1982). A significantly higher percentage of Sephardi-Oriental subgroups than the Ashkenazi subgroup were found to be alcoholics. The differences have been explained to be due to sociological factors in terms of a historic dialectic of differentiation of Jewish minorities from the drinking norms of surrounding majorities. Additional factors like religion and social stress may also play an important role in conditions which foster or thwart alcoholism (Snyder *et al.*, 1982).

Effect of Acculturation

Acculturation processes significantly alter drinking practices of a given minority group even if other variables are important. For instance, genetically determined biological sensitivity to mild doses of alcohol commonly found in the Orientals of Mongoloid heritage has been shown to be a deterrent to alcohol misuse (Agarwal and Goedde, 1990). This adverse response to ingestion of even small amounts of alcohol may protect sensitive individuals from developing alcoholism. However, under altered social and other environmental pressures, American Indians who are known to be of the Mongoloid origin, still misuse alcohol despite the initial aversive reactions they might experience after alcohol drinking. Thus, the environmental factors may be quite important in some of the observed biological and behavioural concomitants in alcoholism.

Availability and Price Factors

Evidently, an individual even with a strong genetic predisposition for alcoholism would not develop the disorder in the absence of alcoholic beverages. Though limiting access to alcohol may not necessarily be an effective way to lessen alcoholism in a particular society, reducing overall consumption may be a good preventive strategy.

PROBLEMS FOCUSING THE EUROPEAN COMMUNITY

The European Community is not a unitary ethnic group but represents the Caucasian race with many ethnic/national subgroups that vary by religion, culture and socioeconomic level. The contemporary European communities have undergone a severe influence of historical processes (various political, social and economic events), migration patterns, isolation and ecological pressure and their interaction. In addition, changing social norms, mores and sanctions exert an influence over these subgroups. Educational level, occupational-generational differences, language, customs, religion and attitudes toward alcohol have also to be taken into consideration. Also, there is a need to distinguish between important within-culture subgroups that are subsumed under the broader groups.

In Europe, British and Northern and Eastern European societies have generally shown a stronger concern in the last 150 years regarding alcohol problems than Central, and particularly Southern European countries (Room, 1989). The societies which admit having alcohol problems often emphasize different nature of the problem. Finnish and Polish literature blames the social disruption associated with drinking, while Germany places great emphasis on drunk driving casualties. French, on the other hand, often focus on long-term medical problems such as cirrhosis.

CONCLUSIONS

Epidemiological studies reported in the past years clearly indicate that race and gender differences in drinking pattern may play an important role in the development of medical conditions associated with alcohol misuse. Indeed, there is a considerable variation in the proportion of drinkers in a given population when divided by ethnicity, gender, age, religious affiliation and socio-economic status. Although some of the putative environmental factors remain obscure in their nature, there is a strong evidence that there is a crucial interplay of nature and nurture, heredity and environment, and biology and culture in the development of alcoholism across ethnic groups and gender. Nevertheless, specific factors which interact with particular genes that predispose to alcoholism require further assessment in order to comprehend better the intricate interaction between predisposing genes and environmental factors in the expression, etiology and treatment of alcohol misuse and alcoholism.

PROPOSALS FOR FUTURE RESEARCH

As compared to a relatively large body of data available on epidemiology of alcohol consumption and alcoholism in general populations and among ethnic minorities in the United States (for references see Midanik and Room, 1992), very little such information is available for Europe in general and EC in particular. From a public health perspective, analysis of the role of gender and ethnicity in alcohol misuse may help to identify biological and social factors which would allow to understand as how to reduce alcohol-related problems in the community.

Specifically, areas needing further research include:

- Identification of cellular and molecular mechanisms related to the apparent increased vulnerability to alcohol misuse and alcohol-related organ damage, including ethnic and gender difference in rates of alcohol metabolism.
- extensive population-based studies of ethnic and gender difference in the patterns of voluntary alcohol consumption.
- identification of trait and state markers that are specific for diagnosis of alcohol misuse and alcohol dependence in ethnic minorities and women.

References

Agarwal, D.P., Benkmann, H.G. and Goedde, H.W. (1995). Alcohol use, abuse, and alcohol-related disorders among ethnic groups in Hungary. Part II. Palocs from Matraderecske. *Anthrop. Anz.* **53**:67–78.

Agarwal, D.P. and Geodde, H.W. (1987). Genetic variation in alcohol metabolizing enzymes: implications in alcohol use and misuse. In: Goedde, H.W., Agarwal, D.P. (eds) *Genetics and Alcoholism.* AR Liss, New York, pp. 121–140.

Agarwal, D.P. and Geodde, H.W. (1990). *Alcohol Metabolism, Alcohol Intolerance and Alcoholism.* Springer-Verlag, Berlin.

Agarwal, D.P. and Geodde, H.W. (1989). Human aldehyde dehydrogenases: their role in alcoholism. *Alcohol,* **6**:517–523.

Agarwal, D.P. and Goedde, H.W. (1992). Medicobiological and genetic studies on alcoholism. Role of metabolic variation and ethnicity on drinking habits, alcohol misuse and alcohol-related mortality. *Clin. Investigat.,* **70**:465–477.

Akutsu, P.D., Sue, S., Zane, N.W.S. and Nakamura, C.Y. (1989). Ethnic differences in alcohol consumption among Asians and Caucasians in the United States: An investigation of the cultural and physiological factors. *J. Stud. Alcohol.,* **50**:261–267.

Armstrong, R.W. (1986). Tobacco and alcohol use among urban Malaysians in 1980. *Interntl. J. Addiction,* **20**:1803–1808.

Blane, H.T. (1993). Ethnicity. In: Galanter M. (ed) *Recent Developments in Alcoholism.* Vol. 11. Plenum Press, New York, pp. 109–122.

Bohman, M., Sigvardsson, S. and Cloninger, C.R. (1981). Maternal inheritance of alcohol misuse. Cross-fostering analysis of adopted women. *Arch. Gen. Psychiatry,* **38**:965–969.

Buchholz, K.K. (1992). Alcohol misuse and dependence from a psychiatric epidemiologic perspective. *Alcohol Health and Research World,* **16**:197–208.

Cadoret, R.J. and Wesner, R.B. (1990). Use of the adoption paradigm to elucidate the role of genes and environment and their interaction in the genesis of alcoholism. In: Cloninger C.R. and Begleiter H. (eds) *Genetics and Biology of Alcoholism.* Banbury Report 33. Cold Spring Harbor Laboratory Press, New York, pp. 31–42.

Caetano, R. (1989). Drinking patterns and alcohol problems in a national sample of US Hispanics. In: Spiegler, D.L.S., Tate, D.A., Aitken, S.S., Christian, C.M. (eds) *Alcohol Use Among US Ethnic Minorities.* Research Monograph No. 18. US Department of Health and Human Services (DHHS) Rockville, USA, pp. 147–162.

Carlini, B.H., Pires, M.L.N., Fernandes, R. and Masur, J. (1986). Alcohol use among adolescents in Sao Paulo, Brazil. *Drug Alcohol Dependence*, **18**:235–246.

Chi, I., Kitano, H.H.L. and Lubben, J.E. (1988). Male Chinese drinking behavior in Los Angeles. *J. Stud. Alcohol.*, **49**:21–25.

Chi, I., Lubben, J.E. and Kitano, H.H.L. (1989). Differences in drinking behaviour among three Asian-American groups. *J. Stud. Alcohol.*, **50**:15–23.

Christian, C.M., Zobeck, T.S. Malin, H.J. and Hitchcock, D.C. (1989). Self-reported alcohol use and misuse among Mexican Americans: Preliminary findings from the Hispanic health and nutrition examination survey adult sample person supplement. In: Spiegler, D.L.S., Tate, D.A., Aitken, S.S., Christian, C.M. (eds) *Alcohol Use Among US Ethnic Minorities*. Research Monograph No. 18. US Department of Health and Human Services (DHHS), Rockville, USA, pp. 425–438.

Cloninger, C.R. (1990). Genetic epidemiology of alcoholism. Observations critical in the design and analysis of linake studies. In: Cloninger, C.R. (ed) Genetics and Biology of Alcoholism. Banbury Report 33. Cold Spring Harbor Laboratory Press, New York, pp. 105–133.

Cloninger, C.R. (1987). Recent advances in family studies of alcoholism. In: Goedde, H.W., Agarwal, D.P. (eds) *Genetics and Alcoholism*. A.R. Liss, New York, pp. 47–60.

Cloninger, C.R., Bohman, M. and Sigvardsson, S. (1981). Inheritance of alcohol misuse. *Arch. Gen. Psychiatry*, **38**:861–868.

Cloninger, C.R., Reich, T., Sigvardsson, S., von Knorring, A.L. and Bohman, M. (1988). Effects of changes in alcohol use in generations on the inheritance of alcohol misuse. In: Rose, R.M., Barret, J.E. (eds) *Alcoholism: A Medical Disorder*. Raven Press, New York, pp. 49–74.

Cotton, N.S. (1979). The familial incidence of alcoholism. A review. Quart *J. Stud. Alcohol.*, **40**:89–116.

Couzigou, P., Begleiter, H., Kiianmaa, K. and Agarwal, D.P. (1993). Genetics and Alcohol: In: Verschuren, P.M. (ed) *Health Issues Related to Alcohol Consumption*. ILSI Europe, pp. 281–329.

de Lint, J. (1976). The epidemiology of alcoholism with specific references to sociocultural factors. In: Everett, M.W., Waddell, J.O., Heath, D.B. (eds) *Cross-cultural Approaches to the Study of Alcohol*. Mouton Publishers, The Hague, pp. 323–339.

Dawson, D.A. and Archer, L. (1992). Gender differences in alcohol consumption: effects of measurement. *Brit. J. Addiction,* **87**:119–123.

Devor, E.J. and Cloninger, C.R. (1989). Genetics of alcoholism. *Annu. Rev. Genet.*, **23**:19–36.

Dinwiddie, S.H. and Cloninger, C.R. (1989). Family and adoption studies of alcoholism. In: Goedde, H.W., Agarwal D.P. (eds) *Alcoholism: Biomedical and Genetic Aspects*. Pergamon Press, New York, pp. 259–276.

Fillmore, K.M. (1990). Risk factors for alcohol problems: Social and ethical considerations with special attention to the workplace. In: Roma, P.M. (ed) *Alcohol: The Development of Sociological Perspectives on Use and Misuse*. Alcohol Research Documentation, Inc. New Brunswick, New Jersey, USA, pp. 289–314.

Frezza, M., Di Padova, C., Pozzato, G., Terpin, M., Baraona, E. and Lieber, C.S. (1990). High blood alcohol levels in women. The role of decreased gastric alcohol dehydrogenase activity and first-pass metabolism. *New Engl. J., Med.*, **322**:95–99.

Gilbert, M.J. (1989). Alcohol related practices, problems and norms among Mexican Americans: An Overview. In: Spiegler, D.L.S., Tate, D.A., Aitken, S.S., Christian, C.M. (eds) *Alcohol Use Among US Ethnic Minorities*. Research Monograph No. 18. US Department of Health and Human Services (DHHS), Rockville, USA, pp. 115–134.

Gilligan, S.B., Reich, T. and Cloninger, C.R. (1988). Etiologic heterogeneity in alcoholism. *Genet. Epidemiol.* **4**:395–414.

Goedde, H.W., Harada, S. and Agarwal, D.P. (1979). Racial differences in alcohol sensitivity: a new hypothesis. *Hum. Genet.*, **51**:331–334.

Goedde, H.W. and Agarwal, D.P. (1989). Acetaldehyde metabolism: Genetic variation and physiological implications. In: Goedde, H.W., Agarwal, D.P. (eds) *Alcoholism: Biomedical and Genetic Aspects*, Pergamon Press, New York, pp. 21–56.

Goedde, H.W., Agarwal, D.P. and Fritze, G (1992). Distribution of ADH2 and ALDH2 genotrypes in different populations. *Hum. Genet.*, **88**:344–346.

Gomberg, E.S.L. (1993). Gender issues. In Galanter, M. (ed) *Recent Developments in Alcoholism*. Vol. 11. Plenum Press, New York, pp. 95–107.

Goodwin, D.W. (1987). Adoption studies of alcoholism. In: Goedde, H.W., Agarwal, D.P. (eds) *Genetics and Alcoholism*. A.R. Liss, New York, pp. 60–70.

Gurling, H.M.D. and Murray, R.M. (1987). Genetic influence, brain morphology, and cognitive deficits in alcoholic twins. In: Goedde, H.W. and Agarwal, D.P. (eds) *Genetics and Alcoholism*. A.R. Liss, New York, pp. 71–82.

Harada, S., Agarwal, D.P. and Goedde, H.W. (1985). Aldehyde dehydrogenase polymorphism and alcohol metabolism in alcoholics. *Alcohol*, **2**:391–392.

Heath, D.B. (1989). Environmental factors in alcohol use and its outcomes. In: Goedde, H.W., Agarwal, D.P. (eds) *Alcoholism: Biomedical and Genetic Aspects*. Pergamon Press, New York, pp. 312–324.

Herd, D. (1989). The epidemiology of drinking patterns and alcohol-related problems among US Blacks. In: Spiegler, D.L.S., Tate, D.A., Aitken, S.S., Christian, C.M. (eds) *Alcohol Use Among US Ethnic Minorities*. Research Monograph No. 18. US Department of Health and Human Services (DHHS), Rockville, USA, pp. 3–50.

Helzer, J.E., Burnam, A. and McEvoy, L. (1991). Alcohol misuse and dependence. In: Robins, L.N., Regier, D.A. (eds) *Psychiatric Disorders in America: The Epidemiological Catchment Area Study*. Free Press, New York, pp. 81–115.

Hesselbrock, M., Hesselbrock, V. and Stabenau, J.R. (1985). Alcoholism in men patients subtyped by family history and antisocial personality. *J. Stud. Alcohol.*, **46**:59–64.

Hill, S.Y. (1992). Absence of paternal sociopathy in the etiology of severe alcoholism: Is there a Type III alcoholism? *J. Stud. Alcohol.*, **53**:161–169.

Hong, O.T. and Isralowitz, R.E. (1989). Cross-cultural study of alcohol behaviour among Singapore college students. *Brit. J. Addiction*, **84**:319–321.

Hughes, K., Yeo, P.P.B., Lun, K.C., Thai, A.C., Wang, K.W. and Cheah, J.S. (1990). Alcohol consumption in Chinese, Malays and Indians in Singapore. *Ann. Acad. Med. Singapore*, **19**:330–332.

Kamien, M. (1975). Aborigines and alcohol: intake, effects and social implications in a rural community in Western New South Wales. *Med. J. Aust.*, **1**:291–298.

Kaufmann, E. (1984). Family system variables in alcoholism. *Alcoholism Clin. Exp. Res.*, **8**:4–8.

Kendler, K.S., Heath, A.C. and Neale, M.C. (1992). A population based twin study of alcoholism in women. *J. Am. Med. Ass.*, **268**:1877–1882.

Klatsky, A.L., Siegelaub, A.B., Landy, C. and Friedman, G.D. (1983). Racial patterns of alcoholic beaverage use. *Alcoholism Clin. Exp. Res.*, **7**:372–377.

Kono, H., Saito, S., Shimada, K. and Nakagawa, J. (1977). Drinking habits of the Japanese. *Actual Drinking Habits and Problem Drinking Tendencies*. Leisure Development Center, Tokyo, pp. 1–15.

Lee, J.A. (1987). Chinese, alcohol and flushing: sociohistorical and biobehavioral considerations. J. *Psycoactive Drugs*, **19**:319–327.

Lubben, J.E., Chi, I. and Kitano, H.H.L. (1989). The relative influence of selected social factors on Korean drinking behavior in Los Angeles. *Adv. Alcohol Substance Misuse*, **8**:1–17.

Lubben, J.E., Chi, I. and Kitano, H.H.L. (1987). Exploring Filipino American drinking behaviour. *J. Stud. Alcohol,* **49**:26–29.

Marshall, M., Forsyth, S.T., Sumanop, F.H. and Piau-Lynch, A. (1985). Alcohol research in Papua New Guinea. Implications for health care workers. *Papua New Guinea Med. J.*, **28**:183–193.

Marshall, M. (1988). Alcohol consumption as a public health problem in Papua New Guinea. *Int. J. Addiction,* **23**:573–589.

Marshall, E.J. and Murray, R.M. (1991). The familial transmission of alcoholism. *Br. Med. J.*, **303**:72–73.

McGue, M., Pickens, R.W. and Svikis, D.S. (1992). Sex and age effects on the inheritance of alcohol problems: a twin study. *J. Abnorm. Psychol.*, **101**:3–16.

Merikangas, K.R. (1990). The genetic epidemiology of alcoholism. *Psychol. Med.*, **20**:11–22.

Mezey, E., Koman, C.J., Diehl, A.M., Mitchell, M.C. and Herlong, H.F. (1988). Alcohol and dietary intake in the development of chronic pancreatitits and liver disease in alcoholism. *Am. J. Clin. Nutr.*, **48**:148–151.

Midanik, L.T. and Room, R. (1992). The epidemiology of alcohol consumption. *Alcohol Health and Research World*, **16**:183–190.

Mishra, L, Sharma, S., Potter, J.J. and Mezey, E. (1989). More rapid elimination of alcohol in women as compared to their male siblings. *Alcoholism Clin. Exp. Res.*, **13**:752–754.

Rahkonen, O. and Ahlström, S. (1989). Trends in drinking habits among Finnish youth from 1973 to 1987. *Brit. J. Addiction*, **84**:1075–1083.

Reed, T.E. (1985). Ethnic differences in alcohol use, misuse, and sensitivity: A review with genetic interpretation. *Soc. Biol.*, **32**:195–209.

Rocha-Silva, L. (1988). Attitudes of urban South Africans towards drinking and drunkenness. *Drug. Alcohol. Depend.*, **21**:203–212.

Room, R. (1989). The epidemiology of alcohol problems: conceptual and methodological issues. In: Ray, R., Pickens, R.W. (eds) *Proceedings of the Indo-US Symposium on Alcohol and Drug Misuse*. National Institute of Mental Health and Neuro Sciences, Bangalore, India, pp. 13–34.

Saito, S.: "Heavy drinkers" and "Problem drinkers" in Japanese general population (1978). *Public Health*, **42**:309–317.

Seitz, H.K., Simanowski, U.A., Waldherr, R., Agarwal, D.P. and Goedde, H.W. (1993). Human gastric alcohol dehydrogenase activity: effect of age, sex, and alcoholism. *Gut*, **34**:1433–1437.

Shibuya, A. and Yoshida, A. (1988). Genotypes of alcohol-metabolizing enzymes in Japanese with alcohol liver disease: A strong association of the usual Caucasian-type aldehyde dehydrogenase gene (ALDH$_2^1$) with the disease. *Am. J. Hum. Genet.*, **43**:744–748.

Snyder, C.R., Phyllis, P., Elder, P. and Elian, P. (1982). Alcoholism among the Jews in Israel: a pilot study. I. Research rationale and a look at the ethnic factor. *J. Stud. Alcohol*, **43**:623–654.

Suwaki, H. and Ohara, H (1985). Alcohol-induced facial flushing and drinking behavior in Japanese men. *J. Stud. Alcohol*, **46**:196–198.

Tarter, R.E., Arria, A.M. and Van, Thiel D.H. (1989). Neurobehavioral disorders associated with chronic alcohol misuse. In: Goedde, H.W., Agarwal, D.P. (eds) *Alcoholism: Biomedical and Genetic Aspects*. Pergamon Press, New York, pp. 113–130.

Tarter, R.E., Kabene, M., Escallier, E.A., Laird, S.B. and Jacob, T. (1990). Temperament deviation and risk for alcoholism. *Alcoholism Clin. Exp. Res.*, **14**:380–382.

Téllez, C. (1984). Chile: alcoholism in a wine-drinking country. *Brit. J. Addiction*, **79**:447–448.

Thomson, N. (1984). Aboriginal health-current status. *Aust. N.Z. J. Med.*, **14**:705–718.

Wolff, P.H. (1973). Vasomotor sensitivity to alcohol in diverse Mongoloid populations. *Am. J. Hum. Genet.*, **25**:193–199.

Vesell, E.S. (1989). Gene-environment interactions in alcoholism. In: Goedde, H.W., Agarwal, D.P. (eds) *Alcoholism: Biomedical and Genetic Aspects*. Pergamon Press, New York, pp. 325–332.

Yamashita, I., Ohmori, T. and Koyama, T. (1990). Biological study of alcohol dependence syndrome with reference to ethnic difference: Report of a WHO collaborative study. *Jpn. J. Psychiatry*, **44**:79–84.

Yeh, E.-K., Huw, H.-G., Chen, C.-C. and Yeh, Y.-L. (1989). Alcoholism: a low risk disorder for Chinese? In: Sun, G.Y. Rudeen, P.K., Wood, W.G, Wei, Y.H., Sun, A.Y. (eds) *Molecular Mechanisms of Alcohol. Neurobiology and Metabolism*. Humana press, Clifton, New Jersey, USA, pp. 335–355.

Yoshida, A., Dave, V., Ward, R.J. and Peters, T.J. (1989). Cytosolic aldehyde dehydrogenase (ALDH1) variants found in alcohol flushers. *Ann. Hum. Genet.*, **53**:1–7.

3 Alcohol and Nutrition

Ramon Estruch

Alcohol Research Unit, Hospital Clinic, Barcelona, Spain

Although only a minority of alcoholics have clinical evidence of malnutrition, they still represent the largest group of patients with treatable nutritional deficiencies in Western countries. Currently, the importance of dietary deficiencies has became lower and malnutrition in most alcoholics is due to maldigestion, malabsorption and several metabolic effects which ethanol has on the storing, activation and excretion of nutrients. Malnourished alcoholics are often those with higher ethanol intake and those who suffer from ethanol-related complications, especially liver disease and neurological disorders.

Epidemiological, clinical and experimental studies have demonstrated that ethanol has a direct effect on most body tissues. However, since not all heavy drinkers exhibit all types of ethanol-related diseases, it has been proposed that other factors such as nutritional deficiencies or genetic variations may enhance or prevent the effects of ethanol on cells. Thus, several studies have suggested that poor nutrition may have an additive effect thereby contributing to the effects of ethanol.

Some diseases in chronic alcoholics are due to specific nutritional deficiencies (i.e. Wernicke encephalopathy). However, since the metabolism of ethanol in the liver alters the activation and degradation of key nutrients, restoring nutritional balance and the use of specific nutrients may also be useful in the treatment of ethanol-related diseases (i.e. alcoholic liver disease) of non-nutritional cause.

INTRODUCTION

Chronic alcoholism has been considered as one of the main causes of malnutrition in Western countries (Darnton-Hill, 1989; Iber, 1990). For most people, the stereotype image of chronic alcoholics is that of a shabby malnourished individual who has not eaten for days, but who has had plenty of alcohol. Furthermore, some previous studies on the nutritional status of alcohol misusers included indigents who consumed large amounts of ethanol and ate little. Other studies have shown biased results due to the inclusion of subjects with advanced clinical consequences of alcoholism such as cirrhosis (Neville *et al.*, 1968); hence, the belief that alcoholics generally suffer from advanced malnutrition.

41

However, alcohol misusers may be found in all strata of society and indeed recent studies have indicated that the nutritional status of chronic alcoholics is not as severely affected as previously thought. In this sense, some studies have concluded that chronic alcoholics without ethanol-related diseases show nutritional parameters similar, or even higher, than those of the general population (Villalta *et al.*, 1989; Nicolás *et al.*, 1993). Thus, the stereo-type image of the chronic alcoholic should be replaced by that of a slightly overweight, clean-shaven businessman, who eats heavily and drinks an average of four whiskies a day. This is the type of alcoholic that a practising physician usually encounters.

CALORIC VALUE OF ETHANOL

Alcoholic beverages contribute significantly to the overall calories found in the diet of most Western countries. Based on epidemiologic consumption data, the estimated alcohol contribution to the diet of the population varies from 4.5 to 5.7 percent of the total calories (Schaefer *et al.*, 1986; Lieber, 1988), but the figure is higher in ethanol consuming populations in whom alcohol accounts from 6 to 18 percent of total energy intake (Dennis *et al.*, 1985). Furthermore, in heavy drinkers ethanol may supply more than 50 percent of dietary energy (Windham *et al.*, 1983; Thomson *et al.*, 1988).

Despite the apparent importance of ethanol as a source of energy, it remains unknown as to whether this energy can be used by the body. To assess the effectiveness of alcohol as an energy source, two approaches have been used, the metabolic studies which directly measure thermogenesis and oxygen consumption and epidemiologic studies, which correlate alcohol intake with body weight and anthropometric measurements.

Experimental Studies

In a bomb calorimeter, ethanol yields 7.1 kcal/g upon complete combustion, but its biologic value may be less, particularly when the dose of ethanol is high and/or the recipient is a chronic alcoholic. In a recent paper (Suter *et al.*, 1992), energy metabolism from ingested ethanol was assessed by metabolic studies measuring thermogenesis and oxygen consumption in eight healthy men who recieved 25 percent of their total energy requirements as ethanol. In this study, ethanol, either added to the diet or substituted other foods, increased 24-hour energy expenditure and decreased lipid oxidation. The conclusion was that habitual consumption of ethanol favours lipid storage and weight gain. Thus, in healthy nonalcoholic volunteers, ethanol is utilized as efficiently as fat or carbohydrate as a source of energy. However, in some studies, chronic alcoholics have lost weight whilst receiving additional calories as ethanol under controlled conditions. In addition, weight loss occurred in volunteers when 35 percent of the carbohydrate calories were replaced by ethanol and was maximal at 50 percent, the highest rate tested (Pirola and Lieber, 1972).

Experimental observations suggest that the caloric use of ethanol may be dose-related. At intakes of less than 25–35 percent of calories, ethanol may be completely utilized as a source of energy, but at higher intakes its utilization may not be complete. When intake is light to moderate, ethanol is metabolized primarily by the alcohol dehydrogenase system with the generation of NADH (from NAD), which leads to ATP synthesis (Lieber, 1988). In contrast, excessive ethanol intake is metabolized predominantly by the microsomal ethanol-oxidizing system, which leads to an increased loss of energy. The NADPH is, in fact, utilized, but no high-energy compound is formed and the reaction only generates heat. Another mechanism to explain energy wasting is the uncoupling of mitochondrial NADH oxidation, perhaps promoted by catecholamine release or a hyperthyroid state (Israel *et al.*, 1975).

Epidemiological Data

The results of the epidemiological studies have been controversial. Some have suggested that drinkers have lower body weights than nondrinkers (Fisher and Gordon *et al.*, 1985; Williamson *et al.*, 1987), whereas in others surveys alcoholics were at, or above, the ideal body weight (Simko *et al.*, 1982; Mills *et al.*, 1983). Likewise, in the Zutphen study a positive correlation was found between alcohol consumption and obesity, which is consistent with effective caloric utilization of ethanol in real-life situations, particularly in light of the lower total calories ingested by obese men in this study (Kromhoult, 1983). Variability in the results of these studies may be due to the difficulty in assessing ethanol intake in free-living subjects and to the fact that some consumers of ethanol add it to their usual food intake, whereas others replace carbohydrates or lipids with ethanol.

DEFINITION AND CLASSIFICATION OF MALNUTRITION

Definition

Malnutrition is a deficiency state which occurs when inadequate proteins, calories or specific nutrients are ingested to meet an individual's nutritional requirements. Malnutrition may be described as a failure to thrive and may be due to decreased intake, increased losses or increased requirements of nutrients. In common practice, gross (protein-calorie) malnutrition and specific deficits of nutrients are differentiated. In the former, a progressive loss of both lean body mass and adipose tissue results from insufficient consumption of protein and energy. However, two syndromes have been distinguished depending on the type of deficient intake, protein or energy (calories): (1) the *Kwashiorkor* syndrome, the clinical syndrome which develops when protein intake is deficient, despite adequate or nearly adequate energy intakes; (2) the *Marasmus* syndrome, the clinical syndrome which results from insufficient consumption of both proteins and calories. These clinical syndromes have been studied extensively in children from developing countries, which show florid manifestations of these deficiencies. In Western nations, although protein-caloric undernutrition is quite common, these clinical syndromes are rarely observed. Thus, in adults, gross malnutrition is classified in protein (*Kwashiorkor-like*) and caloric (*Marasmus-like*) malnutritions (Blackburn *et al.*, 1977), and diagnosed on the basis of sensitive laboratory criteria (see below). Mixed (intermediate) forms of protein-caloric malnutrition are also frequent.

The specific nutrients required for health include 24 organic compounds (9 essential amino acids, 2 fatty acids and 13 vitamins) and 15 inorganic compounds such as calcium, phosphorus, iodine, iron, magnesium, zinc, copper, potassium, sodium, chloride, cobalt, chromium, manganese, molybdenum and selenium.

Classification of Malnutrition

In absence of distinct clinical manifestations, the most sensitive diagnostic measure of caloric (marasmus-like) malnutrition is a history of weight loss. Most authors consider a 10 percent loss of body weight to be clinically significant. Weight loss can also be reported as the ratio between actual to ideal body weight. In common practice, patients are considered to have caloric malnutrition if their actual weight is less than 90 percent of the ideal weight or if the calculated lean body mass is more than 10 percent below the normal value (Blackburn *et al.,* 1977; Farrow *et al.,* 1987).

Most commonly used tests in the diagnosis of protein (Kwashiorkor-like) malnutrition are serum albumin, serum transport proteins, total lymphocyte count, haemoglobin, and skin test antigens (Blackburn *et al.,* 1977). However, in our experience, patients should be considered to be affected by protein malnutrition when three or more of the following parameters are diminished: total lymphocytes, haemoglobin, transferrin, albumin, prealbumin and retinol-binding protein (Nicolás *et al.,* 1993). Diagnosis of mixed (intermediate) malnutrition should be made when tests show both caloric and protein malnutrition.

Finally, chronic alcoholics may present a lack of specific nutrients (vitamins and minerals). Diagnosis of specific deficits should be made using bioassays, microbiologic techniques, chemical analyses and functional enzyme assays.

NUTRITIONAL ASSESSMENT

Since chronic ethanol intake may be associated with many nutritional consequences, complete nutritional assessment should be performed in every alcoholic patient. This evaluation should include a dietary recall history, anthropometric assessment and laboratory analyses (Table 3.1). For each patient a dietary recall history should be obtained by an expert physician or nurse-dietitian through repeated interviews and, whenever possible, data should be verified by relatives and friends. The problem is that sometimes the lack of patient cooperation, urgency of treatment and lack of qualified personnel interfere with proper evaluation (Mahalko *et al.,* 1985). To determine current energy and nutrient intake, dietitians may use a 3-, 5-day, week or month diet history. Since some patients are bingers or eat irregularly, it is better use a dietary history method estimating usual food intake over one week (Carey, 1989) or one month (Staveren *et al.,* 1985). Type, average, quantity per year and frequency of ethanol intake should also be recorded, as well as any signs or symptoms that may be related to nutritional problems such as under- or over-weight, poor oral hygiene, glossitis, vomiting, diarrhea, abdominal pain, edema, enlarged liver or jaundice.

Anthropometric measures should include height, weight, circumference of the upper nondominant arm and tricipital skin fold. The following laboratory parameters should be measured in each case: haemoglobin, total lymphocytes, albumin, transferrin, prealbumin and retinol-binding protein (Burrit and Anderson, 1984). Other interesting laboratory tests are serum electrolytes, liver enzymes, bilirubin, blood urea nitrogen, creatinine, glucose, uric acid, cholesterol and triglycerides. Other authors include an evaluation of cellular immune function made from the response to a battery of four skin tests (purified protein derivative, 5 TU/0.1 ml; histoplasmin, undiluted; trichophytin, 1:500; and Candida, 1:500) (Mendenhall *et al.,* 1984).

Table 3.1 Nutritional parameters commonly assessed in an alcoholic population

Parameter	Normal Value*
Ideal body weight (%)	105.4 ± 11.4
Lean body mass (Kg)	53.1 ± 4.8
Tricipital skin fold thickness (cm)	1.17 ± 0.42
Arm circumference (cm)	28.0 ± 3.2
Arm muscle circumference (cm)	24.3 ± 2.9
Arm muscle area (cm^2)	47.9 ± 9.7
Arm fat area (cm^2)	12.9 ± 4.4
Total protein (g/L)	70.0 ± 7.2
Albumin (g/L)	43.7 ± 5.8
Transferrin (mg/dL)	250 ± 40
Prealbumin (mg/dL)	31.2 ± 6.3
Retinol-binding protein (mg/dL)	5.98 ± 2.11
Hemoglobin (g/L)	145 ± 14.7
Lymphocytes ($\times 10^6$/L)	2300 ± 430
Vitamin A (μg/dl)	26.8 ± 4.9
Vitamin B_1 (% activation)	31.1 ± 20.1
Vitamin B_2 (% activation)	20.1 ± 10.7
Vitamin B_6 (% activation)	27.7 ± 17.5
Vitamin B_{12} (pg/mL)	616 ± 614
Vitamin C (mg/dl)	0.57 ± 0.22
Vitamin E (mg/l)	8.1 ± 0.9
Serum folate (ng/mL)	9.53 ± 5.14
Red-cell folate (ng/mL)	484 ± 163

* Mean ± standard deviation obtained in controls matched for age and sex with chronic alcoholics (Cook, 1991; Nicolás, 1993)

Overall nutrition may be assessed in terms of the proportion of actual to ideal weight. The lean body mass may be calculated from the creatinine-height index (Blackburn *et al.,* 1977) or the circumference of the upper nondominant arm and the thickness of the tricipital skin fold (Bishop *et al.,* 1981). The muscular area of the arm may also be calculated from these last two parameters and is an estimation of the skeletal muscle mass. The fatty area of the arm may be calculated from the tricipital skin fold and is an estimation of the total body fat (Durnin and Wormersley, 1974).

On the other hand, chronic alcoholics may have a lack of specific nutrients (vitamins or minerals). Specific vitamin, mineral and trace element levels may easily be measured. However, it is interesting to note that even the biochemical assessment of vitamin and trace element status are limited to serum/plasma and red cell levels. This is extremely unsatisfactory, providing only indirect evidence of nutritional balance. In chronic alcoholism, vitamin deficiencies are the result of poor diet coupled with malabsortion, excess excretion and impaired activation. As commented above, the vitamin needs of the alcoholic are greater than those of the non-alcoholics. Moreover, the deficit of one vitamin may cause the deficit of another. Thus, folate deficit impairs thiamine absorption, resulting in thiamine deficiency. The main vitamins that may be deficient in chronic alcoholics are folate, pyridoxine, thiamine, nicotinic acid, riboflavin, pantothenic acid, biotin, and vitamins B_{12}, C, D, A, K and E (Morgan, 1982). In addition, chronic alcoholics may also present mineral deficiencies, mainly in zinc, magnesium and selenium (Carey, 1989).

Difficulties in the nutritional assessment of alcoholics

Since many nutritional parameters may be modified by non-nutritional causes in chronic alcoholics, the diagnosis of malnutrition in this population should be cautiously made. Problems often arise when interviewing severe chronic alcoholics for dietary habits (i.e. food frequency questionnaires), specially if the patient has neurological diseases, impaired short term memory and blackouts, or frequent episodes of binges. A family member or a friend may be of great assistance when obtaining dietary information.

Body weight is the most sensitive diagnostic measure to evaluate malnutrition, but changes in weight may be influenced by significant variations in total body water in oedema-forming conditions. Thus, body weight in patients with peripheral oedema (alcoholic cardiomyopathy) or ascites (alcoholic cirrhosis) is inaccurate and should be appropriately corrected. Measurements of tricipital skin fold and midarm perimeter are useful unless arm oedema or paralysis are present. The muscular area of the arm may be considered as an estimation of skeletal muscle mass, but it is not accurate if the patient has muscle atrophy due to alcoholic myopathy or peripheral neuropathy. In such cases, variations of the arm muscle area should not be entirely attributed to malnutrition. Thus, studies of nutritional status of alcoholics with skeletal myopathy or peripheral neuropathy cannot be based on the evaluation of skeletal muscle mass. The amount of creatinine appearing in the urine over 24 hours is also proportional to muscle mass. Again, interpretation of the value of lean body mass calculated from this parameter must, therefore, be carried out cautiously in patients with skeletal myopathy or peripheral neuropathy.

Laboratory analyses are another tool used in the diagnosis of malnutrition, although once again, certain abnormalities that may reflect malnutrition can also have a non-nutritional cause. Most laboratory parameters used in the diagnosis of protein malnutrition such as albumin, prealbumin, retinol-binding protein and transferrin are synthesized in the liver, and therefore low protein nutrition levels may be secondary to chronic liver failure due to cirrhosis. Thus, it is very difficult to make the accurate diagnosis of protein malnutrition in alcoholics with liver disease. In the same manner, interpretation of the studies on the relationship between severity of liver disease and degree of protein malnutrition is very dificult since both entities are measured by the same parameters.

MECHANISMS OF MALNUTRITION IN CHRONIC ALCOHOLICS

Primary Malnutrition

Despite the appreciable contribution to total energy intake, many early studies reported grossly deficient diets in alcoholics and suggested that poor dietary intake was the principal cause of nutritional deficiencies encountered in these patients. However, most of these studies reported alcoholics with evidence of ethanol-related diseases (i.e. liver cirrhosis) or with very poor socioeconomic background (Leevy, 1982; Patek *et al.*, 1975). In contrast, more recent studies performed in alcoholics free of major complicating diseases have reported that the mean daily intake of protein, fat and carbohydrates are similar to intakes in control populations, whereas others have yielded very variable results. Thus, in some studies, alcohol calories tended to be substituted by fat; in others, consumption of simple carbohydrates in the form of sugars was decreased; and, finally, other surveys have found that alcohol calories are added to the diet rather than replacing other foodstuffs (Kromhoult, 1983). In other words, although dietary intake of chronic alcoholics are grossly unbalanced (Sherlock, 1984), the diets of most alcoholics seem adequate in terms of major nutrient intake when compared with a healthy control population (Morgan, 1982). However, in some alcoholics such as those with a low socioeconomic level and/or those with ethanol-related disease, low real calorie intake may play an important role in the genesis of malnutrition (Patek *et al.,* 1975; Estruch *et al.,* 1993).

Secondary Malnutrition

Overall nutritional changes in chronic alcoholics may also be due to the associated maldigestion, malabsorption and several metabolic effects in the storing, activation and excretion of vitamins and minerals (Darnton-Hill, 1989). In the gastrointestinal tract, chronic ethanol intake causes gastritis, delay in gastric emptying and changes in motility, structure and function of the small intestine (Cooke, 1972; Wilson and Hoyumpa, 1979). Significant differences have also been observed in the bacterial flora of the jejunum of chronic alcoholics compared to non-alcoholic controls which may produce functional disturbances of the small intestine (Bode *et al.,* 1984).

Intravenous alcohol inhibits pancreatic exocrine secretion in non-alcoholic patients. Morover, pancreatic exocrine insufficiency has been noted in chronic alcoholics. The most frequent findings are decreases in the output of bicarbonate and pancreatic enzymes after the stimulation of the pancreas with secretin-cholecystokinin, changes which may impair absorption. In addition, nutritional deficiency can adversely affect intestinal and pancreatic function (Mezey and Potter, 1976). Thus, folate-deficient alcoholics show a significantly higher incidence of xylose and vitamin B_{12} malabsorption than folate-replete alcoholics.

On the other hand, ethanol produces wide-ranging effects on metabolism. This toxin inhibits albumin synthesis, impedes protein release from the liver, inhibits gluconeogenesis and impairs vitamin utilization (i.e. thiamine) (Camilo *et al.,* 1981). Other studies have reported that alcoholics, particularly those with liver disease, have a decreased storage of nutrients. As commented above, weight gain is significantly lower when alcohol is consumed rather than isocaloric amounts of carbohydrates (Pirola and Lieber, 1972), suggesting increased energy requirements by the body during alcohol consumption. Oxygen consumption is significantly higher in rats receiving alcohol than in control animals (Pirola and Lieber, 1976). In addition, increased requirements for certain vitamins, particularly those utilized for tissue repair such as folic acid, pyridoxine and vitamin B_{12} have been reported in alcoholic patients. Thus, low serum folic acid levels must be normalized by giving extra folate doses when patients maintain ethanol intake. Finally, ethanol increases fecal loss of nitrogen, as well as urinary loss of zinc, calcium, magnesium and phosphate (Henry and Elmes, 1975).

EVIDENCE OF MALNUTRITION IN CHRONIC ALCOHOLICS

Protein-calorie Malnutrition

Evidence of protein-calorie malnutrition and various vitamin deficiencies have been found in many studies of chronic alcoholics, but even after several decades of study, the prevalence and severity of malnutrition in chronic alcoholics remains uncertain, possibly because of variations in diagnostic criteria or in the age, ethnic composition and/or, nutritional, drug or disease status of the subjects. The populations studied, therefore, have caused great confusion in this issue. Thus, the group of Bonkovsky from Emory University Hospital in Atlanta reported that all hospitalized patients with alcoholic cirrhosis showed evidence of malnutrition (Chawla *et al.,* 1989). Morgan (1982) found that 30 percent of the patients admitted to hospital because of liver disease showed evidence of malnutrition, whereas Goldsmith et al (1983) detected protein-caloric malnutrition in only 8 percent of the upper-middle class alcoholics. In keeping with this last observation, other studies have demonstrated that chronic alcoholics have body weights equal to or even higher than their ideal body weight (Mills *et al.,* 1983; Kromhoult, 1983).

In a recent study performed by our group (Nicolás *et al.,* 1993), we have controlled the possible variables by limiting the selection of the subjects to an ethnically, socially and geographically homogeneous group of 250 chronic alcoholics whose sole motivation for seeking medical attention was their desire to rid themselves of alcohol dependency. All patients studied had stable social and employment histories and supportive relationships with members of their families, who usually accompanied them to the clinic. They were drawn from the middle socioeconomic class, without indigents. In addition, most of the food eaten by the subjects was prepared by female family members and consumed at home.

The dietary histories of these chronic alcoholics showed adequate nutrition. Moreover, although slight differences in the anthropometric parameters between alcoholics and controls were observed, only 25 (10 percent) of the alcoholics showed evidence of energy (caloric) malnutrition, 15 (6 percent), protein malnutrition and 6 (2 percent), mixed malnutrition. Malnourished alcoholics had consumed higher amounts of ethanol, usually more than 20 kg of ethanol/kg of body weight, and reported low caloric intake (ethanol excluded) than well-nourished alcoholics. In addition, ethanol-related diseases were ruled out in all patients and alcoholic cirrhosis was diagnosed in 20 cases (9 percent), skeletal myopathy in 117 (48 percent), dilated cardiomyopathy in 20 (9 percent) and peripheral neuropathy in 41 (16 percent). When patients with ethanol-related disease were excluded, no significant differences were observed in nutritional parameters between chronic alcoholics and controls. Moreover, on multivariate analysis, the only independent factors for the development of malnutrition were the total lifetime dose of ethanol and caloric intake (ethanol excluded) ($p < 0.01$; both), as well as cirrhosis ($p < 0.01$) when protein malnutrition was considered. We conclude that malnutrition is not as frequent as previously thought in middle socioeconomic class alcoholics and its existence may be considered as another consequence of ethanol intake or secondary to alcohol-related diseases. In addition, caloric-protein malnutrition should be suspected in those chronic alcoholics who have consumed high amounts of ethanol (usually a total lifetime dose higher than 20 kg of ethanol/kg of body weight) or present cirrhosis.

Lack of Specific Nutrients

Chronic alcoholics frequently show isolated vitamin deficiencies. Numerous published studies provide evidence of deficiencies of essential nutrients, including the vitamins B_1, B_2, B_6, A, C and E (Leevy, 1982; Aa *et al.,* 1988). Vitamin B_{12} and folate may also be deficient but B_{12} deficiency is relatively uncommon in chronic alcoholism and levels may even be raised (Bonjour, 1980). The percentage of chronic alcoholics with a reduction in these vitamins varies from 6 to 80 percent in different studies (Boyd *et al.,* 1981). In the study performed by our group which included 250 chronic alcoholics, the prevalence of vitamin deficiency was also lower than these previous studies. In fact, the only significant differences observed between alcoholics and controls were in serum folate levels (Estruch *et al.*). In another recent study performed by Cook *et al.* (1991) in London, a wide range of nutritional factors was analyzed in 20 heavy drinkers admitted to hospital for detoxification. It is particularly interesting that none of the parenterally administered vitamins, which are commonly prescribed for alcoholics during detoxification (ascorbid acid, nicotinamide, pyridoxine, riboflavine and thiamine), were found to be reduced in the patient group as compared to controls. Only serum levels of vitamin E were significantly reduced in alcoholics compared with control subjects. Deficiency in trace elements has also been reported in chronic alcoholics, including magnesium, zinc and selenium (Korpela *et al.*, 1985; Bode *et al.*, 1988). Blood lead has been found to be elevated in chronic alcoholics, particularly in those alcoholics who preferentially drink wine (Dally *et al.*, 1989). In the study of Cook *et al.* (1991), alcoholic patients were found to be deficient in magnesium, while a relative excess of serum iron and copper was noted.

Therefore, chronic alcoholics may have isolated deficiencies of vitamins and trace metals. However, their prevalence is not as high as previously thought. Thus, although nutritional supplementation may be necessary in heavy drinkers, the value of traditional routine supplements of vitamins to chronic alcoholics is questionable.

THE ROLE OF MALNUTRITION IN THE PATHOGENESIS OF ETHANOL-RELATED DISEASES

There is epidemiological, clinical and experimental evidence showing the wide-ranging effects of alcohol on all organ tissues. Epidemiological studies have shown a close correlation between ethanol intake and the prevalence of alcohol-related diseases in many countries (Lelbach, 1975; Pequignot *et al.*, 1978). Experimental studies performed in humans (Rubin and Lieber, 1968) and animals (primates) (Lieber *et al.*, 1975) have demonstrated that ethanol is directly hepatotoxic without requiring an element of nutritional deficiency. Thus, Lieber *et al.* (1965) and Rubin and Lieber (1968) gave alcohol to alcoholic and non-alcoholic volunteers and all subjects developed a fatty liver despite adequate dietary intake. Baboons, fed with the Lieber-DeCarli diet, developed the entire spectrum of alcoholic liver disease, i.e. fatty liver, alcoholic hepatitis and even cirrhosis (Rubin and Lieber, 1974). However, only a small proportion of heavy drinkers show alcohol-related diseases. Indeed, between 2 and 30 percent of severe alcoholic misusers develop cirrhosis (Johnson and Williams, 1984). This fact suggests that other factors such as malnutrition, other hepatotoxins, the environment or genetic variations may concur to enhance or prevent tissue damage in chronic alcoholism.

Alcoholic liver disease

The role of malnutrition in the pathogenesis of alcohol-related liver damage has been debated for a long time. Since the earliest clinical descriptions of alcoholic cirrhosis were primarily in derelict alcoholics with severe malnutrition, it was held that liver damage was due to altered nutrition rather than alcohol per se. In fact, alcoholic cirrhosis was known by the term "fatty nutritional cirrhosis" (Jacobs and Sorrell, 1981). Experimental studies showed that rats fed choline-methionine deficient diets and 15 percent ethanol in drinking water, developed fatty liver. Patek and Post (1941) studied chronic alcoholics with cirrhosis and severe malnutrition. In these patients, fed with hypercaloric and hyper-proteic diet and the concomitant administration of modest amounts of alcohol, recovery from alcohol liver injury was not impaired. In follow up studies (Erenoglu *et al.*, 1964), ethanol was administered under controlled conditions to patients recovering from alco-holic liver disease. Concomitant to the administration of 160 g of ethanol a day, some patients received a high-protein diet and others, a low-protein diet. Those patients who were fed with high-protein diet showed steady clinical improvement, but no significant changes in the histologic parameters of liver injury. In contrast, the patients who were fed the low-protein diet did not show either changes or slight deterioration of liver function and histologic features. Similarly, others studies have shown that ethanol in doses of up to 300 g a day does not impede recovery from liver injury (Summerskill *et al.*, 1957). On the other hand, patients who have undergone small bowel bypass for the treatment of obesity develop a liver lesion that is indistinguishable from alcoholic liver injury. The entire spectrum of liver disease ranging from fatty liver to acute hepatitis and even cirr-hosis has been observed in these patients (Peura *et al.*, 1980). Furthermore, liver damage improved by either restoration of intestinal continuity or intravenous hyperalimentation (Baker *et al.*, 1979).

More recently, in a Veterans Administration cooperative study, an association was found between the degree of protein-calorie malnutrition and the severity of illness and mortality (Mendenhall *et al.*, 1984). Two years later, the same investigators showed that protein-calorie malnutrition in patients with alcoholic hepatitis correlated significantly with mortality. They concluded that malnutrition has prognostic significance in alcoholic hepatitis and suggested that nutritional therapy may have a beneficial role in the manage-ment of alcohol-induced liver damage (Mendenhall *et al.*, 1986). At least 12 major con-trolled studies have been performed on this subject (Schneker and Halft, 1993; Mezey *et al.*, 1991) and the predominant conclusions were that nutrition therapy improves nutri-tional status and abnormal liver tests, but does not decrease early mortality. However, preliminary data from another study suggest that the group of moderately malnourished individuals with alcohol liver injury had lower mortality at 1 and 6 months of oral nutri-tional support combined with anabolic steroids, but not the latter alone.

Theoretically, there are a number on mechanisms by which nutrition may affect (modify) alcohol-induced liver damage. First, protein-calorie deficiency may enhance the toxicity of alcohol on the liver. Recent studies have suggested the importance of energy homeostasis, detoxication of oxygen-derived peroxides, membrane integrity and forma-tion and elimination of the metabolites of ethanol, especially acetaldehyde. Nutrients, mainly some amino acids, are essential for the maintenance of these processes, especially when they are "stressed" by ethanol (Schenker *et al.*, 1993). In keeping with this view, glutathione availability and its transfer into the mitochondria seem to be vital to protect the cells from peroxidative injury (Tsukamoto *et al.*, 1990). Moroever, the amount of glu-tathione depends on provision of precursor amino acids (cysteine). In rats exposed to a low calorie diet, hepatic glutathione concentration declined substantially. It is important to note that peroxidation has been associated with development of alcohol-induced hepatic fibrosis (Kamimura *et al.*, 1992) and, by contrast, administration of S-adenosyl-

L-methionine (SAM)(which is a source of cysteine for glutathione production) to baboons exposed to chronic ethanol atenuated part of the alcohol-induced liver injury (Lieber *et al.*, 1990). This improvement was reflected primarily in decreased mitochondrial injury: Liver fat and fibrosis was unaltered. Thus, gluthatione may play a role in alcohol-induced peroxidative injury.

Glycine also has a protective effect in some types of hepatic injury (Dickson *et al.*, 1992) and some studies have emphasized the role of another antioxidant, vitamin E, especially on the mitochondria. In addition, membrane integrity depends on the provision of phospholipids, also derived from some amino acids such as SAM. Indeed, in baboons fed with alcohol for several years, supplementation with oral phospholipids (i.e. polyunsatutaed lecithin) prevented the development of septal fibrosis. Most recently, it was shown that polyunsaturated lecithins selectively inhibited acetaldehyde-mediated hepatic collagen accumulation by stimulating collagenase activity in cultured lipocytes (Li *et al.*, 1992). Finally, malnutrition is indoubtedly of importance in limiting and repairing damage (Morgan, 1982). Hepatic regeneration depends on a cascade of events involving substrates and metabolic pathways for protein synthesis. Protein deprivation may impair repairing processes, since it reduces liver protein stores, RNA and polyamines, and dissagregate ribosomal protein synthesis in the rough endoplasmic reticulum.

Although undoubtedly ethanol has a direct effect on the liver, there is compelling evidence that malnutrition may play a role in the pathogenesis of alcohol-induced liver damage, probably enhancing the effects of the ethanol. In addition, prognosis of alcoholic liver disease has been positively correlated with response to nutritional support and, interestingly, a number of studies have suggested that nutritional support may be beneficial to such patients.

Gastrointestinal tract and pancreas

Chronic alcoholics frequently show gastrointestinal symptoms such as diarrhoea, dyspepsia and nausea. The gastrointestinal tract is exposed to a high alcohol concentration from oral ingestion and also to alcohol absorbed into the blood stream. Indeed, effects of ethanol include increased mucosal permeability, promotion of bacterial overgrowth, altered gut motility and impaired salt, water, vitamin and nutrient absorption (Persson, 1991). On the other hand, malnutrition itself may cause disturbances in the gastrointestinal tract. It has been observed that folate deficiency induces marked morphologic alterations of the mucosa, which normalized after diet supplementation with folate, and it has been proposed that malabsorption and mucosa changes could be the result of folate deficiency or an altered luminal digestion. Up to now, the relative importance of ethanol and malnutrition in the development of structural and functional changes in gastrointestinal tract has not been established.

Although ethanol intake is the main risk factor for the development of acute and chronic pancreatitis in men, epidemiological studies have shown that protein and fat consumption may also be a risk factor of developing chronic pancreatitis (Sarles *et al.*, 1989). Ingestion of ethanol in combination with a high-protein and a high-fat diet enhances concentration of pancreatic enzymes and it has been proposed that increases in exocrine pancreatic secretions result in protein precipitation in pancreatic ducts and contribute to the pathogenesis of pancreatitis. However, other studies have shown that patients with chronic alcoholic pancreatitis have low dietary intake of protein, carbohydrate and fat (Mezey *et al.,* 1988). In other words, the results of the studies on the effects of nutrition on the pathogenesis of chronic pancreatitis in alcoholics are still controversial.

Cardiovascular System

At one time, nutritional deficiency (especially thiamine deficit) was thought to play a role in the pathogenesis of ethanol-induced damage in the heart of chronic alcoholics, but the clinical differences between alcoholic cardiomyopathy (low output failure) and wet beriberi (high output failure), the failure of the former to improve with thiamine treatment and the lack of correlation with nutritional status have led to the current view that large amounts of alcohol are toxic to the myocardium (Dancy *et al.,* 1985; Fernández-Solá *et al.,*1994). In a recent study performed in Barcelona (Spain) (Urbano-Márquez *et al.,* 1989), 50 asymptomatic chronic alcoholics were studied. The daily ethanol consumption was 243 ± 13 g over an average of 16 years and none had clinical or laboratory signs of malnutrition. One third of the alcoholics had a left ventricular ejection fraction of 55% or less, as compared to none of the controls. In addition, six patients (12%) showed a definite dilated cardiomyopathy. The estimated total lifetime dose of ethanol correlated inversely with ejection fraction ($r = -0.58$; $p < 0.001$) and directly with left ventricular mass ($r = 0.59$; $p < 0.001$). According to these results, ethanol seems to be toxic to the cardiac muscle in a dose-dependent manner and nutritional status does not seem to play a role in the development of alcoholic cardiomyopathy.

Haematologic and Immune System

Between 13 and 62 percent of the chronic alcoholics admitted to a General Hospital show hematological abnormalities, mainly anaemia and/or thrombocytopenia (Lindenbaum, 1987). The etiology of these disorders are multifactorial and include acute and chronic effects of ethanol, nutritional deficiencies, alcohol-induced liver disease and infections. Malnourished alcoholics commonly present megaloblastic anaemia due to folic acid deficiency and less frequently to vitamin B_{12} deficit. Folic acid deficiency is usually seen in wine, brandy or whisky drinkers, and less often in beer drinkers, because of the high folate content of this beverage. Chronic alcoholics may also show sideroblastic changes in bone-marrow examination. These changes have been attributed to a defect in haem synthesis secondary to pyridoxine deficiency. Sideroblastic changes have been produced in healthy volunteers given ethanol together with a diet deficient in pyridoxine and folic acid (Chanarin, 1982). Moreover, heavy drinkers with hypophosphatemia due to poor intake and/or urinary losses of phosphates may also present severe haemolysis (Klock *et al.,* 1974).

Chronic alcoholics have a higher incidence of infections (Adams and Jordan, 1984). This fact has been related to toxic the effects of ethanol on haematopoietic and immune systems, alcohol-induced liver disease and concomitant protein-calorie malnutrition. Ethanol consumption by itself may induce changes in the number and function of granulocytes and macrophages (MacGregor, 1986). Recent studies have shown that ethanol may alter T, B, CD4 and CD8 lymphocyte counts and immunoglobulin A (IgA), IgM and IgG levels in a dose-dependent manner. As alcohol consumption increases, higher IgA and IgM levels, relative T and CD4 lymphocytes and the ratio of CD4 and CD8 cells, and lower IgG levels, relative B and CD8 lymphocytes, absolute lymphocyte and lymphocyte subset counts were observed (Mili *et al.,* 1992). Total lymphocyte count, the mean number of CD4 helper/inducer cells and the response to skin testing are also depressed in patients with alcoholic liver disease (Roselle *et al.,* 1988). Finally, protein-calorie malnutrition is the most common form of acquired immunodeficiency. Malnourished patients generally show a depression of phagocytic function and a reduction of total lymphocytes, circulating T lymphocytes and relative CD8 lymphocytes. In addition, deficiencies of riboflavin, thiamine, pantothenic acid, folic acid and vitamin C are associated with an increased susceptibility to infection. Finally, zinc deficiency may produce an impairment in cell-mediated immunity and increase susceptibility to infection.

Chronic alcoholics often present alterations in the number of platelets (thrombocytopenia and thrombocytosis), as well as in their function. These changes are mainly due to a direct effect of ethanol on platelet formation, but they may also be related to severe folate deficiency (Levine *et al.,* 1986).

Nervous System

Ethanol-related neurologic disorders may involve virtually any level of the nervous system, from the cerebral cortex to peripheral and autonomic nerves (Table 3.2) (Charness *et al.,* 1989; Charness, 1993). Not everyone who consumes ethanol to an excess has neurologic complications, nor it is clear why a particular complication occurs in a given person. The neurologic disorders observed in chronic alcoholics has been related to a combination of three factors: a) neurotoxic effects on ethanol and/or its metabolites; b) nutritional factors; and c) individual susceptibility probably related to genetic predisposition.

Although nobody questions the direct effect of ethanol and its oxidative metabolites on the nervous system (King *et al.,* 1988; Harper and Kril, 1990), neurological damage in chronic alcoholics has also been related to the effects of the nonoxidative metabolites of ethanol (fatty-acid ethyl esters) (Laposata and Lange, 1986), changes in neuronal calcium channels (Leslie *et al.,* 1983), the effects of excitatory amino acids on N-methyl-D-aspartate receptors (Lovinger *et al.,* 1989) and an excessive accumulation of hydroxy radicals (Puntarulo and Cederbaum, 1989). Malnutrition and vitamin deficiency

Table 3.2   Neurologic complications observed in chronic alcoholics

Acute intoxication
Ethanol withdrawal
   Tremor
   Visual or auditory illusions and hallucinations
   Tonic-clonic seizures
   Delirium tremens
Diseases related to nutritional deficiencies
   Wernicke-Korsakoff syndrome
   Pellagra
   Nutritional amblyopia
Diseases probably related to toxic effects of ethanol
   Dementia
   Marchiafava-Bignami disease
   Cerebellar degeneration
   Polyneuropathy
   Autonomic neuropathy

may enhance the effects of ethanol on nervous system and/or determine the development of specific nutritional disorders (i.e. Wernicke-Korsakoff syndrome) in alcoholic patients. Finally, genetic factors may also determine the susceptibility of certain alcoholics to neurologic disorders. Thus, some neurologic complications of chronic alcoholics are attributed to specific nutritional deficits (Wernicke-Korsakoff syndrome, pellagra and nutritional amblyopia). Others, such as dementia and Marchiafava-Bignami disease, are due to the toxic effects of ethanol. Central pontine myelinolysis is a rare disorder of the cerebral white matter that usually affects alcoholics but which is related to rapid changes in the levels of water in the brain. Finally, other ethanol-related neurologic complications such as cerebellar degeneration and peripheral and autonomic neuropathy have previously been attributed to nutritional deficiencies, but there is increasing evidence that they are due to the toxic effects of ethanol.

Wernicke-Korsakoff syndrome

Wernicke's encephalopathy is a nutritional disorder caused by a deficiency in thiamine. This is an essential cofactor for several enzymes of the nervous system such as transketolase, alpha-ketoglutarate dehydrogenase, pyruvate dehydrogenase and branched-chain alpha-keto acid dehydrogenase. A deficiency of thiamine produces a diffuse decrease in the use of glucose by the cerebrum. The reduction of pyruvate dehydrogenase activity determines a shift from aerobic metabolism to rapid glycolysis, a sequence similar to the events observed in hypoxic-ischemic injury. It has been proposed that glutamic acid, an excitatory amino acid neurotransmitter, may play a role in the pathogenesis of this disorder (Choi, 1988). Finally, only a subset of thiamine-deficient patients has Wernicke's encephalopathy, those who have inherited or acquired abnormalities of the thiamine-dependent enzyme transketolase (Mukherjee et al., 1987).

One third of the patients present with the classic triad which includes oculomotor abnormalities, gait ataxia and confusional state. Others have a depressed level of consciousness, which, if untreated, progresses through stupor and coma to death. A large proportion of the patients show other ethanol-related diseases such as peripheral neuropathy and liver disease. However, analysis of the autopsy-based series demonstrated a very high incidence of mental status abnormalities, stupor, coma, hypotension and hypothermia in unsuspected cases (Harper et al., 1986). Thus, all alcoholic or malnourished patients with nystagmus, ophtalmoplegia, ataxia, confusion, stupor, coma or hypothermia should be treated with prompt parenteral administration of thiamine. Deficiencies in other vitamins, minerals, and electrolytes, especially magnesium, a transketolase cofactor, should be corrected simultaneously. In addition, it should be remembered that intravenous administration of glucose may precipitate Wernicke's encephalopathy in thiamine-deficient patients. Diagnostic advances, such as CT scanning and magnetic resonance imaging, should increase our knowledge of the natural history of this disorder and facilitate prevention and treatment through earlier detection (Charness and De la Paz, 1987).

Pellagra

This disorder is due to a nicotinic acid deficiency and included dementia, diarrhoea and dermatitis. It should be remarked that nicotinic acid deficient patients may present mental retardation, recent memory loss and melancholia as psychiatric disturbances some weeks or months before the development of other manifestations (Ishii and Nishihara, 1981).

Nutritional amblyopia

Nutritional amblyopia is also known as alcohol-tobacco amblyopia and is diagnosed primarily in chronic alcoholics. This disorder involves retrobulbar neuritis affecting maculopapillary fibers and has been related with a deficiency of thiamine, $vitamin_{12}$ and riboflavine.

Cerebellar degeneration

Almost half of the chronic alcoholics show degeneration of Purkinje cells in the cerebellar cortex and especially in the midline cerebellar structures (anterior and superior vermis). However, only a smaller proportion of chronic alcoholics complain of ataxia which affects mainly gait and less frequently limbs (Charness *et al.,* 1989).

The similarity of the cerebellar lesions with Wernicke's encephalopathy may suggest that this disorder could be related to thiamine deficiency. However, there is some evidence that suggests that it may be due to the direct toxic effects of ethanol, although experimental studies in animals in which cerebellar degeneration is induced by ethanol in the absence of nutritional deficiency, show a different pattern of cerebellar pathology, which primarily involves the granule and molecular-layer interneurons (Ferrer *et al.,* 1984; Tavares *et al.,* 1987).

Peripheral and autonomic neuropathy

Alcoholic neuropathy is a gradually progressive disorder due to the involvement of sensory, motor, and autonomic nerves. The clinical abnormalities are typically symmetric and affect the lower limbs. Autonomic disturbances include orthostatic hypotension, diarrhoea, impotence and sweating disorders. Although these symptoms are less common, their presence has been associated with increased mortality (Johnson and Robinson, 1988).

Alcoholic polyneuropathy has also been attributed to associated malnutrition or a specific lack of thiamine. However, studies conducted in experimental animals (Bosch *et al.,*1979) and in chronic alcoholics (Villalta *et al.,* 1989) have suggested that peripheral neuropathy is secondary to a toxic effect of ethanol or its metabolites. In a study performed in our Unit (Estruch *et al.,* 1993), although patients with peripheral neuropathy exhibited significantly lower anthropometric parameters than their counterparts, no relationship was observed between peripheral neuropathy and nutrition status in the multivariate analysis. The only risk factor for the development of peripheral neuropathy was the total lifetime dose of ethanol. The higher prevalence of malnutrition among the patients with alcoholic neuropathy may be explained by the fact that malnourished chronic alcoholics with polyneuropathy had a significantly higher total lifetime dose of ethanol.

Although alcohol has profound direct effects on the central and peripheral nervous system, several chronic alcoholics exhibit a number of neurological disorders which are related to nutritional deficiencies. Thus, further studies are required to delimitate the relative importance of ethanol and nutrition.

THERAPEUTIC IMPLICATIONS OF NUTRITIONAL DISORDERS IN ALCOHOLICS

According to the results of the most recent studies, only a minority of alcoholics have clinically manifest nutritional problems, but they still represent the largest group of patients with treatable nutritional deficiencies in Western countries. Patients with the highest risk of presenting nutritional disorders are those with the highest ethanol intake (total lifetime of alcohol consumption >20 Kg of ethanol/Kg of body weight) and those who had ethanol-related diseases, especially liver disease. These patients should be supplemented with balanced hypercaloric diets, vitamins and minerals.

Since the levels of vitamins and trace minerals are relatively normal in asymptomatic chronic alcoholics, the value of nutritional supplementation in all cases is questionable. Only patients with clinical evidence of malnutrition, high ethanol intake and/or ethanol-related diseases should be treated with vitamins such as thiamine, nicotinamide, pyridoxine and riboflavine. Alcoholic patients receiving intravenous infusions of glucose have a high risk of presenting Wernicke's encephalopathy and should be treated parenterally with thiamine. Previous studies have reported that the serum levels of vitamin E are significantly reduced in alcoholics as compared to controls, however, the need for supplementating alcoholics with this vitamin remains to be clarified.

Nutritional treatments for alcoholic liver disease are still experimental. Since the metabolism of ethanol in the liver alters the activation and degradation of key nutrients which may enhance the effects of ethanol or its metabolites on liver cells, alcoholics with liver disease should be advised of the importance of maintaining an adequate nutritional balance. Preliminary results suggest that malnourished alcoholics with liver disease have a lower mortality when treated with oral nutritional support combined with anabolic steroids. The role of specific nutrients such as gluthatione, cysteine, SAM, glycine, phospholipids or lecithins in the treatment of these patients needs to be clarified in future trials.

Chronic alcoholics with dilated cardiomyopathy do not require treatment with thiamine unless beriberi cardiomyopathy (high output failure) is suspected. All alcoholics with haematological abnormalities, mainly anaemia and/or thromobocytopenia should be treated with folic acid and vitamin B_{12}.

More interesting are the nutritional disorders of the central and peripheral nervous system. Wernicke's encephalopathy is the main nutritional disorder in alcoholics being due to a thiamine deficiency. Pellagra is another vitamin deficiency commonly seen in chronic alcoholics. All alcoholics or malnourished patients with neurological symptoms should be immediately treated with parenteral thiamine and nicotinamide, as well as other vitamins and electrolytes. The role of nutritional factors in other neurological diseases in alcoholics is more controversial. However, although the main risk factor in developing peripheral or autonomic neuropathy is the total lifetime dose of ethanol, a high proportion of alcoholics with neuropathy show evidence of malnutrition. It is our current point of view that all alcoholics with such a complication be supplemented with vitamins.

CONCLUSIONS AND PROPOSALS FOR FUTURE RESEARCH

Chronic alcoholism still represents the most important cause of malnutrition in Western countries. The aetiology of malnutrition in chronic alcoholics is multifactorial. With the improvement of dietary intake of the population, the importance of primary malnutrition (dietary deficiencies) has become lower and that of secondary malnutrition, greater. Thus, malnutrition in most alcoholics is mainly due to maldigestion, malabsorption and several metabolic effects of ethanol in the storing, activation and excretion of nutrients. Therefore, malnourished alcoholics are often those with higher ethanol intake and/or those who suffer from ethanol-related diseases, mainly alcoholic liver disease.

Over time, alcoholism and malnutrition have been discussed jointly with regards to the pathogenesis, the prognosis and even the therapy of the ethanol-related diseases. Epidemiological, clinical and experimental studies have demonstrated that ethanol has a direct toxic effect on most tissues and organs. However, since not all heavy drinkers exhibit all the varieties of ethanol-related diseases, it has been proposed that other factors (nutritional deficiencies, other hepatotoxins, enviromental circumstances and genetic variations) may enhance, or prevent, the effects of ethanol on the cells and tissues.

Experimental studies have demonstrated the effects of nutrients in the area under the blood ethanol concentration versus time curve (Derr and Draves, 1990). Thus, removal of all vitamins, fat and proteins from the diet resulted in a significant increase in the area under the blood alcohol concentration versus time curve. Moreover, the ingestion of a food, containing all the nutrients in the proportions which are recommended for the humans, simultaneously with the ingestion of each ethanol drink, results in significantly lower blood alcohol levels and hence would reduce toxicity to organs and tissues. In keeping with this last observation, in a recent study performed in our Unit (Nicolás *et al.*, 1993; Estruch *et al.*, 1993), no significant differences were observed in nutritional status between those patients without ethanol-related diseases and controls. These findings may be interpreted to show that more adequate nutrition protects against certain kinds of organ injury, since other studies which included more malnourished populations have shown higher rates of cirrhosis (Simko *et al.*, 1982). However, in the multivariate analysis, there was no significant positive or negative relationship between malnutrition and ethanol-related diseases. The only independent risk factor for developing malnutrition and ethanol-related disease was the total lifetime dose of ethanol. We concluded that malnutrition in alcoholics must be considered as another consequence of ethanol intake or as secondary to alcohol-related diseases.

However, an additive effect of poor nutrition which may contribute to the effects of ethanol has not be ruled out in our studies, especially in relation to alcoholic liver disease. Since little, if any, metabolism of ethanol occurs in extra-hepatic organs, the pathogenesis of the extra-hepatic complications of alcoholism seems to be related to the direct toxic effect of ethanol or its metabolites. Since malnutrition often accompanies alcoholic liver disease and no specific therapy, other than removal of the toxic agent, is available, the possible value of restoring nutritional balance and the use of specific nutrients seems worthy of study.

Proposals for future research

1. Long-term follow-up studies of a large number of alcoholic and non-alcoholic subjects to determine the relationship between ethanol intake and nutritional status over time.
2. To determine the risk factors of malnutrition and vitamin deficiencies according to socioeconomic status, ethnic characteristics, dietary habits, ethanol intake and alcohol-related diseases.

3. Specific deficiencies of substances such as vitamins and trace metals are readily detected. However, good and reproducible methods for assessing overall nutritional status are lacking. New tools of nutritional assessment are needed.

4. All parenterally administered vitamins, commonly prescribed during detoxification, were found to be normal in chronic alcoholics. Thus, it would be interesting to evaluate the actual need for routine administration of vitamins to chronic alcoholics.

5. To perfom a multicenter study on Wernicke's encephalopathy to determine the prevalence, risk factors, genetic predisposition, clinical findings and treatment of this disorder in Europe.

6. To assess the possibility of fortifying alcoholic beverages with fat-soluble analogues of thiamine to prevent Wernicke-Korsakoff syndrome.

7. New trials on the effects of special nutrients (S-adenosyl-L-methionine, polyunsaturated lecithin, in patients with various stages of alcoholic liver disease are of interest.

References

Aa, G.E., Johnson, B.J., Bjmeboe, A., Bachewug, J-E., Morland, J. and Dream, C.A. (1988). Diminished serum concentration of vitamin E in alcoholism. *Annals of Nutrition and Metabolism*, **32**:56–61.

Adams, H.G. and Jordan, J. (1984). Infecctions in the alcoholics. *Medical Clinics in North America*, **68**:179–200.

Baker, A.L., Elson, C.O., Jaspan, J. and Boyer, J.L. (1979). Liver failure with steatonecrosis after jejunoileal bypass: Recovery with parenteral nutrition and reanastomosis. *Archives of Internal Medicine*, **139**:289–292.

Bishop, C.W., Bowen, P.E. and Ritchey, S.J. (1981). Norms for nutritional assessment of American adult by upper anthropometry. *American Journal of Clinical Nutrition*, **34**:2530–2539.

Blackburn, G.L., Bistrain, B.R., Maini, B.S., Schlamm, B.A. and Smith, M.F. (1977). Nutritional and metabolic assessment of the hospitalized patient. *Journal of Parenteral Nutrition*, **1**:11–22.

Bode, J.C., Bode, C., Heidlebach, R., Dürr, H.K. and Martini. G.A. (1984). Jejunal microflora in patients with chronic alcohol abuse. *Hepatogastroenterology*, **31**:30–34.

Bode, J.C., Hanisch, P., Henning, H., Koening, W., Ritcher, F-W. and Bode, C. (1988). Hepatic zinc content in patients with various stages of alcoholic liver disease and in patients with chronic active and chronic persistent hepatitis. *Hepatology*, **8**:1605–1609.

Bonjour, J.P. (1980). Vitamins and alcoholism. II. Folate and vitamin B_{12}. *International Journal for Vitamin and Nutrition Research*, **50**:96–121.

Bosch, E.P., Pelham, R.W., Rasool, C.G., Chatterjee, A., Lash, R.W., Brown, L., Munsat, T.L. and Bradley, W.G. (1979). Animal models of alcoholic neuropathy: morphological, electrophysiological and biochemical findings. *Muscle and Nerve*, **2**:133–144.

Boyd, D.H., Maclaren, D.S. and Stoddard, M.E. (1981). The nutritional status of patients with alcohol problems. *Acta Vitaminologica et Enzymologica*, **3**:75–82.

Burrit, M.F. and Anderson, C.F. (1984). Laboratory assessment of nutritional status. *Human Pathology*, **15**:130–133.

Camilo, M.E., Morgan, M.Y. and Sherlock, S. (1981). Erythrocyte transketolase activity in alcoholic liver disease. *Scandinavian Journal of Gastroenterology*, **16**:273 –279.

Carey, G.B. (1989). Nutrition and Alcoholism: Problems and therapies. *Occupational Medicine*, **4**:311–326.

Cook, C.C.H., Walden, R.J., Graham, B.R., Gillham, C., Davis, S. and Prichard, B.N.C. (1991). Trace element and vitamin deficiency in alcoholic and control subjects. *Alcohol and Alcoholism*, **26**:541–548.

Cooke, A.R. (1972). Ethanol and gastric function. *Gastroenterology*, **62**:501–502.

Chanarin, I. (1982). Haemopoiesis and alcohol. *British Medical Bulletin*, **38**:81–86.

Charness, M.E. and De la Paz, R.L. (1987). Mamilary body atrophy in Wernicke's encephalopathy: antemortem identification using magnetic resonance imaging. *Annals of Neurology*, **22**:595–600.

Charness, M.E. (1993). Brain lesions in alcoholics. *Alcoholism: Clinical and Experimental Research*, **17**:2–11.

Charness, M.E., Simon, R.P. and Greenberg, D.A. (1989). Ethanol and the nervous system. *New England Journal of Medicine*, **321**:442–454.

Chawla, R.K., Wolf, S.C., Kutner, M.H. and Bonkovsky, H.L. (1989). Choline may be an essential nutrient in malnourished patients with cirrhosis. *Gastroenterology*, **97**:1514–1520.

Choi, D.W. (1988). Glutamate neurotoxicity and diseases of the nervous system. *Neuron*, **1**:623–634.

Dally, S., Girre, C., Hispard, E., Thomas, G. and Fournier, L. (1989). High blood level lead in alcoholics: wine vs. beer. *Drug and Alcohol Dependence*, **23**:45–48.

Dancy, M., Blaud, J.M., Leech, G. and Gaitionde, M.K. (1985). Preclinical left ventricular abnormalities in alcoholics are independent of nutritional status, cirrhosis and cigarrette smoking. *Lancet*, **1**:1122–1125.

Darnton-Hill, I. (1989). Interactions of alcohol, malnutrition and ill health. *World Review of Nutrition and Dietetics (Basel)*, **59**:95–125.

Dennis, B.H., Haynes, S.G., Anderson, J.D., Liu-Chi, S.B.L., Hosking, J.D. *et al.* (1985). Nutrient intakes among selected north american populations in the lipid research clinic prevalence study: composition of energy intake. *American Journal of Clinical Nutrition*, **41**:312–329.

Derr, R.F. and Draves, K. (1990). Prevention of alcohol toxicity by adequate nutrients: Mechanism and potential application. *Nutrition Research*, **10**:1285–1297.

Dickson, R.C., Bronk, S.J. and Gores, G.J. (1992). Glycine cytoprotection during lethal hepatocellular injury from adenosine triphosphate depletion. *Gastroenterology*, **102**:2098–2107.

Durnin, J.V. and Womersley, J.K. (1974). Body fat assessed from total density and its estimation from skinfold thickness: measurements on 481 men and women aged from 16 to 72 years. *British Journal of Nutrition*, **32**:77–97.

Erenoglu, E., Edreira, J.G. and Patek, A.J.Jr. (1964). Observations on patients with Laennec's cirrhosis receiving alcohol while on controlled diets. *Annals of Internal Medecine*, **60**: 814–823.

Estruch, R., Nicolás, J.M., Villegas, E., Junqué, A. and Urbano-Márquez, A. (1993). Relationship between ethanol-related diseases and nutritional status in chronic alcoholic men. *Alcohol and Alcoholism*, **28**:543–550.

Farrow, F.A., Rees, J.M. and Worthington-Roberts, B.S. (1987). Health, developmental and nutritional status of adolescent alcohol and marijuana abusers. *Pediatrics*, **79**:218–223.

Fernández-Solá, J., Estruch, R., Grau, J.M., Paré, J.C., Rubin, E. and Urbano-Márquez, A. (1994). The relation of alcoholic myopathy to cardiomyopathy. *Annals of Internal Medicine*, **120**:529–536.

Ferrer, I., Fabregas, I., Pineda, M., Gracia, I. and Ribalta, T. (1984). A Golgi study of cerebellar atrophy in human chronic alcoholism. *Neuropathology and Applied Neurobiology*, **10**:245–253.

Fisher, M. and Gordon, T. (1985). The relation of drinking and smoking habits to the diet: the lipid research clinic prevalence study. *American Journal of Clinical Nutrition*, **41**:623–630.

Goldsmith, R.H., Iber, F.L. and Miller, P.A. (1983). Nutritional status of alcoholics of different socioeconomic class. *Journal of the American College of Nutrition*, **2**:215–220.

Harper, C.G., Giles, M. and Finlay-Jones, R. (1986). Clinical signs in the Wernicke-Korsakoff complex: a retrospective analysis of 131 cases diagnosed at necropsy. *Journal of Neurology, Neurosurgery and Psychiatry*, **49**:341–345.

Harper, C.G. and Kril, J.J. (1990). Neuropathology of alcoholism. *Alcohol and Alcoholism*, **25**:207–216.

Henry, R.W. and Elmes, M.E. (1975). Plasma zinc in acute starvation. *British Medical Journal*, **4**;625–626.

Iber, F.L. (1990). Alcoholism and associated malnutrition in the elderly. *Progress in Clinical and Biological Research*, **326**:157–173

Ishii, N. and Nishihara, Y. (1981). Pellagra among chronic alcoholics: clinical and pathological study of 20 necropsy cases. *Journal of Neurology, Neurosurgery and Psychiatry*, **44**:209–215.

Israel, Y., Kalant, H., Orrego, H., Khanna, J.M., Videla, L. and Phillips, J.M. (1975). Experimental alcohol-induced hepatic necrosis: Suppression by propylthiouracil. *Proceedings of the National Academy of Sciences of United States of America*, **72**:1137–1141.

Jacobs, R.M. and Sorrell, M.F. (1981). The role of nutrition in the pathogenesis of alcoholic liver damage. *Seminars in Liver Disease*, **1**:244–253.

Johnson, R.H. and Robinson, B.J. (1988). Mortality in alcoholics with autonomic neuropathy. *Journal of Neurology, Neurosurgery and Psychiatry*, **51**:476–480.

Johnson, R.D. and Williams, R. (1984). Genetic and enviromental factors in the individual susceptibility to the development of alcoholic liver disease. *Alcohol and Alcoholism*, **30**:137–160.

Kamimura, S., Gaal, K., Britton, R.S. *et al.* (1992). Increased 4-hidroxynonenal levels in experimental alcoholic liver disease. Association of lipid peroxidation with liver fibrogenesis. *Hepatology*, **16**:448–453.

King, M.A., Hunter, B.E. and Walker, D.W. (1988). Alterations and recovery of dendritic spine density in rat hippocampus following long-term ethanol ingestion. *Brain Research*, **459**:381–385.

Klock, J.C., Williams, H.E. and Mentzer, W.C. (1974). Hemolytic anemia and somatic cell dysfunction in severe hypophosphatemia. *Archives of Internal Medicine*, **134**:360–364.

Korpela, H., Kumpulainen, J., Luoma, P.V., Arranto, A.J. and Sotaniemi, E.A. (1985). Decreased serum selenium in alcoholics as related to liver structure and function. *American Journal of Clinical Nutrition*, **42**:147–151.

Kromhoult, D. (1983). Energy and macronutrient intake in lean and obese middle-aged men (the Zutphen Study). *American Journal of Clinical Nutrition*, **37**:295–299.

Laposata, E.A. and Lange, L.G. (1986). Presence of nonoxidative ethanol metabolism in human organs commonly damage by ethanol abuse. *Science*, **231**:497–499.

Leevy, C.M. (1982). Thiamine deficiency and alcoholism. *Annals of the New York Academy of Sciences*, **378**:316–326.

Lelbach, W.K. (1975). Cirrhosis in the alcoholic and its relation to the volume of alcohol abuse. *Annals of the New York Academy of Sciences*, **252**:85–105.

Leslie, S.W., Barr, E., Chandler, J. and Farrar, R.P. (1983). Inhibition of fast- and slow- phase depolarization-dependent synaptosomal calcium uptake by ethanol. *Journal of Pharmacology and Experimental Therapy*, **225**:571–575.

Levine, R.F., Spivak, J.L., Maegler, R.C. and Sieber, F. (1986). Effect of ethanol on thrombopoiesis. *British Journal of Haematology*, **62**:345–354.

Li, J., Kim, C-I, Leo, M.A. *et al.* (1992). Polyunsaturated lecithin prevents acetaldehyde-mediated hepatic collagen accumulation by stimulating collagenase activity in cultured lipocytes. *Hepatology*, **15**:373–381.

Lieber, C.S. (1988). Biochemical and molecular basis of alcohol-indiced injury to liver and other tissues. *New England Journal of Medicine*, **319**:1639–1650.

Lieber, C.S. (1988). The influence of alcohol on nutritional status. *Nutrition Reviews*, **46**:241–254.

Lieber, C.S., Jones, D.P. and DeCarli, L.M. (1965). Effects of prolonged ethanol intake: Production of fatty liver despite adequate diets. *Journal of Clinical Investigation*, **44**:1009–1021.

Lieber, C.S., DeCarli, L.M. and Rubin, E. (1975). Sequential production of fatty liver, hepatitis, cirrhosis in sub-human primates fed ethanol with adequate diets. *Proceedings of the National Academy of Sciences of USA*, **72**:437–441.

Lieber, C.S., Casini, A., DeCarli, L.M. *et al.* (1990). S-adenosyl-L-methionine attenuates alcohol-induced liver injury in the baboon. *Hepatology*, **11**:165–172.

Lindenbaum, J. (1987). Hematologic complications of alcohol abuse. *Seminars in Liver Disease*, **7**:169–178.

Lovinger, D.M., White, G. and Weight, F.F. (1989). Ethanol inhibits NMDA-activated ion current in hippocampal neurons. *Science*, **243**:1721–1724.

MacGregor, R.R. (1986). Alcohol and inmune defense. *Journal of American Medical Association*, **256**:1474–1479.

Mahalko, J.R., Jonhson, L.K., Gallagher, S.K. and Milne, D.B. (1985). Comparison of dietary histories and seven-day food records in a nutritional assessment of older adults. *American Journal of Clinical Nutrition*, **42**:542–553.

Mendenhall, C.L., Anderson, S., Weesner, R.E., Goldberg, S.J. and Crolic, K.A. (1984). Protein-Calorie Malnutrition Associated with Alcoholic Hepatitis. *American Journal of Medicine*, **76**:211–222.

Mendenhall, C.L., Tosch, T., Weesner, R.E., Garcia-Pont, P., Goldberg, S.J., Kiernan, T., Seeff, L.B., Sorrell, M., Tamburro, C., Zetterman, R., Chedid, A., Chen, T. and Rabin L. (1986). VA cooperative study on alcoholic hepatitis II: prognostic significance of protein-calorie malnutrition. *American Journal of Nutrition*, **43**:213–218.

Mezey, E. and Potter, J.J. (1976). Changes in exocrine pancreatic function produced by altered dietary protein intake in drinking alcoholics. *Johns Hopkins Medical Journal*, **138**:7–12.

Mezey, E., Kolman, C.J., Diehl, A.M., Mitchell, M.C. and Herlong, H.F. (1988). Alcohol and dietary intake in the development of chronic pancreatitis and liver disease in alcoholism. *American Journal of Clinical Nutrition*, **48**:148–151.

Mezey, E., Caballeria, J., Mitchell, M.C., Parés, A., Herlong, F. and Rodés, J. (1991). Effect of parenteral amino acid supplementation on short-term and long-term outcomes in severe alcoholic hepatitis: a randomized controlled trial. *Hepatology*, **14**:1090–1096.

Mili, F., Flanders, W.D., Boring, J.R., Annest, J.L. and DeStefano, F. (1992). The associations of alcohol drinking and drinking cessation to measures of the immune system in middle-aged men. *Alcoholism: Clinical and Experimental Research*, **16**:688–694.

Mills, P.R., Shenkin, A., Anthony, R.S., McLelland, A.S., Main, A.N.H., MacSween, A.S. and Russell, R.I. (1983). Assessment of nutritional status and in vivo inmune response in alcohol liver disease. *American Journal of Clinical Nutrition*, **38**:849–859.

Morgan, M.M. (1982). Alcohol and Nutrition. *British Medical Bulletin*, **38**:21–29.

Mukherjee, G.C., Svoronos, S., Ghazanfari, A. *et al.* (1987). Transketolase abnormality in cultured fibroblasts from familial chronic alcoholic men and their male offspring. *Journal of Clinical Investigation*, **79**:1039–1043.

Neville, J.N., Eagles, J.A., Samson, G. and Olson, R.E. (1968). Nutritional status of alcoholics. *American Journal of Clinical Nutrition*, **21**: 1320–1340.

Nicolás, J.Mª., Estruch, R., Antunez, E., Sacanella, E. and Urbano-Márquez, A. (1993). Nutritional status in chronic alcoholic men from the middle socioeconomic class and its relation to ethanol intake. *Alcohol and Alcoholism*, **28**:551–558.

Patek, A.J. and Post, J. (1941). Treatment of cirrhosis of the liver by a nutritious diet and supplements rich in vitamin B-complex. *Journal of Clinical Investigation*, **20**:481–505.

Patek, A.J.Jr., Toth, I.G., Saunders, M.G., Castro, G.A.M. and Engel, J.J. (1975). Alcohol and dietary factors in cirrhosis. An epidemiological study of 304 alcoholic patients. *Archives of Internal Medicine*, **135**:1053–1057.

Pequignot, F., Tuyns, A.J. and Berta, B.J. (1978). Ascitic cirrhosis in relation to alcohol consumption. *International Journal of Epidemiology*, **7**:113–120.

Persson, J. (1991). Alcohol and the small intestine. *Scandinavian Journal of Gastroenterology*, **26**:3–15.

Peura, D.A., Stromeyer, F.W. and Johnson, L.F. (1980). Liver injury with alcoholic hyaline after intestinal resection. *Gastroenterolgy*, **79**:128–130.

Pirola, R.C. and Lieber, C.S. (1972). The energy cost of the metabolism of drugs, including ethanol. *Pharmacology*, **7**:185–196.

Pirola, R.C. and Liber, C.S. (1976). Hypothesis: energy wastage in alcoholism and drug abuse: possible role of hepatic microsomal enzymes. *American Jornal of Clinical Nutrition*, **29**:90–93.

Puntarulo, S. and Cederbraum, A.I. (1989). Chemiluminiscence from acetaldehyde oxidation by xanthine oxidase involves generation and interaction with hydroxy radicals. *Alcoholism (New York)*, **13**:84–90.

Roselle, G.A., Mendenhall, C.L., Grossman, C.J. and Weesner, R.F. (1988). Lymphocyte subset alterations in patients with alcoholic hepatitis. *Journal of Clinical and Laboratory Immunology*, **26**:169–173.

Rubin, E. and Lieber, C.S. (1968). Alcohol-induced hepatic injury in non-alcoholic volunteers. *New England Journal of Medicine*, **278**:869–876.

Rubin, E. and Lieber, C.S. (1974). Fatty liver, alcoholic hepatitis and cirrhosis produced by alcohol in primates. *New England Journal of Medicine*, **290**:128–135.

Sarles, H., Bernard, J.P. and Johnson, C. (1989). Pathogenesis and epidemiology of chronic pancreatitis. *Annual Reviews of Medicine*, **40**:453–468.

Schaefer, E.J., Rees, D.G. and Siguel, E.N. (1986). Nutrition, lipoproteins and atherosclerosis. *Clinical Nutrition*, **5**:99–111.

Schenker, S. and Halff, G.A. (1993). Nutritional therapy in alcoholic liver disease. *Seminars in liver disease*, **13**:196–209.

Sherlock, S. (1984). Nutrition and the alcoholic. *Lancet*, **I**:436–438.

Simko, V., Connell, A.M. and Banks, B. (1982). Nutritional status in alcoholics with and without liver disease. *American Journal of Clinical Nutrition*, **35**:197–203.

Staveren, W.A., Boer, J.O. and Burema, J. (1985). Validity and reproducibility of a dietary history method estimating the usual food intake during one month. *American Journal of Clinical Nutrition*, **42**:554–559.

Summerskill, W.H.J., Wolfe, S.J. and Davidson, C.S. (1957). Response to alcohol in chronic alcoholics with liver disease. *Lancet*, **1**:335–340.

Suter, P.M., Schutz, M.S. and Jequier, E. (1992). The effect of ethanol on fat storage in healthy subjects. *New England Journal of Medicine*, **326**:983–987.

Tavares, M.A., Paula-Barbosa, M.M. and Cadete-Leite, A. (1987). Chronic alcohol consumption reduces the cortical layer volumes and the number of neurons of the rat cerebellar cortex. *Alcoholism (New York)*, **11**:315–319.

Thomson, M., Fulton, M., Elton. R.A., Brown, S., Wood, D.A. and Oliver, M.F. (1988). Alcohol consumption and nutrient intake in middle-aged Scottish men. *American Journal of Clinical Nutrition*, **47**:139–145.

Tsukamoto, H., Goal, K. and French, S.W. (1990). Insights into the pathogenesis of alcoholic liver necrosis and fibrosis: Status report. *Hepatology*, **12**:599–608.

Urbano-Marquez, A., Estruch, R., Navarro-López, F., Grau, J.Mª., Mont, Ll. and Rubin, E. (1989). Effects of alcoholism on skeletal and cardiac muscle. *New England Journal of Medicine*, **320**: 409–415.

Villalta, J., Estruch, R., Antunez, E., Valls, J. and Urbano-Márquez, A. (1989). Vagal neuropathy in chronic alcoholics: relation to ethanol consumption. *Alcohol and Alcoholism*, **24**, 421–428.

Williamson, D.F., Forman, M.R., Binkin, N.J., Gentry E.M., Remington, P.L. and Trowbridge, F.L. (1987). Alcohol and body weight in United States adults. *American Journal of Public Health*, **77**:1324–1330.

Wilson, F.A. and Hoyumpa, A.M.Jr. (1979). Ethanol and small intestine transport. *Gastroenterology*, **76**:388–403.

Windham, C.T., Wyse, B.S. and Hansen, R.G. (1983). Alcohol consumption and nutrient density of diets in the Nationwide Food Consumption Survey. *Journal of American Dietary Association*, **82**:364–373.

4 Alcohol and the Liver

D. Sherman, J. Koskinas and Roger Williams

Institute of Liver Studies, King's College School of Medicine and Dentistry, London SE5, UK

Alcoholic liver disease (ALD) is one of the most important consequences of alcohol misuse. Mortality from cirrhosis in a population parallels per capita ethanol consumption. There is increasing evidence for a wide variation in susceptibility of individuals to alcohol-induced liver damage, some of which may be due to inherited variations in ethanol metabolism. Although the pathophysiology of ALD is poorly understood, the mechanisms by which ethanol is thought to cause liver damage are reviewed. Finally, the principles of management of alcoholic hepatitis and cirrhosis, including the controversial issue of liver transplantation, are discussed.

INTRODUCTION

Alcoholic liver disease (ALD) accounts for a substantial proportion of alcohol-related morbidity and mortality throughout Europe, and is one of the most important consequences of chronic alcohol misuse. This review will consider the epidemiology of ALD, the basis of individual susceptibility, the major theories of pathogenesis, and recent advances in treatment including liver transplantation.

The most commonly used classification of ALD is based upon histological criteria, as clinical presentation varies widely. *Fatty liver* is present in at least 90% of chronic alcohol misusers, but is almost invariably asymptomatic. This review will therefore concentrate on more severe forms of damage. *Alcoholic hepatitis* is an intermediate stage, and is characterised histologically by hepatocellular necrosis, an acute inflammatory infiltrate and the presence of an eosinophilic material, Mallory's hyaline. Some patients with this lesion may be totally asymptomatic, but more commonly the presentation varies from a mild illness with hepatomegaly and jaundice to an acute, life-threatening syndrome with encephalopathy, hepatorenal failure, coagulopathy, fever, leucocytosis and gastrointestinal bleeding. Despite many randomized studies over the past 20 years, attempts to find effective treatments for the acute illness have had only limited success, so that management is still based upon abstinence and supportive measures. Abstinence is usually accompanied by improvement, but in a minority the hepatitis may persist or even progress (Galambos, 1972).

Cirrhosis usually follows alcoholic hepatitis, but may also arise without a clinically apparent stage of hepatitis. Paradoxically, many patients presenting with acute alcoholic hepatitis (up to 50% in some series) have underlying cirrhosis already. End-stage cirrhosis manifests clinically with the consequences of hepatocellular failure and portal hypertension, particularly variceal bleeding, ascites, oedema, encephalopathy and general debility. A small proportion of patients with longstanding cirrhosis develop *hepatocellular carcinoma*, for which the prognosis is extremely poor.

Historical Overview and epidemiology

The association between heavy drinking and liver damage was probably first noticed in Biblical times by Hippocrates, but was first documented by Matthew Baillie (1793). An autopsy study by Jolliffe and Jellineck conducted between 1884 and 1992 suggested that between 50 and 75% of cirrhosis was caused by alcohol (Jollife and Jellinek, 1941). More recent epidemiological studies have, in fact, yielded similar figures (Saunders *et al.*, 1981). However, until the 1960s it was thought that the nutritional deficiencies that accompany alcoholism, rather than alcohol itself, were the cause of the liver damage. Basic research on both animals and humans over the past 30 years has not only confirmed the primary aetiological role of alcohol, but also has revealed the importance of a number of secondary factors, including malnutrition.

In any adult population, there is a rough correlation between the per capita alcohol consumption and the prevalence of, or mortality from, cirrhosis. Analyses of trends in per capita alcohol consumption and cirrhosis mortality in various countries between 1930 and 1960 have shown a strong correlation (with coefficients of 0.43 to 0.89) between these two variables (Grant *et al.*, 1988). Although it was previously thought that a time lag of up to 20 years existed before increases in ethanol consumption were reflected by increases in the prevalence of cirrhosis, this concept has been questioned by epidemiologists in view of parallel increases in some populations (Terris, 1967). As a result it is now thought that in populations with a large 'reservoir' of heavy drinkers, cirrhosis rates may respond rapidly to increases in consumption due to the rapid development of severe liver disease in individuals who already have sub-clinical liver damage (Skog, 1980, 1985).

In current times cirrhosis and alcoholic hepatitis remain major causes of death in Western societies, particularly in men of working age. In England and Wales death rates for cirrhosis almost doubled between 1950 and 1980 (Paton, 1988). Figure 4.1 and 4.2 illustrate the relationship between death rates for all causes of cirrhosis and alcohol consumption in a number of European countries in the mid 1970's and mid 1980's, respectively (Paton, 1988; Royal College of Physicians, 1991). Deaths from alcohol-induced cirrhosis will account for only one half to two thirds of the total, but such figures are likely to be underestimates. It can be seen that alcohol consumption rose in 11 out of the 12 countries during the period from 1975 to 1986/7, with parallel increases in the recorded mortalities from cirrhosis in most countries.

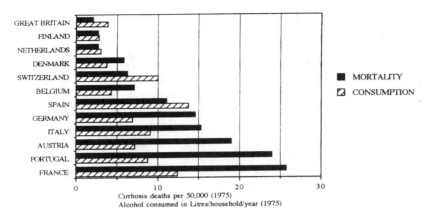

Figure 4.1   Death Rates from Cirrhosis and Alcohol Consumption in various European Countries in the mid-1970's.

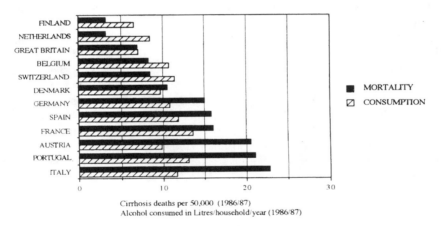

Figure 4.2   Death Rates from Cirrhosis and Alcohol Consumption in various European Countries in the mid-1980's.

Such statistics are prone to sampling error, under-reporting of alcohol-related deaths and other inaccuracies, and should therefore be interpreted with caution, but they do illustrate a trend of increasing consumption and mortality from alcoholic liver disease throughout Europe. The lack of close correlation between the two may reflect differences in the demographic make-up of populations, drinking patterns, and the type of beverage consumed. In addition, the incidence of non-alcoholic causes of cirrhosis (eg. high incidence of hepatitis B and C viral hepatitis in Mediterranean countries) is likely to have contributed to the rise in all-cause cirrhosis mortality in some countries such as Italy.

BASIS OF INDIVIDUAL SUSCEPTIBILITY

Background

Despite the correlation between drinking levels and the development of alcoholic liver disease in populations, there is striking variability in individual susceptibility to liver damage from alcohol misuse. Only 8 to 30% of long-term alcohol misusers develop alcoholic cirrhosis (Grant *et al.*, 1988), and a minority of individuals do not progress beyond the stage of fatty liver despite persistent drinking. As shown by classic case-control studies performed in the 1970s, some of this variation is accounted by differences in amount, duration and pattern of drinking. Lelbach (1975) demonstrated that the prevalence of cirrhosis increases in a linear fashion according to the duration of misuse, although in this study only 50% of those consuming in excess of 200g per day for over 20 years developed cirrhosis. The studies of Pequignot (1974, 1978) in France attempted to find a minimum level of intake above which the risk of cirrhosis was significantly increased. It was suggested that this level was 61 to 80g/day for men, and as low as 21 to 40g/day for women. In addition Pequigot and co-workers proposed a risk model using 3 categories of consumption: (a) low risk — less than 80g/day; (b) moderate risk — 80 to 160 g/day; (c) high risk-more than 160g/day.

However, some studies have not shown this relationship. For example, Sorenson *et al.* (1984) found that the risk of alcoholics with early liver damage progressing to cirrhosis was 2% per year, and that this risk was independent of intake in those individuals consuming more than 80g/day. Interestingly, retrospective studies suggest that a minority of chronic misusers who develop cirrhosis show a high level of alcohol dependency. Wodak *et al.* (1981) demonstrated that two thirds of cirrhotic patients referred to a specialist liver unit had SADQ (Severity of Alcohol Dependence Questionnaire) scores indicating moderate or low levels of dependency. Susceptibility to acute severe forms of alcoholic hepatitis is also unpredictable, although many patients have been drinking heavily prior to presentation. Evidence from these and other studies has led to the search for other environmental and genetic factors that may contribute to the development of alcoholic liver disease.

Genetic factors

The increased susceptibility of women to the effects of alcohol on the liver is well known (Morgan and Sherlock, 1977). A number of factors are responsible, including increased bio-availability of ethanol due to a lower body water content, altered immune responsiveness, and possibly reduced 'first pass' ethanol metabolism by the gastric mucosa (Frezza *et al.*, 1990). There is also evidence that some racial groups, particularly Asian of Indian origin, develop liver damage more rapidly (Mendenhall *et al.*, 1989). Attempts to find reliable biological markers initially focused upon the specific and highly polymorphic Human Leucocyte Antigen (HLA) system, which is determined by a number of genes on the short arm of chromosome 6 (Eddleston and Davis, 1982). A large number of studies followed in the early 1980s, examining many different antigens in diverse populations. The most frequent findings was of an association with HLA B8, which in one study was connected with more rapid development of cirrhosis (Saunders *et al.*, 1982).

Table 4.1 Candidate genes for susceptibility to alcoholic liver disease

	Chromosome
Specific for alcoholic liver disease	4q21–q25
Alcohol dehydrogenase (ADH$_1$, ADH$_2$, ADH$_3$)	9, 12
Aldehyde dehydrogenase (ADLH$_1$, ALDH$_2$)	10
Cytochrome P4502E1	
Non-specific for alcoholic liver disease	
Class I and II HLA antigens	6p21
Type 1 collagen: COL1 A1	17q21
COL1 A 2	7q22
alpha-1-antitrypsin	14q31–q32.3
Specific for alcoholism/addiction	
Dopamine D$_2$ receptor	11q22–q23
? Adenylate cyclase, Monoamine oxidase etc.	

The advent and widespread application of molecular biological techniques over the past 10 years have superceded these studies, and techniques such as the polymerase chain reaction have greatly simplified the characterization of genes that have already been cloned. In addition, these techniques have the added advantage that they do not necessarily require liver biopsy material for study, as DNA is readily extracted from white cells in peripheral blood. The genes most likely to play a major role in the pathogenesis of alcoholic liver disease ('candidate' genes) are listed in Table 4.1.

Ethanol metabolism and molecular approaches

Considerable progress in the understanding of ethanol metabolism has been made over the past 15 years, and knowledge of the biochemistry and molecular biology of the major enzyme systems involved is now being applied to the genetics of alcoholic liver disease. Ninety percent of alcohol reaching the liver in the portal blood is oxidised to acetaldehyde by isoenzymes of alcohol dehydrogenase (ADH) and thence to acetate by aldehyde dehydrogenase (ALDH) isoenzymes. The cytochrome P450IIE1 system (Microsomal Ethanol Oxidising System) provides an alternative pathway, accounting for up to 10% of ethanol oxidation in chronic misusers due to enzyme induction (Leiber, 1988). The activities of these enzymes, and their distributions within the liver lobule, are likely to play an important role in determining the degree and pattern of liver damage as they determine the rates of formation and elimination of acetaldehyde, which mediates both direct and indirect toxicity (Lauterburg and Bilzer, 1988).

Both ADH and ALDH show considerable polymorphism (ie. variation), and have been studied extensively at the biochemical and molecular level. Five ADH genes encode the genetic information for over 20 possible ADH isoenzymes, each with different kinetic properties. The most important sites of genetic variation are in the alcohol dehydrogenase genes ADH$_2$ and ADH$_3$, each of which occurs in more than one variant (allele) (Bosron and Li, 1986). Each allele encodes isoenzymes which have small differences in their amino acid sequence, but which differ greatly in their capacities to metabolize ethanol. The advent of PCR has enabled the development of relatively simple but precise genotyping methods to distinguish different ADH_2 and ADH_3 alleles from peripheral blood samples. Since most European Caucasians possess similar ADH_2 genotypes, studies have concentrated on comparisons of ADH_3 genotypes in patients with ALD and normal controls. Three studies have produced conflicting results, and have not shown a clear association with susceptibility to ALD (Couzigou et al., 1990; Day et al., 1991; Ward et al., unpublished data). Using an alternative approach we have recently identified a Restriction Fragment Length Polymorphism (RFLP) within the ADH_2 gene which shows a genetic association with severe alcoholic liver disease (Sherman et al., 1993).

Two major isoenzymes of ALDH have been identified that play a major role in hepatic acetaldehyde metabolism, of which the mitochondrial form ($ALDH_2$) is the most important. The $ALDH_2$ gene is of considerable interest as it occurs in 2 polymorphic forms. The 'wild type' gene encodes the active enzyme, whereas a 'mutant' form encodes an inactive enzyme, due to a point (single base) mutation in its genetic sequence. This mutant allele is extremely rare in Caucasians, but 40% of Orientals possess the mutation and therefore the inactive enzyme (Goedde et al., 1989). The result of this 'inborn error' of acetaldehyde metabolism is a marked reduction in the capacity of the liver to metabolize acetaldehyde. Affected individuals develop a marked facial 'flushing reaction' after a single drink of alcohol, as high blood acetaldehyde levels produce generalised vasodilatation. Studies in Japanese have shown that individuals possessing of two copies of the mutant allele, which is inherited in an autosomal dominant manner, are protected against both alcoholism and alcoholic liver disease (Shibuya and Yoshida, 1988). Conversely, heterozygotes may be more susceptible to liver damage than those with normal ALDH activity (Enomoto et al., 1991). However the mutant allele, and therefore the inactive enzyme, occur in low frequency in Caucasian populations, which suggests that genetic variations of the alcohol dehydrogenases are likely to be of greater importance. Further research into this area may yield important clues into the genetic basis of individual susceptibility.

Environmental factors

Alcohol often exacerbates other liver diseases, and conversely environmental factors other than the consumption of ethanol itself may contribute to the development of alcoholic liver disease. One of the most important of these is viral hepatitis, which has a higher incidence in Mediterranean countries such as Italy. Although there is evidence for an increased prevalence of hepatitis B (HBV) markers in both alcohol misusers and patients with alcoholic liver disease (Saunders et al., 1983), HBV does not appear to be a major exacerbating factor for alcoholic liver disease in most European populations. However, one study from Italy showed that chronic carriers of HBV who misuse alcohol have a more rapid rate of progression of liver damage (Villa et al., 1982).

There has also been considerable interest in Hepatitis C (HCV) infection. A number of assays are available for HCV antibodies, but the less specific of these produce false positive results in alcoholic hepatitis due to the co-existent polyclonal hypergammaglobulinaemia, which may in turn become negative in abstinence (Mendenhall et al., 1991; Wands and Blum, 1991). Some reports suggest that the presence of HCV antibody is associated with more severe histology (Pares et al., 1990). In general, the frequency with which co-existent HBV or HCV infection causes more rapid progression of alcoholic liver disease is related to their population prevalences, so that this is likely to occur more commonly in Mediterranean than in Northern European countries.

Recent studies have shown that protein-calorie malnutrition is found in the majority of patients with acute alcoholic hepatitis and cirrhosis (Mendenhall *et al.*, 1984), and aggravates liver injury in many cases. Multiple factors are involved, including reduced dietary intake, malabsorbtion, increased catabolism and altered energy processing. In addition, chronic exposure to certain drugs may exacerbate alcoholic liver disease (Leiber, 1988). Although approximately 30% of patients with ALD show increased amounts of liver iron (Chapman *et al.*, 1982), it is unclear whether iron overload contributes to the process of liver damage.

PATHOGENESIS OF ALCOHOLIC LIVER DISEASE

The role of ethanol in either causing liver injury or perpetuating hepatocyte damage has been the subject of debate. Ethanol metabolism i.e. breakdown, centrilobular hypoxia, activation of the inflammatory cascade, immunologic reactions and fibrogenesis are important factors contributing to pathogenesis of alcoholic liver disease.

Ethanol metabolism causes a shift in redox potential of the cytosol altering intermediary metabolism and promoting production of free radicals (Dicker and Cederbaum, 1990). Disturbances in the lipid metabolism result in accumulation of triglycerides in the hepatocytes (Leiber and Spritz, 1966). Acetaldehyde, the main product of ethanol metabolism, inhibits tubulin polymerization leading to disruption of protein trafficking and export mechanisms (Tuma *et al.*, 1991). Changes in the plasma membrane constitution and fluidity interferes with hormone receptors, membrane transport and receptor mediated endocytosis (Tuma *et al.*, 1990). Covalent binding of acetaldehyde specifically inhibits enzymes with catalytically active lysine residues (Mauch *et al.*, 1986) and stimulates collagen gene transcription (Casini *et al.*, 1991). In addition, alcohol can increase oxygen consumption worsening the oxygen gradient from portal to central vein (Iturriaga *et al.*, 1980). Cytochrome P-450IIE1, the ethanol-inducible microsomal cytochrome, is located selectively in the centrilobular zone and uses more oxygen for ethanol oxidation than the acetaldehyde dehydrogenase pathway (Tsukamoto *et al.*, 1990).

The role of endotoxin and the cytokine cascade in alcoholic liver disease has been well studied in animal models and clinical studies (Bhagwandeen *et al.*, 1987). Increased levels of IL-6 and TNF in serum are found in patients with alcoholic hepatitis and higher levels of TNF-α are associated with increased mortality (Bird *et al.*, 1990). Furthermore, in severe AH circulating and tissue levels of IL-8 — the major leucocyte chemoattractant — are highly elevated and tissue levels are correlated with the degree of neutrophil infiltration (Sheron *et al.*, 1993). Humoral and cellular immune responses are also operating in alcoholic liver disease. Elevated levels of globulins and particularly lg A are commonly found in alcoholics and deposition of lg A1 on the hepatocyte plasma membrane is a characteristic finding of alcohol-mediated liver damage (Van de Wiel *et al.*, 1988; Swerdlow and Chowdury, 1983).

Humoral and cellular responses to Mallory bodies have also been described (Kanagasundaram *et al.*, 1987). Acetaldehyde binds to different intracellular proteins generating strongly immunogenic adducts (Tuma and Sorrel, 1985). Circulating antibodies to synthetic acetaldehyde adducts have been demonstrated in animals fed alcohol chronically and in alcoholic patients (Worral *et al.*, 1989; Hoerner *et al.*, 1986). Acetaldehyde modified hepatic cytosolic protein is recognised by lg A antibodies in patients sera

(Koskinas *et al.*, 1992) and acetaldehyde adducts were detected in the livers of alcoholics (Niemela *et al.*, 1990). Furthermore, other studies have shown that lymphocytes from patients with alcoholic liver disease appear to immunologically recognize their own hepatocytes and mount either a cytotoxic or a lymphoproliferative response (Actis *et al.*, 1993). Additionally, heat shock proteins (HSP) are expressed in liver tissue in patients with alcoholic hepatitis and circulating lg A anti-HSP-60 correlate with hepatic expression of HSP-60 (Koskinas *et al.*, 1993).

Alcoholic fibrogenesis follows chronic alcohol consumption and matrix deposition occurs earliest around central veins and in the subendothelial space of Disse, known as "capillarization of the sinusoids". Activated lipocytes are the cellular source of almost all extracellularmatrix proteins found in alcoholic fibrosis (Bissell, 1992; Bachem, 1990). Various autocrine and paracrine mediators (cytokines) play a role in initiation and perpetuation of lipocyte activation and *in vitro* experiments have shown that acetaldehyde is fibrogenic (Friedman, 1990).

TREATMENT OF ALCOHOLIC LIVER DISEASE

The cornerstones of therapy in alcoholic hepatitis are abstinence, adequate diet, correction of vitamin deficiencies and management of complications. In addition several therapeutic approaches have been studied in order to reduce short term mortality and stop progression to cirrhosis.

Several trials have shown that corticosteroids appear to reduce short term mortality in a subgroup of patients with acute alcoholic hepatitis, namely those patients with prolongation of prothrombin time, increased levels of bilirubin and hepatic encephalopathy (Carithers *et al.*, 1989; Reynolds *et al.*, 1989). There is no evidence that corticosteroid therapy, even though it is associated with more frequent and rapid recovery, can prevent progression to cirrhosis. Infusions of insulin and glucagon have been used in an attempt to stimulate liver regeneration. The results are conflicting and the resulting insulin-induced hypoglycaemia can be dangerous (Feher *et al.*, 1987; Bird *et al.*, 1991). There is also a question as to whether these stimulants of regeneration can be taken up and used by injured hepatocytes.

Propylthiouracil (PTU) has also been given with the rationale to reduce hypermetabolism and protect the vulnerable zone III of the hepatic lobule from hypoxic injury. Again there are conflicting results as to short term benefits and whether PTU improves mortality, although in a 2 year controlled clinical trial of 310 patients with alcoholic liver disease there was a 48% reduction in the cumulative mortality rate from 0.25 (placebo group) to 0.13 (PTU group) ($p < 0.05$), with the most pronounced therapeutic benefit found in patients with alcoholic hepatitis (Israel *et al.*, 1979; Orrego *et al.*, 1987).

Anabolic-androgenic steroids have been studied with overall poor results (Copenhagen Study Group, 1986). In addition, long term therapy could be a factor in the development of hepatocellular carcinoma (Maddrey, 1986).

Orthotopic Liver Transplantation

The role of orthotropic liver transplantation in end-stage alcoholic liver disease has become increasingly accepted over the past 10 years. The most common clinical indications are ascites and oedema resistant to conventional therapy, repeated episodes of variceal bleeding, recurrent encephalopathy or a poor quality of life due to liver failure, and small hepatocellular carcinomas detected early on ultrasound screening. Patients with acute alcoholic hepatitis are rarely considered because of the accompanying multi-organ failure and the difficulties in assessing the likelihood of future abstinence. The assessment includes careful screening for other alcohol-related end-organ damage, particularly cardiomyopathy, pancreatic and CNS disease, as well as consideration of the psychosocial background.

Series from the major centres have shown that recipient one-year survival rates are compatible with the results obtained in other chronic liver diseases (Starzl *et al.*, 1988). However, this form of treatment is always likely to be available for only a small proportion of patients with end-stage ALD. During the 1980s, very small numbers of such patients were transplanted because of concerns regarding relapse of alcohol misuse, poor rehabilitations, failure to comply with immunosuppressive treatment or failure to attend regularly for follow-up. More recently, transplant centres have paid even greater attention to patient selection and the complex ethical issues involved.

Twenty two patients (approximately 4% of the total) were transplanted in the King's College/Cambridge series between 1980 and 1989 (Bird *et al.*, 1990). Although 6 had hepatomas, 66% survived at least one-year, a figure which compares favourably with the other major series of 73 patients reported by the Pittsburgh group, in which one-year survival was 74% (Kumar *et al.*, 1990). Selection criteria with respect to alcohol misuse were more stringent in the series from King's, all but three patients having been abstinent for at least 3 months prior to transplantation. A return to alcohol consumption was seen in only 3 patients (13%), in comparison with a reported recidivism rate of 12% in the Pittsburgh series. Two recent reports from transplant programmes in Ann Arbor, Michigan (Lucey *et al.*, 1992) and Madison, Wisconsin (Knetchle *et al.*, 1992) have shown similarly favourable results.

A review of the European Liver Transplant Registry reveals that relatively few liver transplants were performed for end-stage ALD before 1989 (Figure 4.3), comprising between 3 and 6% of all transplants in countries with major transplant programmes. There has been considerable expansion in overall transplant activity over the past 4 years, with some countries showing a marked increase in the number of transplants performed for ALD eg. Spain, France and Germany, whereas in the UK the proportion has increased only slightly. This almost certainly reflects differences in referral patterns, criteria for selection, as well as differences in the prevalence of ALD (Figure 4.2).

A recent study from Michigan (Lucey *et al.*, 1992), in which a cohort of 54 patients judged unsuitable for transplantation were followed up for 2 years, illustrated the importance of patient selection. The pre-operative assessment included an alcoholism 'prognosis score', based upon the acceptance of an alcohol problem by the patient and his family, the prognosis for future abstinence and social stability (Beresford *et al.*, 1990). No fixed period of abstinence was required. The 17 patients who were psychiatrically unsuitable showed a significantly lower survival at one year than those transplanted (65% compared with 78%, respectively). The low rates of return to drinking seen in this transplanted group were attributed to careful individual selection and structured post-transplant supervision. Clearly the ethical arguments for and against liver transplantation for alcoholic liver disease will continue (Neuberger, 1989). Given the likelihood of a persistent shortage of donor organs, continuation of transplant programmes for ALD will benefit if low rates of alcohol misuse in recipients can be demonstrated.

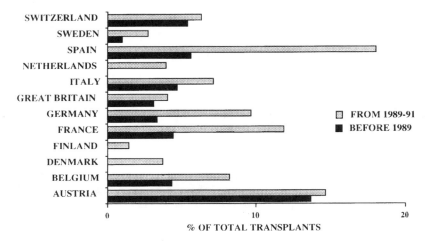

Figure 4.3   Proportion of Liver Transplants Performed for Alcohol-Induced Cirrhosis in Europe.

FUTURE RESEARCH STRATEGIES

The management of alcoholic liver disease should aim towards:

(1) Early diagnosis and psychiatric evaluation to identify prognostic factors promoting abstinence.

(2) Better understanding of the mechanisms involved in the pathogenesis of alcohol-induced liver injury, including the basis of individual susceptibility to alcoholic hepatitis and cirrhosis.

(3) Specific strategies to eliminate factors that can cause superimposed injury (drugs, viruses, etc.)

(4) New therapeutic approaches should be planned. Cytoprotective drugs such as ursodeoxycholic acid and prostaglandins may have a role. Proline analogues and propyl hydroxylase inhibitors can interfere with matrix production. Gamma interferon and cytokine inhibitors can inhibit lipocyte activation and proliferation.

(5) Selection criteria for orthotropic liver transplantation and in particular the development of a consensus upon transplantation for acute alcoholic hepatitis.

(6) An integrated public health approach to alcohol consumption, with improved public education of 'safe' drinking limits.

References

Actis, G., Mieli-Bergani, G., Portmann, B., Eddleston, A.W., Davis, M. and Williams, R. (1983). Lymphocyte cytotoxicity to autologous hepatocytes in alcoholic liver disease. *Liver*, **3**:8–12.

Bachem, M.G. (1990). Cellular sources of noncollagenous matrix proteins: role of fat storing cells in fibrogenesis. *Semin Liv Dis.*, **10**:30–46.

Baillie, M. (1783). The morbid anatomy of the most important parts of the human body. Johnson, J., Nicol, G. (Eds). London, St. Paul's Churchyard and Pall Mall, pp. 141.

Beresford, T.P., Turcotte, J.G., Merion, R., Burtch, G., Blow, F.C., Campbell, D. *et al.* (1990). A rational approach to liver transplantation for the alcoholic patient. *Psychosomatics*, **31**:241–254.

Bhagwandeen, B.S., Apte, M., Manwarring, L. and Dickeson, J. (1987). Endotoxin induced hepatic necrosis in rats on an alcohol diet. *J. Pathol.*, **152**:47–53.

Bird, G.L.A., I'Grady, J.G., Harvey, F.H., Calne, R.Y. and Williams, R. (1990). Liver transplantation in patients with alcoholic cirrhosis: selection criteria and rates of survival and relapse. *Br. Med. J.*, **301**:15–17.

Bird, G.L., Sheron, N., Goka, A.K., Alexander, G.J. and Williams, R. (1990). Increased plasma tumour necrosis factor in severe alcoholic hepatits, *Ann. Intern. Med.*, **112**:917–920.

Bird, G., Lau, J.Y.N., Koskinas, J., Wicks, C. and Williams, R. (1991). Insulin and glucagon infusion in acute hepatitis: a prospective randomised controlled trial. *Hepatology*, **14**:1097–1101.

Bissell, D.M. (1992). Lipocyte activation and hepatic fibrosis. *Gastroenterology*, **102**:1803–1805.

Bosron, W.F. and Li, T-K. (1986). Genetic polymorphism of human liver alcohol and aldehyde dehydrogenases, and their relationship to alcohol metabolism and alcoholism. *Hepatology*, **6**:502–510.

Carithers, R.L., Herlong, H.F., Diehl, A.M., Shaw, E.W., Combes, B., Fallon, H.J. and Maddrey, W.C. (1989). Methylprednisolone therapy in patients with severe alcoholic hepatitis: a randomised multicentre trial. *Ann. Int. Med.*, **110**:685–690.

Casini, A., Cunningham, M., Rojkind, M. and Leiber, C.S. (1991). Acetaldehyde increases procollagen type I and fibronectin gene transcription in cultured rat fat storing cells through a protein synthesis-dependent mechanism. *Hepatology*, **13**:758–765.

Chapman, R.W., Morgan, M.Y., Laulicht, M., Hoffbrand, A.V. and Sherlock, S. (1982). Hepatic iron stores and markets of iron overload in alcoholics and patients with idiopathic haemachromatosis. *Dig. Dls. Sci.*, **27**:909–916.

The Copenhagen Study Group for Liver Diseases. Testosterone treatment of men with alcoholic cirrhosis: a double blind study. *Hepatology*, 1986; **6**:807–813.

Couzigou, P., Fleury, B., Groppi, A., Cassaigne, A., Begueret, J. Iron, A., and the French Group for Research on Alcohol and the Liver. (1990). Genotyping study of alcohol dehydrogenase class I polymorphism in French patients with alcoholic cirrhosis. *Alcohol and Alcohol*, **25**:623–626.

Day, C.P., Bashir, R., James, O.F.W., Bassendine, M.F., Crabb, D.W., Thomasson, H.R. *et al.* (1991). Investigation of the role of polymorphisms at the alcohol and aldehyde dehydrogensase loci in genetic predisposition to alcohol-related end-organ damage, *Hepatology*, **14**:798–801.

Dicker, E. and Cederbaum, A.I. (1990). Generation of reactive oxygen species and reduction of ferric chelates in the presence of a reconstituted system containing ethanol, NAD and alcohol dehydrogenase. *Alcoholism: Clin. Exp. Res.*, **14**:283–244.

Eddleston, A.W.L.F. and Davis, M. (1982). Histocompatibility antigens in alcohoic liver disease. *Brit. Med. Bull.*, **38**:13–16.

Enomoto, N., Takase, S., Takada, N. and Takada, A. (1991). Alcoholic liver disease in heterozygotes of mutant and normal aldehyde dehydrogenase-2 genes. *Hepatology*, **13**:1071–1075.

Feher, J., Cornides, A., Romany, A. *et al.* (1987). A prospective multi-center study of insulin and glucagon infusion therapy in acute alcoholic hepatitis. *J. Hepatol.*, **5**:224–231.

Frezza, M., Di Padova, C., Pozzato, G., Terpin, M., Baraona, E. and Leiber, C.S. (1990). High blood alcohol levels in women: the role of decreased gastric alcohol dehydrogenase activity and first pass metabolism. *N. Eng. J. Med.*, **322**:95–99.

Friedman, S.L. (1990). Acetaldehyde and alcoholic fibrogenesis — fule to the fire but not the spark. *Hepatology*, **12**:609–612.

Galambos, J.T. (1972). Natural history of alcoholic hepatitis III. Histological changes. *Gastroenterology*, **63**:1026–1035.

Goedde, H.W., Harada, S. and Agarwal, D.P. (1979). Racial differences in alcohol sensitivity; a new hypothesis. *Hum. Genet.*, **51**:331–334.

Grant, B.F., Dufour, M.C. and Harford, T.C. (1988). Epidemiology of alcoholic liver disease. *Semin. Liv. Dis.*, **8**:12–25.

Hoerner, M.U., Behrens, U.J., Worner, T. and Leiber, C.S. (1986). Humoral immune response to acetaldehyde adducts in alcoholic patients. *Res. Commun. Chem. Pathol. Pharmacol.*, **54**:3–12.

Israel, Y., Walfish, P.G., Orrego, H. *et al.* (1979). Thyroid hormones in alcoholic liver disease: effect of treatment of with 6-n-propylthoiuracil. *Gastroenterology*, **76**:116–122.

Iturriaga, H., Ugare, H. and Israel, Y. (1980). Hepatic vein oxygenation, liver blood flow, and the rate of ethanol metabolism in recently abstinent alcoholic patients. *Eur. J. Clin. Invest.*, **10**:211–218.

Jollife, N. and Jellinek, E.M. (1941). Vitamin deficiencies and liver cirrhosis in alcoholism, Part VII; Cirrhosis of the liver. *Q. J. Stud. Alcohol.*, **2**:544–483.

Kanagasundaram, N., Kakamu, S., Chen, T. and Leevy, C.M. (1977). Alcoholic hyalin antigen and antibody in alcoholic hepatitis. *Gastroenterology*, **73**:1368–1373.

Knetchle, S.J., Fleming, M.F., Barry, K.L., Steen, D., Pirsch, J.D., Hafez, G.R. *et al.* (1992). Liver transplantation for alcoholic liver disease. *Surgery*, **112**:694–703.

Koskinas, J., Kenna, J.G., Bird, G.L., Alexander, G.J.M. and Williams, R. (1992). Immunoglobulin A antibody to a 200-kilodalton cytosolic acetaldehyde adduct in alcoholic hepatitis. *Gastroenterology*, **103**:1860–1867.

Koskinas, J., Winrow, V.R., Bird, G.L., Lau, J.Y.N., Portmann, B.C., Blake, D.R., Alexander, G.J. and Williams, R. (1993). Hepatic 60-kD heat shock protein responses in alcoholic hepatitis. *Hepatology*, **17**:1047–1051.

Kumar, S., Stauber, R.E., Gavaler, J.S., Basista, M.H., Dindzans, V.J., Schade, R.R. *et al.* (1990). Orthotopic liver transplantation for alcoholic liver disease. *Hepatology*, **11**:159–164.

Lauterburg, B.H. and Bilzer, M. (1988). Mechanisms of acetaldehyde hepatotoxicity. *J. Hepatol*, **7**:384–390.

Leiber, C.S. and Spritz, N. (1966). Effects of prolongued ethanol intake in man; Role of dietary, adipose, and endogenously synthesized fatty acids in the pathogenesis of the alcoholic fatty liver. *J. Clin. Invest.*, **45**:1400–1411.

Leiber, C.S. (1988). Biochemical and molecular basis of alcohol-induced injury to liver tissues. *N. Eng. J. Med.*, **319**:1639–1650.

Leiber, C.S. (1988). Metabolic effects of ethanol and its interaction with other drugs, hepatotoxic agents, vitamins and carcinogens: A 1988 update. *Semin. Liv. Dis.*, **8**:47–68.

Lelbach, W.K. (1975). Cirrhosis in the alcoholic and its relation to the volume of alcohol abuse. *Ann. NY Acad. Sci.*, **252**:85–105.

Lucey, M.R., Merion, R.M., Henley, K.S., Campbell, D.A., Turcotte, J.G., Nostrant, T.T. *et al.* (1992). Selection for and outcome of liver transplantation in alcoholic liver disease. *Gastroenterology*, **102**:1736–1741.

Maddrey, W.C. (1986). Is therapy with testosterone or anabolic-androgenic steroids useful in the treatment of alcoholic liver disease? *Hepatology*, **6**:1033–1035.

Mauch, T.J., Donohue, T.M., Zetterman, R.K., Sorrell, M.F. and Tuma, D.J. (1986). Covalent binding of acetaldehyde selectively inhibits the catalytic of lysine-dependent enzymes, *Hepatology*, **6**:263–269.

Mendenhall, C.L., Anderson, S., Weesner, R.E., Goldberg, S.J., Crolic, K.A., and the VA Cooperative Study Group. (1984). Protein-calorie malnutrition associated with alcoholic hepatitis. *Am. J. Med.*, **76**:211–222.

Mendenhall, C.J., Gartside, P.S., Roselle, G.A., Grossman, C.J., Weesner, R.E., Chedid, A. *et al.* (1989). Longevity among ethnic groups in alcoholic liver disease. *Alcohol and Alcohol*, **24**:11–19.

Mendenhall, C.L., Seeff, L., Diehl, A.M., Ghosn, S.J., French, S.W. *et al.*, and the VA Cooperative Study Group. (1991). Antibodies to hepatitis B virus and hepatitis C virus in alcoholic hepatitis and cirrhosis; their prevalence and clinical relevance. *Hepatology*, **14**:581–589.

Morgan, M.Y. and Sherlock, S. (1977). Sex-related differences among 100 patients with alcoholic liver disease. *Br. Med. J.*, **i**:939–941.

Neuberger, J.M. (1989). Tranplantation for alcoholic liver disease. *Br. Med. J.*, **i**:299–693.

Niemela, O., Juvonen, T. and Parkkila, S. (1990). Immunohistochemical demonstration of acetaldehyde-modified epitopes in human liver after alcohol consumption. *J. Clin. Invest.*, **87**:1367–1374.

Orrego, H., Blake, J.E., Blendis, L.M. *et al.* (1987). Long term treatment of alcoholic liver disease with propylthiouracil. *N. Eng. J. Med.*, **317**:1421–1427.

Pares, A., Barrera, J.M., Caballeria, J., Ercilla, G., Bruguera, M., Caballeria, L. *et al.* (1990). Hepatitis C virus antibodies in chronic alcoholic liver patients: association with severity of liver injury. *Hepatology*, **12**:1295–1299.

Paton A. (Ed). (1988). ABC of alcohol,. *British Medical Journal,* London.

Pequignot, G., Chabert, C., Eydoux, H., Coucoul, M.A. (1974). Augmentation du rieque de cirrhose en fonction de la ration d'alcool. *Revue de L'Alcool*, **20**:191–202.

pequignot, G., Tuyns, A.G and, Berta, J.L. (1978). Ascitic cirrhosis in relation to alcohol consumption. *Int. J. Epidemiol.*, **7**:113–10.

Reynolds, T.B., Benhamou, J.P., Blake, J., Nacarato, R. and Orrego, H. (1989). Treatment of acute alcoholic hepatitis. *Gastroenterol Int.*, **2**:208–216.

Royal College of Physicians, Faculty of Public Health Medicine. Alcohol and the Public Health. Macmillan, London 1991.

Saunders J.B., Walters J.R.F., Davies P. and Paton A. (1981). A 20-year prospective study of cirrhosis. *Br. Med. J.*, **282**:263–266.

Saunders, J.B., Haines, A., Portmann, B., Wodak, A.D., Powell-Jackson, P.R., Davis, M. and Williams, R. (1982). Accelerated development of alcoholic cirrhosis in patients with HLA B8. *Lancet*, **i**:1381–1384.

Saunders, J.B., Wodak, A.D., Morgan-Capner, P., White, Y.S., Portmann, B., Davis, M., Williams, R. (1983). Importance of markers of hepatitis B virus in alcoholic liver disease. *Br. Med. J.*, **286**:1851–1854.

Sherman, D.I.N., Ward, R.J., Warren-Perry, M., Williams, R. and Peters, T.J. (1993). Association of an RFLP marker for the alcohol dehydrogenase-2 gene with alcohol-induced liver damage. *Br. Med. J.*, **307**:1388–1390.

Sheron, N., Bird, G.L., Koskinas, J., Portmann, B., Ceska, M., Lindley, I. and Williams, R. (1993). Circulating and tissue levels of the neutrophil chemotaxin interleukin-8 are elevated in severe acite alcoholic hepatitis, and tissue levels correlate with neutrophil infiltration. *Hepatology*, **18**:41–46.

Shibuya, A. and Yoshida, A. (1988). Genotypes of alcohol metabolizing enzymes in Japanese with alcoholic liver disease: a strong association of the usual Caucasian-type aldehyde dehydrogenase gene (ALDH21) with the disease. *Am. J. Hum. Genet.*, **43**:744–748.

Skog O-J. (1980). Liver cirrhosis epidemiology: some methodological problems. *Br. J. Addict.*, **75**:227–243.

Skog O-J. (1985). The collectivity of drinking cultures: a theory of the distribution of alcohol consumption. *Br. J. Addict.*, **80**:83–99.

Sorenson, T.I.A., Bentsen, K.D., Eghoje, K., Orholm, M., Hoybye, G. and Christofferson, P. (1984). Prospective evaluation of alcohol abuse and alcoholic liver inury in men as predictors of development of cirrhosis. *Lancet*, **ii**: 241–244.

Starzl, T.E., Van Thiel, D., Tzakis, A.G., Iwatsuki, S., Todo, S., Marsh, W. *et al.* (1988). Orthotopic liver transplantation for alcoholic cirrhosis. *JAMA*, **260**: 2542–2544.

Swerdlow, M.A. and Chowdury, L.N. (1983). IgA subclasses in liver tissue in alcoholic liver disease. *Am. J. Clin. Pathol.*, **80**:283–289.

Terris M. (1967). Epidemiology of cirrhosis of the liver; National mortality data. *Am. J. Public Health*, **57**:2076–2088.

Tsukamoto, H., Gaal, K. and French, S.W. (1990). Insights into the pathogenesis of alcoholic liver necrosis and fibrosis: status reprot. *Hepatology*, **12**:599–608.

Tuma, D.J. and Sorrel, M.F. (1985). Covalent binding of acetaldehyde to hepatic proteins: role in alcoholic liver injury. In Aldehyde Adducts in alcohllism, M.A. Collins, Ed. *Prog. Clin. Biol. Res.* Vol, **183**:3–17. Alan R. Liss, Inc. New York, NY.

Tuma, D.J., Casey, C.A. and Sorrell, M.F. (1990). Effects of ethanol on hepatic protein trafficking; impairment of receptor mediated endocytosis. *Alcohol Alcoholism*, **25**:117–125.

Tuma, D.J., Smith, S.L. and Sorrell, M.F. Acetaldehyde and microtubules. *Ann NY Acad. Sci.*, 1991; **625**:786–792.

Van de Wiel, A., van Hattum, J., Schurman, J-J. and Kater, L. (1988). Immunoglobulin A in the diagnosis of alcoholic liver disease. *Gastroenterology*, **94**:457–462.

Villa, E., Barchi, T., Grisendi, A., Bellentani, S., Rubbiani, L., Ferreti, I. *et al.* (1982). Susceptibility of chronic symptomless HBsAg carriers to ethanol-induced hepatic damage. *Lancet*, **ii**: 1243–1244.

Wands, J.R. and Blum, H.E. (1991). Hepatitis B and C virus and alcohol-induced liver injury. *Hepatology*, **14**:730–733.

Ward, R.J., Sherman, D.I.N., Coutelle, C., Williams, R. and Peters, T.J. Unpublished data.

Wodak, A.D., Saunders, J.B., Ewusi-Mehsah, I., Davis, M. and Williams, R. (1981). Severity of alcohol dependence in patients with alcoholic liver disease. *Br. Med. J.*, **287**:1420–1422.

Worral, S., De jersey, J., Shanley, B.C. and Wilce, P.A. (1989). Ethanol induces the production of antibodies to acetaldehyde modified epitopes in rats. *Alcohol Alcoholism*, **24**:217–223.

5 Alcohol Misuse and the Skin

Elisabeth M. Higgins

Department of Dermatology, King's College Hospital, London, England

Although it has long been recognised that the skin may be affected in advanced liver disease, it has now been demonstrated that skin disease is also a feature of alcohol misuse. Psoriasis, cutaneous infections and discoid eczema often occur in heavy drinkers without biochemical evidence of alcohol toxicity. The true aetiology of the cutaneous disease therefore may be missed unless specifically sought. There is a close link between drinking and activity of the skin disease, especially with reference to treatment resistance. Ethanol has far reaching effects on cutaneous physiology, in particular vascular responses and immunomodulation. Both these factors may be implicated in the pathogenesis of alcohol related skin disease, but the exact mechanisms are yet to be clarified.

INTRODUCTION

Historically the skin has been regarded as a source of physical signs reflecting established alcoholic liver disease. It is now becoming apparent that the skin may be affected at a much earlier stage of alcohol misuse. Moreover, awareness of these associations can serve to highlight at risk patients early in their disease, often before features of dependency ensue.

Much of the work relating to the systemic effects of alcohol, especially studies investigating possible mechanisms, has come from America, but only a few studies have been specifically directed at the effects on the skin. Work is now emerging from Europe, emphasizing that the importance of this association is becoming more widely appreciated.

THE SKIN IN ESTABLISHED LIVER DISEASE

A Historical Perspective

The classical stigmata of alcoholism have been well documented since the last century, and are more widely recognised than the signs associated with alcohol misuse.

Although they may occur in hepatic disease from any cause, they are more common in alcoholic liver disease (Strauss *et al.*, 1990). Two English reviews have highlighted many of the stigmata of alcoholic cirrhosis (Sarkany, 1988; Higgins and du Vivier 1992). The cutaneous signs of alcoholism include palmar erythema, spider naevi and nail dystrophies, and arise as a result of the far reaching effects of alcohol on the cutaneous vasculature.

Palmar erythema

Warm hands with a prominent rim of erythema are common in established liver disease. The erythema begins on the hypothenar border of the hand, but as the condition advances, spreads to involve the finger tips, finally becoming confluent. Comparable changes may be present on the soles. Although traditionally seen as a sign of chronic liver disease, a British survey has shown that palmar erythema occurs in 20% of alcohol misuse patients (Higgins and du Vivier, 1994a).

Spider neavi

These lesions occur within the territory drained by the superior vena cava, most commonly on the face and anterior chest wall. They consist of an enlarged central arteriole from which small vessels radiate in a spoke-like manner. Spider naevi are more common in patients with oesophageal varices, and have been found to be of predictive value in assessing the future risk of variceal bleeds. In a prospective study from the USA, the number, size and distribution of spider naevi were shown to correlate with the risk of oesophageal haemorrhage (Foutch *et al.*, 1988). Patients with more than 20 spider naevi have more than a 50% chance of variceal bleeding. The risk is increased if the spiders are found at atypical (eg oropharyngeal) sites, but is highest of all (>80% risk) for patients with large (>15 mm diameter) spiders.

Nails changes

The observation that patients with cirrhosis developed white nails (leuconychia) was first reported nearly four decades ago (Terry, 1954). However, the nails of drinkers may become abnormal at a much earlier, pre-cirrhotic stage. Red lunulae have been described in patients who are alcohol misusers, with no evidence of cirrhosis (Wilkerson and Wilkin, 1989). Like many of the cutaneous effects of alcohol (Higgins and du Vivier, 1992a), these changes are thought to be vascular in origin, due to increased arteriolar blood flow through the nail bed (Wilkerson and Wilkin, 1989).

Porphyria Cutanea Tarda (PCT)

PCT is due to a deficiency of the enzyme uroporphyrinogen decarboxylase, which results in the interruption of the haem synthesis pathway. The resultant accumulation of uroporphyrin renders that patient photosensitive. PCT may be precipitated in susceptible (heterozygote) individuals by alcohol. The patient presents with skin fragility and blistering on sun exposed sites, which heal to leave characteristic scarring and milia. Treatment is by means of regular venesection to deplete iron stores, but abstinence from alcohol may be all that is required in some cases.

Flushing/Facial erythema

Alcohol has potent vasodilatatory properties (Hatake *et al.*, 1991), which may be mediated through increased prostacyclin synthesis (Guivernau *et al.*, 1987) or via inhibition of prostaglandins (Auggard, 1983). Chronic ingestion of alcohol leads to the loss of vasoregulatory control mechanisms, and a persistent facial erythema. This plethoric facies can be a useful factor in prompting the examining physician to ask about alcohol consumption and to pursue the possibility of alcohol misuse. Acute alcohol ingestion is associated with flushing (Johnson *et al.*, 1986) and flushing is one of the most commonly reported effects of drinking amongst alcoholics (Watson *et al.*, 1985). Some individuals, particularly within certain racial groups have an inherited predisposition to flush following alcohol ingestion. Other side effects, including tachycardia and flushing, can be so unpleasant as to limit alcohol consumption in affected individuals (Ohmori *et al.*, 1986). Patch tests in which ethanol is applied to the skin can be used to predict the flushing response. Susceptible subjects develop erythema at the site of alcohol application (Wilkin and Fortner, 1985). In these individuals it is the metabolites of ethanol, rather than alcohol itself which are responsible for the response (Wilkin, 1988). Historically, alcohol induced flushing was considered to be an Oriental trait, but studies amongst an English student population have demonstrated that between 20–30% also flush after alcohol, although to a lesser degree (Ward *et al.*, 1991). However, the enzyme defect is different in the two groups. Oriental flushing is associated with abnormal $ALDH_2$ activity and accumulation of acetaldehyde, whereas Caucasian flushing may be secondary to reduced $ALDH_1$, with normal levels of circulating acetaldehyde (Ward *et al.*, 1991).

THE PRESENT POSITION

Interest in the influence of alcohol on the skin has been increasing over the last decade. Alcohol has now been linked to a variety of skin diseases, in particular psoriasis and cutaneous infections. There is marked variation in the drinking habits of different populations, but the link between psoriasis and alcohol has been defined in America, Scandinavia and Europe.

Psoriasis

Psoriasis is an inflammatory skin disorder characterised by hyperproliferation of the epidermis with dilated dermal capillaries. The disease is common affecting 2% of Northern Europeans and although the exact aetiology of the disorder is unknown it is thought to have an immunological basis. There is a strong genetic component to the disease, which can be precipitated by a multitude of factors including drugs, infection and trauma. There is now unequivocal evidence that alcohol should be considered in the list of agents known to exacerbate psoriasis. However, there is not as yet any information to suggest a specific genetic predispostion to alcohol-related skin disease as opposed to other forms of psoriasis.

Studies from EEC Countries

U.K.

There has been a suspicion for many years that alcohol can cause a deterioration in psoriasis (Berge *et al.*, 1970), but the earliest studies found no evidence of any increase in the alcohol intake of psoriatics (Delaney and Leppard, 1974). Subsequently several studies have identified a definite association between heavy drinking and psoriasis (Monk and Neill, 1986; Higgins *et al.*, 1993a). While the incidence of alcohol misuse is undoubtedly rising in the UK, it cannot alone account for the discrepancy between the early and more recent studies. It is more probably explained by the current use of specially designed questionnaires, which are more sensitive in detecting alcohol misuse. Monk and Neill examined 100 patients with psoriasis and found a high incidence (16%) of alcohol misuse (Monk and Neill, 1986). 2/45 women drank more than 40 g/day and 14/55 men drank more than 80 g/day. In addition they found that alcohol misuse correlated with the severity of the psoriasis. 22% of men with severe psoriasis were drinking heavily compared with only 9% of those with mild disease (Monk and Neill, 1986).

A more recent study has shown an even higher prevalence (39%) of alcohol misuse in psoriatic patients (Higgins *et al.*, 1992b). Heavy drinking is a common factor in the development of psoriasis in both men (48%) and women (21%) (Higgins *et al.*, 1992b). It would appear that it is alcohol misuse rather than alcohol dependency which is associated with psoriasis, as only 4/148 (3%) patients showed any features of dependency (Higgins *et al.*, 1993a). These studies were carried out at a large hospital serving a local population with a highly varied ethnic mix. Psoriasis is not as common in Asians or Afro-Caribbean races, and the majority of patients studied were therefore Caucasian. Although the results were less dramatic, alcohol misusers were identified in all the racial groups studied. (Table 5.1)

It is important to identify those patients who are drinking heavily, as alcohol appears to be able to drive the disease process and precipitate or perpetuate the disease in a genetically susceptible subject. In the USA, alcohol misusers have been shown to be more resistant to treatment of their psoriasis (Gupta *et al.*, 1993), a finding supported by British observers (Higgins and du Vivier, 1994b). However, identifying these individuals requires a high index of suspicion, since the majority of psoriatics who are drinking heavily have no evidence of hepatic toxicity on standard biochemical screening tests (Higgins *et al.*, 1993a).

Table 5.1 Racial classification of psoriatics studied

Race	Total Number		Drinkers		% (%M) (%F)	
Caucasian	135	(79M) (56F)	55	(43M) (12F)	41%	(54%) (21%)
Afro-Caribbean	7	(5M) (2F)	2	(1M) (1F)	25%	(20% (50%)
Asian	5	(4M) (1F)	1	(1M) (0F)	20%	(25%) (0)
Oriental	1	(0M) (1F)	1	(0M) (1F)	100%	(0) (100%)

Not only has the psoriasis of drinkers been found to be more severe (Monk and Neill, 1986), but the psoriasis appears to be of a specific character — very inflamed and occuring at atypical (flexural) sites (Higgins and du Vivier, 1994a). Awareness of these findings can alert the physician to the underlying alcohol problem and so facilitate treatment.

It has been suggested in the past that smoking is an important factor in the aetiology of psoriasis (O'Doherty and Macintyre, 1985; Mills *et al.*, 1992), but investigators have ignored the question of concommitant drinking. More critical studies examining all confounding variables have shown that both alcohol misuse and smoking were more common in psoriatic patients than controls, but that it is alcohol which is the independent risk factor in the development of psoriasis (Higgins *et al.*, 1993b).

Many groups have studied the effect of stress on psoriasis (Seville, 1977; Ramsay and O'Reagan 1988). Stress can precipitate psoriasis and psoriatics often experience feelings of anxiety and stigmatization (Ginsburg and Link, 1989) and psychotherapy can be a valuable adjunct to treatment (Price *et al.*, 1991). A Welsh group have developed a scoring system to assess the social, emotional and physical impact of psoriasis on the patient's life: the Psoriasis Disability Index [PDI] (Finlay and Kelly, 1987). Turning to alcohol is a recognised stress response, and in the past this relief drinking has been offered as the explanation for those patients with skin disease who are drinking heavily. However, careful chronological studies have shown that drinking preceeds the development of psoriasis (Poikolainen *et al.*, 1990) or causes existing psoriasis to worsen (Vincenti and Blunden, 1987) in the majority of cases. Furthermore there is no difference in the PDI scores between psoriatics who misuse alcohol and those who do not (Higgins and du Vivier, 1994a), implying that those patients who drink heavily do not feel more stigmatised/disabled by their disease than their non-drinking counterparts.

Psoriasis has been found to occur with a prevalence ten times greater than that of the general population in a group of patients attending an alcohol misuse clinic, confirming the strong association with ethanol (Higgins *et al.*, 1992b).

ITALY

In a multicentre case-controlled study to investigate possible risk factors in psoriasis conducted by six hospitals in Northern Italy who examined 215 patients with psoriasis, a positive family history was identified as the strongest risk factor for the development of psoriasis (Naldi *et al.*, 1992). The risk of developing psoriasis was higher amongst smokers than those who had never smoked (Naldi *et al.*, 1992). Using multiple logistic regression analysis, the risk of psoriasis was found to be higher for alcohol drinkers than teetotallers (Naldi *et al.*, 1992). There was a trend for the adjusted odds-ratio to be higher with increasing number of drinks per day, but this trend did not reach significance (Naldi *et al.*, 1992). However, in contrast to the British study (Higgins *et al.*, 1993b), the adjusted odds ratio found smoking to be a greater risk factor than alcohol for psoriasis (Naldi *et al.*, 1992).

FRANCE

Chaput *et al.* have investigated the prevalence of psoriasis in patients with alcoholic cirrhosis admitted to a liver unit. Psoriasis was more common than expected, but it was the magnitude of drinking rather than the extent of liver damage which was associated with psoriasis. 5.3% of patients drinking more than 50g/day had psoriasis compared with only 0.7% of those drinking less than 50g/day (Chaput *et al.*, 1985).

II Other Countries

SCANDINAVIA

A Finnish study found alcohol to be a risk factor for psoriasis in young and middle-aged men (Poikolainen *et al.*, 1990). Using self-administered questionnaires, they found no association between psoriasis and age, sex, social class or smoking. However, alcohol intake and episodes of intoxication were individually identified as risk factors (Poikolainen *et al.*, 1990). In contrast to the UK study (Monk and Neill, 1986) they did not find any correlation between drinking and the severity of psoriasis. They calculated that the odds ratio for developing psoriasis in an individual drinking 100 g/day was 2.2 (Poikolainen *et al.*, 1990). Heavy drinking preceeded the development of psoriasis, and psoriatics tended to drink more heavily with time than controls (Poikolainen *et al.*, 1990).

A potential flaw in this study was that it relied upon recall data (often from many years previously) but in recognition of this problem, and in an attempt to improve the accuracy of the sample, the study was limited to adult men under the age of 50 years. Experience from the UK would suggest that while the association is stronger in men, alcohol is still a significant risk factor in women (Higgins and du Vivier, 1994a).

Another study looked at part of a general population survey in Norway, in which 10,576 randomly selected families took part in a questionnaire conducted by non-medical personnel (Braathan *et al.*, 1989). From this large group, 149 (1.4%) individuals with psoriasis were identified and their data analysed separately. Psoriatics were found to smoke and drink more frequently than controls (Braathan *et al.*, 1989). Fewer patients with psoriasis were total abstainers than in the general population (Braathan *et al.*, 1989). Alcohol consumption was noted to be particularly high in men with psoriasis. The authors concluded that the increased consumption of alcohol reflected the isolation felt by patients with psoriasis, and suggested that instead of turning to counsellors or other forms of paramedical support, they indulged in relief drinking (Braathan *et al.*, 1989). This conflicts with data from Finland (Poikolainen *et al.*, 1990) and the UK (Higgins and du Vivier, 1994a).

USA

The adverse effect of alcohol in the perpetuation of psoriasis and decreased response to treatment was initially described by a group in Michigan (Gupta *et al.*, 1993). A study from the Mayo clinic also found a higher incidence of heavy drinking amongst in-patients with psoriasis (11%) than those admitted for the treatment of other skin disorders (3%) (Morse *et al.*, 1985). However, a questionnaire designed to detect alcohol dependency was used. As other studies have now shown that alcohol dependency is rare in psoriasis (Higgins *et al.*, 1993a), this study may have underestimated the prevalence of alcohol misuse.

Putative mechanisms in the interaction between alcohol and psoriasis

Psoriasis is now considered to be an immunological disorder in which T-helper cells play a central role. Additional factors are the prominant collections of neutrophils which form microabscesses within the epidermis, and the dilated capillaries in the dermis. Research has yet to address the mechanism by which alcohol can precipitate psoriasis, but ethanol has immunosuppressant properties, so increasing susceptibility to infection, and it is a powerful vasodilator (Higgins and du Vivier, 1992a).

Other Skin Diseases

A. Seborrhoeic Dermatitis

A hypersensitivity to the pityrosporum yeast has been implicated in the pathogenesis of the adult variety of this form of eczema. Although the condition is common, florid forms are associated with immunosuppression (Mathes and Douglas, 1985). Alcohol is known to affect both humoral (MacGregor, 1986) and cell-mediated immunity (Dehne *et al.*, 1989). Studies have now demonstrated an increased incidence of seborrhoeic dermatitis in patients who drink alcohol to excess (Higgins *et al.*, 1992b; Barba *et al.*, 1982). In a case-controlled study, Barba *et al.* examined 84 patients with alcohol-related disease and found that one third of patients with chronic pancreatitis secondary to alcohol had seborrhoiec dermatitis compared to only 4% of controls had features of seborrhoeic dermatitis. There was no increase in the prevalence of seborrhoeic dermatitis among patients with alcoholic cirrhosis, suggesting that the malnutrition associated with pancreatitis could be responsible (Barba *et al.*, 1982). However this is refuted by a more recent English study, which found a high (16%) incidence of seborrhoeic dermatitis in patients with alcohol misuse but no evidence of pancreatitis (Higgins *et al.*, 1992b).

B. Cutaneous Infections

Both bacterial and fungal infections of the skin are more common in alcohol misusers. Over half the patients attending an alcohol misuse clinic were found to have some form of skin infection (Higgins *et al.*, 1992b), presumably as a consequence of the immuno-suppressive properties of ethanol. Fungal infections, particularly tinea pedis have been identified in 33% of heavy drinkers (Higgins *et al.*, 1992b), which is three times the esti-mated frequency in the general population. Bacterial infections, e.g. folliculitis (Higgins *et al.*, 1992b) and acne (Higgins and du Vivier, 1994) are also common in alcohol mis-users, and all infections tend to be more resistant to treatment in the heavy drinker.

C. Discoid Eczema

This well circumscribed eczematous condition is most commonly seen on the limbs of middle-aged men and requires potent topical steroids for control. Classically the condition has been considered a variant of endogenous eczema, but has now been shown to have a strong association with alcohol misuse (Higgins and du Vivier, 1992a), possibly through a mechanism of enhanced susceptibility to infection. It is particularly difficult to eradicate the skin disease until the patient substantially reduces their alcohol intake or becomes abstinent. In contrast to psoriasis, the majority of patients with discoid eczema who are drinking have abnormal hepatic toxicity tests (Higgins and du Vivier, 1992a). It appears that the association between alcohol and discoid eczema is specific and not applicable to patients with atopic eczema, who have a low incidence of alcohol misuse (<4%) (Higgins *et al.*, 1993b).

D. *Acrodermatitis enteropathica*

Zinc deficiency can result in a florid, erosive dermatitis affecting the perioral and perianal areas and the extremities. The eruption is most characteristically seen in premature babies, but it may occur as an acquired phenomenon in adults who drink heavily and become malnourished (West and Anderson, 1986).

E. *Alcohol and skin cancer*

There is a considerable overlap between diseases of the skin and those affecting the oral and genital mucosae. Alcohol has been strongly implicated in the pathogenesis of carcinoma of the oropharynx (Adami *et al.*, 1992; Negri *et al.*, 1993), but there is very limited literature examining any possible relationship between alcohol and cutaneous malignancy. To date, the evidence would suggest that there is no link (Adami *et al.*, 1992). However, initial studies have focused on malignant melanoma. Basal cell and squamous cell carcinomas of the skin are much more common, and in light of the evidence from oral cancers, it would be of interest to examine the possible role of alcohol in the aetiology of cutaneous squamous cell carcinoma.

POSSIBLE MECHANISMS

The cutaneous effects of alcohol described above are far reaching. The common factors in the pathogenesis of the various diseases are an altered immune defence and enhanced vascular responsiveness. It would seem likely therefore that the effects of alcohol are mediated through one or other of these processes, either alone or in combination.

Immunological Effects of Alcohol

There has been an exponential rise in research investigating the properties of alcohol over the last decade, much of it from North America. Although immunoglobulin activity is impaired in alcoholics (MacGregor, 1986), the most pronounced effect of alcohol on the immune response is the selective inhibition of T-cell function (Levallois, 1989).

Cytokines are central to the regulation of T-lymphocyte activation and a French study has shown that IL-2 production from murine splenocytes is enhanced by low concentrations of ethanol, but inhibited by higher concentrations (Levallois, 1989). Cell-mediated immunity is rapidly but reversibly impaired by alcohol (Dehne *et al.*, 1989). Inhibition of cell-mediated immunity occurs at low doses of alcohol, before dependency develops (Jerrels *et al.*, 1989). In patients with alcoholic cirrhosis cutaneous tests of delayed hypersensitivity are greatly decreased (Snyder *et al.*, 1978). The effect of alcohol on the immune system has been considered a secondary effect of malnutrition in alcoholics. However, studies from Italy have examined lymphocyte function in chronic alcoholics of good nutritional status and demonstrated that alcohol has a direct effect on T-cell activation (Stefani *et al.*, 1978). Alcohol has now been shown to enhance leucocyte chemotaxis (Ternowitz, 1989), a process central to the development of many inflammatory processes, but particularly psoriasis. Finally, alcohol enhances the expression of MHC class I antigens on the lymphocyte cell surface, a factor thought to play a pivotal role in the subsequent development of alcohol-related disease (Singer *et al.*, 1989).

The Vascular Effects of Alcohol

Chronic ethanol ingestion stimulates the relaxation of blood vessel walls (Hatake *et al.*, 1991) and impairs vasoconstrictive responses (Malinowski *et al.*, 1990) in alcohol-fed rats. In humans, Malpas *et al.* have demonstrated that alcohol ingestion produces an increase in forearm blood flow and raises peripheral skin temperature (Malpas *et al.*, 1990). No such response is observed in quadraplegics, suggesting that alcohol-induced vasodilatation is a central phenomenon. Regional differences in cutaneous blood flow can be demonstrated in patients with alcoholic cirrhosis (Okumura *et al.*, 1990), a factor which may explain the preferential distribution of alcohol-associated skin disease at certain body sites.

THERAPEUTIC IMPLICATIONS

The majority of studies of alcohol-related skin disease have shown no correlation between dose-dependency and the severity (extent) of the skin disease, but there would appear to be a relationship to disease activity. This is particularly true with respect to psoriasis and porphyria cutanea tarda, in which reduction in alcohol intake improves treatment response and may even induce remission of the skin disease. It is important to recognise alcohol-related treatment resistance as it has important economic implications in terms of patient morbidity (including time off work) and in respect of prescribing costs for continued therapy.

CONCLUSIONS

The problem of alcohol misuse affects many disciplines (Potamianos *et al.*, 1988; McGarry *et al.*, 1994) not immediately (or traditionally) considered relevant to alcohol studies. Awareness of the role of alcohol in the development of other diseases needs to be increased. In particular, it has been demonstrated that there is a close link between alcohol and a variety of skin diseases. Dermatology forms a significant part of the medical case-load of any community, accounting for more than 10% of the patients seen in general practice. The influence of alcohol in the development of skin disease is probably under-recognised. Awareness of these associations is important not only from the point of view of improving response to treatment, but also for the future counselling of the patient with respect to the risk of developing other alcohol-related problems. The dermatology clinic has been shown to be a valuable and appropriate place to detect alcohol misuse, and the relationship between alcohol and the skin should become more clearly defined in the future.

PROPOSALS FOR FUTURE RESEARCH

Alcohol clearly has a profound effect on a variety of biological processes in the skin, leading in some instances to the subsequent development of overt skin disease. Future research should be directed at elucidating these mechanisms further. In particular attention should be focused on:

i)   Epidemiological studies to define fully the relationship between alcohol and skin disease.

ii) Studies of the effect of ethanol on the skin immune system.

iii) Studies to investigate any possible genetic predisposition to alcohol-associated skin disease.

iv) Assessment of the impact of abstinence on the outcome of treatment.

Such a programme will not only enhance our understanding of the pathogenesis of many dermatological diseases, but will also have socio-economic implications for the well-being of the population.

References

Adami, H.-O., McLaughlin, J.K., Hsing and A.W. *et al.* (1992). Alcoholism and cancer risk: a population-based cohort study. *Cancer Causes and Control*, 3:419–425.

Auggard, E. (1983). Ethanol, essential fatty acids and prostaglandins. *Pharmacol. Biochem. Behav.*, 18 (suppl); 401–7.

Barba, A., Piubello, I. and Vantini, R. *et al.* (1982). Skin lesions in chronic alcoholic pancreatitis. *Dermatologica,* 164:322–326.

Berge, G., Lundquist, A., Rorman, H. and Akerman, M. (1970). Liver biopsy in psoriasis. *Br. J. Dermatol.*, 82:250.

Braathan, L.R., Botten, G. and Bjerkedal, T. (1989). Psoriatics in Norway. *Acta Derm Venereol*, Suppl., 142:9–12.

Chaput, J.-C., Poynard, T., Naveau, S., Penso, D., Durrmeyer, O. and Suplisson, D. (1985). Psoriasis, alcohol and liver disease. *Br. Med. J.*, 291:25.

Dehne, N.E., Mendenhall, C.L. and Roselle, G.A. (1989). Cell mediated immune responses associated with short term alcohol intake: time course and dose ependency. *Alcoholism Clinical and Experimental Research*, 13:201–5.

Delaney, T.J. and Leppard, B. (1974). Alcohol intake and psoriasis. *Acta DermatoVenereol.*, 54:237–8.

Finlay, A.Y. and Kelly, S.E. (1987). Psoriasis — an index of disability. *Clin. Exp. Dematol.*, 12:8–11.

Foutch, P.G., Sullivan, J.A., Gaines, J.A. and Sanowski, R.A. (1988). Cutaneous vascular spiders in cirrhotic patients; correlation with haemorrhage from oesophageal varices. *Am. J. Gastroenterol.*, 83:723–6.

Ginsburg, I.H. and Link, B.G. (1989). Feelings of stigmatization in patients with psoriasis. *J. Am. Acad. Dermatol.*, 20:53–63.

Guivernau, M., Baraona, E. and Lieber, C.S. (1987). Acute and chronic effects of ethanol and its metabolites on vascular production of prostacyclin in rats. *J. Pharmacol. Exp. Ther.*, 240:56–64.

Gupta, M.A., Schork, N.J., Gupta, A.K. and Ellis, C.N. (1993). Alcohol intake and treatment responsiveness of psoriasis: A prospective study. *J. Am. Acad. Dermatol.*, 28:730–2.

Hatake, K., Wakabayashi, I., Kakashita, E., Taniguchi, T., Ouchi, H. and Hishida, S. (1991). Development of tolerance to inhibitory effect of ethanol on endothelium-dependent vascular relaxation in ethanol fed rats. *Alc. Clin. Exp. Res.*, 15:112–5.

Higgins, E.M. and du Vivier, A.W.P. (1992a). Alcohol and the skin. *Alc. Alcohol.*, 27:595–602.

Higgins, E.M., du Vivier, A.W.P. and Peters, T.J. (1992b). Skin disease and alcohol misuse. *Alc. Alcohol*, 27 (suppl):95.

Higgins, E.M., du Vivier, A.W.P. and Peters, T.J. (1993a). Drinking habits of patients with psoriasis. *Clin. Sci.*, 84:33P.

Higgins, E.M., du Vivier, A.W.P. and Peters, T.J. (1993b). Smoking, drinking and psoriasis. *Br. J. Dermatol.*, 129:749–750

Higgins, E.M. and du Vivier, A.W.P., (1994a). Cutaneous disease and alcohol misuse. *Br. Med. Bull.* 50:85–98.

Higgins, E.M. and du Vivier, A.W.P., (1994b). Alcohol misuse and treatment resistance in skin disease. *J. Am. Acad. Dermatol.*, 30:1048.

Jerrels, T.R., Peritt, D., Marietta, C.A. and Eckardt, M.J. (1989). Mechanisms of suppression of cellular immunity induced by ethanol. *Alc. Clin. Exp. Res.*, 13:490–3.

Johnson, R.H., Eisenhofer, G. and Lambie, D.G. (1986). The effects of acute and chronic ingestion of ethanol on the autonomic nervous system. *Drug Alc. Depend.*, 18:319–28.

Levallois, C., Ronahi, N., Balmes, J.L. and Mani, J.C., (1989). Effects of ethanol *in vitro* on some parameters of the immune response. *Drug. Alc. Dep.*, 24:239–44.

MacGregor, R.R. (1986). Alcohol and immune defense, *JAMA*, 256:1474–1479.

Malinowska, B., Pietraszek, M., Chabielska, E., Pawlak, D., Buczko, W. (1990). The effect of ethanol and serotonin on blood vessels in the rat. *Polish journal of Pharmacology and Pharmacy*, **42**:333–42.

Malpas, S.C., Robinson, B.J. and Malina, T.J.B. (1990). Mechanism of ethanol-induced vasodilation. *J. Appl. Physiol.*, **68**:731–4.

Mathes, B.M. and Douglas, M.C. (1985). Seborrhoeic dematitis in patients with AIDS. *Journal of the American Academy of Dermatology*, **13**:947–51.

McGarry, G.W., Gatehouse, S. and Hinnie, J. (1994). Relation between alcohol and nose bleeds. *Br. Med. J.*, **309**; 640

Mills, C.M., Srivastava, E.D. and Harvey, I.M. *et al.* (1992). Smoking habits in psoriasis: a case-controlled study. *Br. J. Dermatol.*, **127**:18–21.

Monk, B. and Neill, S.M. (1986). Alcohol consumption and psoriasis. *Dermatologica*, **173**:57–60.

Morse, R.M., Perry, H.O. and Hurt, R.D. (1985). Alcoholism and Psoriasis. *Alc. Clin. Exp. Res.*, **9**:396–399.

Naldi, L., Parazzinin, F. and Brevi, A. *et al.* (1992). Family history, smoking habits, alcohol consumption and risk of psoriasis. *Br. J. Dermatol.*, **127**:212–217.

Negri, E., La vecchia, C., Franchesci, S. and Tavani, A. (1993). Attributable risk for oral cancer in N. Italy. *Cancer Epidemiol. Biomed. Review.*, **2**:1189–193.

O'Doherty, C.J. and Macintyre, C. (1985). Palmoplantar pustulosis and smoking. *Br. Med. J.*, **291**:861–4.

Ohmori, T., Koyami, T., Chen, C.C., Yeh, E.K., Reyes, B.V. and Yamashita, I. (1986). The role of aldehyde dehydrogenase isoenzyme variance in alcohol sensitivity, drinking habits formation and the development of alcoholism in Japan, Taiwan and the Phillipines. *Prog. in Neuropsychopharm.*, **10**:229–235.

Okumura, H., Aramaki, T. and Katsuta, Y. *et al.* (1990). Regional differences in peripheral circulation between upper and lower extremities in patients with cirrhosis. *Scand. J. Gastroenterol.*, **25**:883–9.

Poikolainen, K., Rennal, A.T., Karvonen, J., Lanharanta, J. and Karkkainen, P. (1990). Alcohol intake; a risk factor for psoriasis in young and middle aged men? *Br. Med. J.*, **300**: 780–783.

Potamianos, G., Gorman, D.M., Duffy, S.W. and Peters, T.J. (1988). Alcohol consumption by patients attending out-patients clinics. *Int. J. Soc. Psych.*, **34**:97–101.

Price, M.L., Mottahedin, I. and Mayo, Pr. (1991). Can psychotherapy help patients with psoriasis? *Clin. Exp. Dermatol.*, **16**:114–117.

Ramsay, B. and O'Reagan, M. (1988). A survey of the social and psychological effects of psoriasis. *Br. J. Dermatol.*, **118**:195–201.

Sarkany, I. (1988). The skin — liver connection. *Clinical and Experimental Dermatology*, **13**:152–9.

Seville, R.H. (1977). Psoriasis and stress. *Br. J. Dermatol.*, **97**:297.

Singer, D.S., Parent, L.J. and Kolber, M.A. (1989). Ethanol: an enhancer of transplantation antigen expression. *Alc. Clin. Exp. Res.*, **13**:480–4.

Snyder, N., Bessoff, J., Dwyer, J. and Conn, H.O. (1978). Depressed Cutaneous delayed hypersensitivity in alcoholic hepatitis. *Am. J. Digest. Dis.*, **23**:353–8.

Strauss, E., Lacet, C.M., Caly, W.R., Fukishhima, J.T. and Gayotto, L.C. (1990). Cryptogenic cirrhosis; clinico-biochemical comparison with alcoholic and viral aetiologies. *Arqu. de Gastroent.*, **27**:46–52.

Ternowitz, T. Monocyte and neutrophil chemotaxis in psoriasis. (1989). *Dan. Med. Bull.*, **36**: 1–14.

Terry, R.C. (1954). White nails in hepatic cirrhosis. *Lancet*, **i**:248–9.

Vincenti, G.E. and Blunden, S.M. (1987). Psoriasis and alcohol misuse. *J. Roy. Army. Med. Cor.*, **133**:77–8.

Ward, R.J., McPherson, A.J.S., Warren-Perry, M., Dave, V., Hsu, L., Yoshida, A. and Peters, T.J. (1991). Biochemical and genetic studies in ALDH1-deficient subjects. In *Alcohol: A molecular perspective* (Ed. Palmer T.N.), Plenum Press, New York.

Watson, C.G., Anderson, D.H. and Jacobs, L. (1995). Factor analysis of the after-effects of drinking in alcoholics. *J. Clin. Physiol.*, **41**:111–7.

West, B.L. and Anderson, P.C., (1986). Alcohol and aquired acrodermatitis enteropathica. *J. Am. Acad. Dermatol.*, 15:1305.

Wilkerson, M.G. and Wilkin, J.K. (1989). Red lunulae revisited. A clinical and histopathological examination. *J. Am. Acad. Dermatol.*, **20**:453–7.

Wilkin, J.K. and Fortner, G. (1985). Cutaneous vascular sensitivity to lower aliphatic alcohols and aldehydes in Orientals. *Alc. Clin. Exp. Res.*, **9**:522–5.

Wilkin, J.K. (1988). 4-Methylpyrazole and the cutaneous vascular sensitivity to alcohol in Orientals. *J. Inv. Dermatol.*, **91**:117–9.

6 HIV and Alcohol Abuse

Thomas J. McManus and Peter Weatherburn

Department of Genitourinary Medicine, King's Healthcare NHS Trust, London, SE5,
Project Sigma, University of Essex

Alcohol ingestion has been shown to influence human behaviour in general and can influence sexual behaviour in particular. It has been hypothesised that alcohol can alter a person's ability to maintain a safe sexual lifestyle. Health educators advise that excessive drinking can lead to unsafe sexual behaviour in some circumstances. While this is undoubtedly true, the effect of alcohol on such behaviour is more complex than just a straightforward lack of control. Alcohol can, in some circumstances, be used as a means to help negotiate safer sex. Advanced HIV infection is associated with immune deficiency. Alcohol is just one of many substances that has been shown *in vitro* and in animal studies to alter immune function. However, an adverse effect to alcohol on HIV disease progression has not been substantiated in observations in humans.

INTRODUCTION

Human Immunodeficiency Viruses I and II (HIV I and II) have been found in Europe. HIV I is by far the more prevalent virus. Infection with Human Immunodeficiency viruses leads to development of the Acquired Immune Deficiency Syndrome (AIDS). AIDS, as the name suggests, is a breakdown of the body's natural immune system. The rate of progression from the acquisition of HIV to AIDS is variable and at present unpredictable. Evidence from San Francisco (Buchbinder *et al.*, 1992) suggests that 50% of men who acquired HIV infection from homosexual activity had developed AIDS 10 years after seroconversion. It is uncertain why different people have differing rates of progression to AIDS. The type of virus, the destruction of the immune system, acquisition of other infections and aspects of lifestyle have all at some point been put forward as reasons for progression to symptomatic infection.

It may be helpful, before entering into the main discussion of this paper, to outline the extent of the HIV problem in Europe (see Table 6.1). At the end of 1991 there were 81,091 people known to have AIDS in Europe (statistics from WHO). This is clearly a gross underestimate of the extent of the HIV problem in Europe as many people with HIV infection have not had an HIV antibody test. The figures represent only confirmed cases of AIDS that have been reported to the relevant surveillance teams.

Although many publications have examined the impact of alcohol consumption on various aspects of HIV infection. The prime focus of this research, at least in terms of research output, has been on the possible relationship between alcohol use and an increased likelihood of engagement in "unsafe sexual behaviour" (see Bolton *et al.*, 1993; Leigh and Staff, 1993; Weatherburn *et al.*, 1993 for reviews). Drawing on evidence from the 1970s, as well as more recent data, there is debate concerning the impact of alcohol consumption on immune function (Flavin and Francis, 1987; Dunne, 1989; Haverkos, 1990) and more specifically, on the possible impact of alcohol as a co-factor for the development of AIDS or HIV related symptomatic disease (Kaslow *et al.*, 1989; Coates *et al.*, 1990).

Table 6.1 Statistics from the World Health Organization (Reported AIDS Cases in Europe)

	Date of report	Total	1991 No. of cases*
France	17.12.92	21487	7.1
Spain	17.12.92	14991	8.7
Italy	17.12.92	14783	5.2
Germany	17.12.92	8893	2.4
United Kingdom	17.12.92	6510	2.0
Switzerland	17.12.92	2591	6.6
Netherlands	17.12.92	2330	2.9
Romania	17.12.92	2073	2.1
Belgium	17.12.92	1224	2.3
Denmark	17.12.92	1072	3.9
Portugal	17.12.92	1007	2.1
Austria	17.12.92	825	2.4
Sweden	17.12.92	743	1.5
Greece	17.12.92	689	1.4
Yugoslavia[a]	30.04.92	313	0.3
Ireland	17.12.92	294	1.8
Norway	17.12.92	283	1.3
Israel	17.12.92	192	0.6
Poland	17.12.92	118	0.1
Finland	17.12.92	112	0.5
Hungary	17.12.92	105	0.2
Russian Federation[b]	30.09.92	94	0.0
Turkey	17.12.92	89	0.0
Luxembourg	17.12.92	55	3.2
Czechoslovakia	17.12.92	32	0.0
Malta	17.12.92	25	1.9
Iceland	17.12.92	22	2.3
Bulgaria	17.12.92	15	0.0
Monaco	17.12.92	9	7.4
Belarus[b]	30.09.92	5	0.0
Lithuania[b]	30.09.92	2	0.0
Latvia[b]	30.09.92	2	0.0
San Marino	17.12.92	1	0.0
Albania	30.09.92	0	0.0

* Rate/reported cases/100000; 1992 reporting generally incomplete
[a] Refers to Republics and areas of the former Socialist Federal Republic of Yugoslavia (Bosnia and Herzegovina, Croatia, Macedonia, Montenegro, Serbia, Slovenia)
[b] Covers Republics and areas of former Soviet Union

In order to understand the impact of alcohol consumption on the potential course of the HIV pandemic we must examine all three of these debates, namely the relationship between alcohol and unsafe sex, the impact of alcohol on the immune system and the possibility that alcohol alters disease progression. Firstly, the likelihood that alcohol facilitates engagement in sexual practices that enable HIV to be transmitted from one individual to another will be examined, as will the evidence relating to the effects of alcohol consumption on immune function, especially its ability to weaken a HIV infected person's natural immune defence mechanisms. Finally, the impact of alcohol on disease progression among persons who have asymptomatic and symptomatic HIV will be discussed.

ALCOHOL USE AND ENGAGEMENT IN "UNSAFE" SEX

There are a large number of papers reporting the effects of alcohol use on "unsafe" sex. The populations studied have mainly been what we consider are convenience groups such as adolescents, college students, gay men and heterosexual women. (see Bolton *et al.*, 1993; Leigh and Staff, 1993 for reviews) The general conclusion is that drinking alcohol is related to the practice of unsafe sex. If a person is under the influence of alcohol she/he is more likely to engage in acts which could result in the transmission of HIV.

It is often assumed that this finding is a description of a self evident fact. Indeed health educators have promoted the safe use of alcohol as a major part of the "safe sex" campaign. It is important to look at the results of this research in more detail. The published work contains a number of limitations (Bolton *et al.*, 1993; Weatherburn *et al.*, 1993). The first arises as a result of the widespread assumption that there is, or could be, just one straightforward relationship between alcohol use and sexual behaviour, irrespective of factors such as culture, gender or sexual orientation. Thus, despite evidence that the relationship varies according to gender and sexual orientation (Stall *et al.*, 1990; Trocki and Leigh, 1991), results from samples of homosexual and heterosexual men and women are commonly considered together.

Examination of the available literature shows that evidence for any relationship between alcohol misuse and unsafe sex is not truly proven. From our extensive review of papers pertaining to gay and bisexual men (Weatherburn *et al.*, 1993) only eight (Stall *et al.*, 1986; McKirnan *et al.*, 1989; Kelly *et al.*, 1991; Valdisserri *et al.*, 1988; McKirnan *et al.*, 1989; Ilaria *et al.*, 1991; Calzavara *et al.*, 1991; Stall *et al.*, 1986) find a significant relationship, fifteen (Bolton *et al.*, 1993; Connell *et al.*, 1990; Willoughby *et al.*, 1991; Siegel *et al.*, 1991; McCusker *et al.*, 1989; Ostrow *et al.*, 1990; Martin *et al.*, 1990; Doll *et al.*, 1989; Stall *et al.*, 1991; Zielinski *et al.*, 1989; Gold *et al.*, 1991; Gold *et al.*, 1992; Harrison *et al.*, 1989; Leigh, 1990; Leigh, 1993) fail to do so and a further four are equivocal (Trocki, 1991; Prieur, 1990; McCusker *et al.*, 1990; Ekstrand *et al.*, 1990). Furthermore, all those papers which use critical incident (Doll, 1989; Gold *et al.*, 1991; Gold *et al.,* 1992; Harrison *et al.*, 1989) or diary techniques (Leigh, 1993) to test directly the relationship between alcohol use and unsafe sex, fail to find any association.

Secondly, the vast majority of literature has methodological limitations (Weatherburn *et al.*, 1993). The most important is the conflation of alcohol and other drugs (including such diverse substances as marijuana, cocaine and amyl and butyl nitrites) in one global measure (Valdisserri *et al.*, 1988; McKirnan, 1989; Stall *et al.*, 1990; Kelly *et al.*, 1991;

Connell *et al.*, 1990) assuming that all drugs are used in similar circumstances and to obtain similar effects. A third problem arises with the comparison of past sexual behaviour with gross measures of prior alcohol consumption (typically drinking sessions per time period) (Doll *et al.*, 1989; McKirnan and Peterson, 1989; McKirnan *et al.*, 1989; McCusker *et al.*, 1989; Siegel *et al.*, 1989; Zielinski *et al.*, 1989; Connell *et al.*, 1990; Ekstrand and Coates, 1990; Martin *et al.*, 1990; McCusker *et al.*, 1990; Ostrow *et al.*, 1990; Prieur, 1990; Calzavara *et al.*, 1991; Ilaria *et al.*, 1991; Stall *et al.*, 1991; Willoughby *et al.*, 1991). Since both of these variables represent measures of past behaviour, any association tells us little about the actual relationship since not only are there likely to be many intervening factors, but also the alcohol use need never have coincided with the unsafe behaviour. Similar confusion and contradiction is found in papers relating to the effect of alcohol consumption on ("unsafe") sexual behaviour among samples of heterosexuals (Bolton *et al.*, 1993; Leigh and Staff, 1993).

Though a proven causal relationship between alcohol use and engagement in "unsafe" sex may still have to be proven, this does not mean that no association between alcohol use and sexual behaviour exists. Even though alcohol does not appear to have a direct and specific impact on the propensity to engage in "unsafe" sexual behaviour, it is possible that there is some relationship between the two. Accepting this possibility it is important to recognise the potential explanations for, and implications of, any such association.

Ostrow (1986) discussed at length some possible explanations for any potential gross association between alcohol use and sexual behaviour. They put forward a number of hypotheses termed: "null"; "aphrodisiac"; "personality"; "social context"; "multifactorial" and "disinhibition". Each of these mechanisms (with the partial exception of "social context" and "null" — see below) assumes that alcohol use predisposes or leads to unsafe behaviour and leads the authors to suggest a different intervention strategy.

Stall *et al.*, (1986) also concentrated on the disinhibition hypothesis. This hypothesis they postulated "asserts that culturally learned responses to substance use are causal of the content of inebriated behaviour", such that the physiological effects of alcohol "are often interpreted in a way that encourages participation in high risk activity [that is] being drunk serves as an acceptable excuse for risky sexual behaviour". They suggested that health educators should disseminate their discovery of the relationship between alcohol use and unsafe sex accompanied by information which emphasised that disinhibition was not an acceptable excuse for unsafe sex.

Health education campaigns in many countries have traditionally stressed that "alcohol and drugs affect your judgement and make you more likely to take risks" ("Travel Safe" campaign of the UK Department of Health, 1993). Campaigns which mention alcohol rarely stress that alcohol is not a valid excuse for engaging in unsafe sex. As a result, such programmes may have provided individuals with an easy self-justification for engaging in unsafe sex by allowing them to abrogate responsibility for behaviours which they and their peers find unacceptable. Furthermore such campaigns, by providing a ready-made agenda for intervention absolve those involved in health education from addressing the complex and intractable problems of negotiation and interaction which are central to the problem of "unsafe" sex.

Given the centrality of alcohol to the social lifestyles of a large proportion of individuals (perhaps especially to those who are young and/or single and hence the most sexually active) it may be that one explanation for any association between alcohol use and "unsafe" sex is the result of "social context" (Stall *et al.*, 1986). Qualitative work by Weatherburn and *Project Sigma* (1992) suggests that alcohol is an important factor in the sexual lifestyle of more than a fifth of gay and bisexual men. Alcohol is an entrenched part of the gay social scene and may be used as a means to facilitate social and sexual lifestyles. Thus, alcohol is used in a premeditated way to enhance sexual desire or performance and/or overcome sexual and social inhibitions. Some gay men stress that they use alcohol to enable them to engage in sexual negotiations that they might otherwise be too shy to attempt. Crucially these include the negotiations of safer sex.

Alternatively, any correlation between alcohol use and "unsafe" sexual behaviour might arise because of some unexamined third factor, correlated with both alcohol use and unsafe sex. This possibility has been examined, though usually in the guise of the "risky personality", that there are individuals who are accustomed or addicted to the taking of risks and this manifests itself in high levels of alcohol use and unsafe sexual behaviour. People with HIV infection may use alcohol as a means of coping with their condition. An attempt to forget or deny the dreadful prognosis associated with HIV infection can often be facilitated by the use of alcohol or other drugs.

Finally, any relationship between alcohol use and sexual behaviour might be spurious, a methodological artefact. If the methodological problems discussed earlier are accepted this remains a possibility. The failure of any study which has looked directly at the specific interaction between alcohol use and unsafe behaviour to confirm the hypothesis must lead us to conclude that the early findings measured the contextual effect of alcohol use and sex. If a relationship between alcohol and sexual behaviour really exists this needs to be clarified (Temple *et al.*, 1993). Not least because such findings will be essential to professionals involved in intervention programmes aimed at stopping the spread of HIV.

ALCOHOL USE AND IMMUNE FUNCTION

It has been noted that alcoholics have an increased susceptibility to infections. Some studies have attributed this to defects in host immune defence mechanisms (MacGregor *et al.*, 1874; Pickrell, 1938; McFarland *et al.*, 1963; Brayton *et al.*, 1970; Hsu and Leavy, 1971; Strans *et al.*, 1971; Bernstein *et al.*, 1974; Lundy *et al.*, 1975; Gluckham *et al.*, 1977; Lui, 1980; Stimmel, 1987). The lifestyle of the chronic alcoholic might however contribute to the inability to fight off infection (Gluckham *et al.*, 1977) as they are more likely than the normal population to experience malnutrition and cirrhosis and delay seeking medical help.

In HIV infection defects in both cellular and humoral immune systems are known to occur (Fauci *et al.*, 1991). However, the rate of development of these abnormalities and related infections varies from individual to individual. The reason for the collapse of the immune system is basically unknown but several potential mechanisms leading to the function and quantitative depletion of CD4 lymphocytes have been found.

These mechanisms include:

- Direct HIV-mediated cytopathic effects (single cell killing)
- HIV-mediated formation of syncytia
- Virus-specific immune responses

- HIV specific cytolytic T lymphocytes
- Antibody-dependent cellular toxicity
- Natural killer cells
- Autoimmune mechanisms
- Anergy caused by inappropriate cell signalling through gp120-CD4 interaction
- Superantigen-mediated perturbation of T-cell subgroups
- Programmed cell death (apoptosis)

Earlier explanations for the collapse of the immune system concentrated on the "overload" theory. It was thought that individuals who were exposed to other infections were more likely to activate their immune system and eventually overload it. In such an environment immune cells harbouring HIV would become activated, HIV production would increase and the number of immune cells able to recognise and fight off infections would gradually decrease. A number of toxins, in addition to viruses and bacteria, were implicated in this "poisoning" of the immune system. Recreational drugs, in particular, were thought to have an adverse effect on the immune system. Alcohol was investigated as possibly having a negative influence on the immune system.

Stimmel (1987) has demonstrated that alcohol has an adverse effect on the immune system of laboratory animals. Dunne (1989), citing the work of other authors, suggests that lymphocyte production and function may be altered by heavy alcohol consumption. Liu (1980) reported a decrease in lymphocytes in 19 of 82 subjects who ingested excessive amounts of alcohol. It cannot be assumed, however, that alcohol alone was responsible for the lymphopenia and other studies have shown that nutritional deficiencies are common in alcoholics and can have a detrimental effect on the synthesis, development and proliferation of lymphocytes (Cunningham-Randle, 1982). Bernstein *et al.* (1974) reported an observed reduction in circulating T lymphocytes in association with alcoholics liver disease. Other abnormalities of immune response found in alcoholic include inhibition of granulocyte chemotoxins, inhibition of the establishment of delayed hypersensitivity and antibody response to a new antigen and impaired lymphocyte transformation (McFarland *et al.*, 1963; Brayton, *et al.*, 1970; Hsu and Leavy, 1971; Strans *et al.*, 1971; MacGregor *et al.*, 1974 and Lundy *et al.*, 1975).

Many of these studies have been of "problem" drinkers and alcoholics with cirrhosis. One study by Lundy *et al.*, (1975) suggested that the inhibition of sensitisation of new antigens require continued alcohol exposure throughout the sensitisation period and that abstinence may allow some defects to reverse.

Theoretically in HIV infection the multiple immune defects may be aggravated in an alcoholic or if alcohol intake increases. Conversely if alcohol intake decreases or ceases this change could be reflected in an improvement in immune function. No work to date has correlated immune dysfunction with an HIV infected person's alcohol intake, but the management of a person with HIV disease can be complicated by excess alcohol use.

Haematological abnormalities found in association with alcohol can often be a part of HIV disease e.g. anaemia and thrombocytopenia (Zon and Groopman, 1988; Karpatkin, 1988; Seadden *et al.*, 1989; Fauci *et al.*, 1991). In patients with overt AIDS, anaemia occurs in 66% to 85% (Seadden *et al.*, 1989; Zon and Groopman, 1988). The cause of the anaemia is complex and multifactorial but includes direct effects of HIV on erythroid precursors (Fauci *et al.*, 1991). Alcohol can have a direct toxic effect on the bone marrow. Thrombocytopenia is the most common platelet abnormality in HIV infected patients. Again the cause is unclear but platelet-associated immunoglobulin is present (Karpatkin, 1988). Thrombocytopenia can occur in chronic alcoholics and may occur without accompanying folate deficiency.

Macrocytosis is a particularly common haematological disorder in chronic alcoholics. Zidovudine antiretroviral therapy results in macrocytosis in almost all patients for whom it is prescribed (Richman, 1987). Clinicians expect to see a macrocytosis after zidovudine therapy and such an effect usually heralds a satisfactory response to the drug. Clearly management in chronic alcoholics could be problematic.

Peripheral neuropathy can complicate the various stages of HIV-1 infection. The most common neuropathy in AIDS patients is a distal, predominantly sensory and axional neuropathy (McKhann and McDonald, 1986). In some patients the sensory symptoms resemble closely those due to the neuropathy found in alcoholics (Blass and Gibson, 1971; Asbury *et al.*, 1984). Some of the less commonly used antiretroviral agents, e.g. dideoxyinosine and dideoxycytidine have pancreatitis as one of their associated toxicities precluding their use in chronic alcoholics (Richman, 1987).

DISEASE PROGRESSION AMONG PERSONS WITH HIV INFECTION

Among the many reasons suggested for the variation in disease progression among people with HIV infection is the influence of "co-factors". A co-factor has been defined (Haverkos, 1990) as a "non-HIV related influence that operates in conjunction with HIV to affect disease progression". Other viruses, such as cytomegalovirus and Epstein-Barr virus, bacterial infections, inhaled amyl nitrite and other substances of abuse, have all been mentioned as important factors. As yet no firm evidence of their role in disease progression has been established. Many researchers do not agree with the concept of co-factors as a major influence in disease progression and the early certainty that amyl nitrite was a cause for disease progression in gay men, although investigated thoroughly, has not been proven.

Taking into account the work that has been done on the effects of alcohol on the immune system it is not surprising that the ingestion of alcohol was considered as a possible factor in disease progression in HIV infected individuals. The question posed was do HIV positive people with an excessive alcohol intake fair less well than other persons with HIV infection?

Kaslow *et al.* (1989) in a multicentre cohort study of homosexual men (MACS) found that prior use of alcohol was not associated with low mean CD4 helper cell counts at enrolment to the study. Continued alcohol ingestion in the seropositive cohort did not influence progression to AIDS or CD4 cell depletion. Conversely, continued heavy drinking was associated with a lower prevalence of persistent generalised lymphadenopathy.

Similar findings were reported from the Netherlands (Van Griensven *et al.*, 1990) where 286 HIV antibody positive homosexual men were followed up between 1984 and 1988. No relation could be found between alcohol use and disease progression. A similar America study (Coates *et al.*, 1990) examining co-factors which influence progression to AIDS in a cohort of 249 homosexual men found no significant association between the use of alcohol or recreational drugs with risk of progression to clinically defined AIDS. Only estimated duration of infection with HIV was associated with increasing risk of disease progression. Despite the variation in methodology used in the various studies, there appears at present to be no evidence that alcohol intake influences the rate of HIV disease progression.

CONCLUSIONS AND PROPOSALS FOR FURTHER RESEARCH

From our review of the data concerning the impact of alcohol use on the likelihood of engagement in sexual practices which are "unsafe" it is obvious that any relationship is complicated and very poorly understood. There is an argument that, contrary to popular belief, the consumption of alcohol does not appear to make individuals more likely to engage in "unsafe" sex. However, it does not necessarily follow that there is no association between alcohol consumption and sexual behaviour, more generally, but this is probably related to other factors such as lifestyle or social context variables. Further research is necessary but it needs to concentrate on the specific effects of alcohol consumption within the context of sexual interaction.

While alcohol has been shown to affect immune function *in vivo*, *in vitro* and in laboratory animals, there is no clear evidence that it plays any part in individuals' susceptibility to other infections after HIV infection. Even though the evidence concentrates mainly on small samples of "problem drinkers" none of these very specific studies proved that alcohol consumption increased vulnerability to infection.

Finally, the few large scale cohort studies that have been published seem to indicate that alcohol has no impact on disease progression among persons with HIV infection. Clearly such research is in its infancy. A valuable study would be one which identifies the alcohol intake of people, especially gay men, with HIV infection at various stages of disease. It may be that major life events influence the ingestion of alcohol. Such a study would help to define more clearly any effect alcohol may have on disease progression and whether disease progression influences alcohol intake. Well designed sequential studies might also be used to answer these problems.

References

Asbury, A.K., Gilliatt, R.W. *et al.* (1984). Peripheral Nerve Disorders — a Practical Approach. *Bulleworth and Co., Publ., London.*

Buchbinder, S.P., Katz, M.H., Hessol, N.A., O'Malley, P.M., Barhart, J.L. and Holmberg, S.D. (1992). Healthy long-term positives: men infected with HIV for more than 10 years with CD4 counts greater than 500 cells. *VIII International Conference on AIDS/VII STD World Congress, 1992:* Abstract No. TUC 0572.

Bolton, R., Vincke, J., Mak, R. and Dennhy, E. (1993). Alcohol and Risky Sex: In Search of an Elusive Connection. *Medical Anthropology* (in press), 1992, Vol 14. pp 323–63.

Bernstein, I.M., Webster, K.H., Williams, Jnr. R.C. and Strickland, R.G. (1974). Reduction in circulating T-lymphocyte in alcoholic liver disease. *Lancet,* **2**:488–90.

Blass, J.P. and Gibson, J.E. (1971). Deleterious aberrations of a thiamine-requiring enzyme in four patients with Wernicke — "Korsakoff's Syndrome". *NEJM,* **297**:1367–70.

Brayton, R.G., Stokes, P.E., Schwarts, M.S. *et al.* (1970). Effect of alcohol and various diseases on leukocyte mobilization, phagocytosis and intracellular bacterial killing. *NEJM,* **282**:123–8.

Calzavara, L., Coates, R., Raboud, J. *et al.* (June 1991). Recreational Drug Use and High-Risk Sexual Behaviour in a Toronto Sexual Contact Study Cohort. *Presented at VII International Conference on AIDS, Florence, Italy.*

Coates, R.A., Farewell, V.T., Raboud, J., Read, S.E., MacFadden, D.K., Calzavara, L.M., Johnson, J.K., Shepherd, F.A. and Fanning, M.M. (1990). Cofactors of progression of Acquired Immunodeficiency Syndrome in a cohort of male sexual contact of men with Human Immunodeficiency Virus disease. *Am. J. Epidemiool*, **32**:717–772.

Connell, R.W., Crawford, J., Dowsett, G.W. *et al.* (1990). Danger and Context: Unsafe Anal Sexual Practice among Homosexual and Bisexual Men in the AIDS Crises. *ANZJS*, **26(2)**:187–208.

Cunningham-Rundles, S. (1982). Effects of nutritional status on immunological functions. *Am. J. Clin. Nutrition*, **35**:1202–10.

Dunne, F.J. (1989). Alcohol and the immune system. *British Medical Journal*, **298**:543–544.

Doll, L. (April 1989). Alcohol Use as a Co-factor for Disease and High-risk Behaviour. *Presented at NIAA Alcohol and AIDS Network Conference, Tuscon, Arizona.*

Ekstrand, M.L. and Coates, T.J. (1990). Maintenance of Safer Sexual Behaviour and Predictors of Risky Sex: The San Francisco Men's Health Study. *AJPH*, **80(8)**:973–977.

Flavin, D.K. and Francis, R.J. (1987). Risk-taking behaviour, substance abuse disorder and the Acquired Immune Deficiency Syndrome. Advances in *Alcohol and Substance Abuse*, **6**:23–32.

Fauci, A.S. (moderator), Schnittman, S.M., Poli, G. *et al.* (1991). Immunopathogenic mechanisms in human immunodeficiency virus (HIV). infection. *Ann. Intern. Med.*, **114**:678–93.

Gluckham, S.J., Dvorak, V.C. and McGregor, R.R. (1977). Effects of ethyl alcohol on human peripheral lymphocytes. *Archives of Internal Medicine*, **137**:1539–1543.

Gold R.S., Skinner M.J., Grants P.J. and Plummer D.C. (1991). Situational Factors and Thought Processes Associated with Unprotected Intercourse in Gay Men. *Psychology and Health*, **5**:259–278.

Gold, R.S. and Skinner, M.J. (1992). Situational Factors and Thought Processes Associated with Unprotected Intercourse in Young Gay Men. *Unpublished Manuscript.*

Harrison, J.S., Doll, L.S., Weller, P. *et al.* (June 1989). Condom Use can Occur Despite use of Alcohol and Drugs. *Presented at V International Conference on AIDS, Montreal, Canada.*

Haverkos, H.W. (1990). The search for cofactors in AIDS, including an analysis of the association of nitrite inhalant abuse and Kaposi's Sarcoma. In: Alcohol, Immunomodulation and AIDS Seminar. D., Watson R.R., Pawlowski, A. (Eds). *New York*: Alan R. Liss.

Hsu, C.C.S. and Leavy, C.M. (1971). Inhibition of PHA-stimulated lymphocyte transformation by plasma from patients with advanced alcoholic cirrhosis. *Clin. Exp. Immunol.*, **8**:749–60.

Ilaria, G., Weiss, D.J., Clotz, D. *et al.* (June 1991). Association of drug taking and high risk sexual behaviour in 774 gay men in New York City: Implications for Prevention. *Poster at VII International Conference on AIDS, Florence, Italy.*

Karpatkin, S. (1988). Immunologic thrombocytopenic purpura in HIV-seropositive homosexuals, addicts and haemophiliacs. *Semin Haematol*, **25**:219–229.

Kaslow, R.A., Blackwlder, W.C., Ostrow, D.G., Yerg, D., Palenicek, J., Coulson, A.H. and Valdiserri, R.D. (1989). No evidence for a role of alcohol or other psychoactive drugs in accelerating immunodeficiency in HIV-1 positive individuals. A report from the multicenter AIDS cohort study. *JAMA*, **261**:2324–3429.

Kelly, J.A., St. Lawrence, J.S. and Brasfield, T.L. (1991). Predictors of vulnerability to AIDS risk behaviour relapse. *Journal of Consulting and Clinical Psychology*, **59(1)**:163–166.

Leigh, B.C. (1990). The relationships of substance use during sex to high-risk sexual behaviour. *Journal of Sex Research*, **27**:199–213.

Leigh, B.C. and Staff R. (1993). Substance use and risky sexual behaviour for exposure to HIV: Issues in methodology, interpretation and prevention. *Journal of Abnormal Psychology* (in press).

Leigh, B.C. (1993). Alcohol consumption and sexual activity as reported with a prospective diary technique. *Journal of Abnormal Psychology* (in press).

Liu, Y.K. (1980). Effects of alcohol on granulocytes and lymphocytes. *Seminars in Haematology*, **17**:130–6.

Lundy, J., Roaf, J.H., Deakins, S. *et al.* (1975). The acute and chronic effects of alcohol on the human immune system. *Surg. Gynaecol. Obstet.*, **141**:212–8.

Martin, J.L. and Hasin, D.S. (1990). Drinking, alcoholism, and sexual behaviour in a cohort of gay men. *Drugs and Society*, **5(1–2)**:47–67.

MacGregor, R.R., Spagnuolo, P.J. and Lentuek, A.L. (1974). Inhibition of granulocyte adherence by ethanol, prednisone and aspirin, measured with an assay system. *NEJM*, **291**:642–6.

McCusker, J., Stoddard, A.M. Zapka, J.G. *et al.* (1989). Predictors of AIDS-Preventative behaviour among homosexually Active Men. *AIDS*, **3(7)**:443–448.

McCusker, J., Westenhouse, J., Stoddard, A.M. *et al.* (1990). Use of drugs and alcohol by homosexually active men in relation to sexual practices. *Journal of Acquired Immune Deficiency Syndromes*, **3**:729–736.

McFarland, W. and Libre, E.P. (1963). Abnormal leukocyte response in alcoholism. *Ann. Intern. Med.*, **59**:865–877.

McKhann, G.M. and McDonald, W.I. (1986). Diseases of the Nervous System. Clinical Neurobiology. Ed. by Asbury A.K., *Wilken Heineman Medical Book (RMO), London.*

McKirnan, D.J. and Peterson, P.L. (1989). AIDS-risk Behaviour among Homosexual Males: The Roles of Attitudes and Substance Abuse. *Psychology and Health*, **3**:161–171.

McKirnan, D.J. and Peterson, P.L. (June 1989). Tension reduction expectancies underlie the effect of alcohol use on AIDS-risk behaviour among homosexual males. *Poster at V International Conference on AIDS, Montreal, Canada,* (abstract TD010).

Molgaard, C.A., Nakamure, C., Howell, M. and Elder, J.P. (1988). Assessing alcoholism as a risk factor for acquired immunodeficiency Syndrome (AIDS). *Social Science and Medicine*, **27**:1147–1152.

Ostrow, D.G. (1986). Barriers to the recognition of links between drug and alcohol abuse and AIDS. In Acquired Immune Deficiency Syndrome and Chemical Dependency, *Washington D.C.: US Government Printing Office pp. 15–20* (DHHS Pub. No. ADM 87–1513).

Ostrow, D.G., Van Raden, M.J., Fox, R. *et al.* (1990). Recreational drug use and sexual behavior change in a cohort of homosexual men. *AIDS*, 1904:759–765.

Pickrell, K.L. (1938). "The effect of alcoholic intoxication and other anaesthesia on resistance to pneumococcal infection". *Bull Johns Hopkins Hosp.*, **63**:238–60.

Prieur, A. (1990). Gay men: Reasons for continued practice of unsafe sex. AIDS education and prevention **2**:11–117.

Richman, D. (1987). AZT Collaborative Working Group: The toxicity of azidothymidine in the treatment of patients with AIDS and AIDS-related complex. *N. Engl. J. Med.*, **317**:192–7.

Seadden, D.T., Zon, L.I. and Groopman, J.E. (1989). Pathophysiology and management of HIV-associated haematologic disorders. *Blood*, **74**:1455–63.

Siegel, K., Mesagno, F.P., Chen, J-Y. and Christ G. (1989). Factors distinguishing homosexual males practising risky and safer sex. *Social Science and Medicine*, **28(6)**:561–569.

Stall, R., McKusick, L., Wiley, J., Coaes, T. and Ostrow, D. (1986). Alcohol and drug use during sexual activity and compliance with safe sex guidelines for AIDS: The AIDS Behavioural Research Project. *Health Education Quarterly*, **13**:359–371.

Stall, R., Heurtin-Robert, S., McKusick, L. *et al.* (1990). Sexual risk for HIV transmission among singles-bar patrons in San Francisco. *Medical Anthropology Quarterly*, **4**:115–128.

Stall, R., Barrett, D., Bye, L. *et al.* (1991). A comparison of younger and older gay men's HIV risk-taking behaviours: The communication technologies 1989 Cross-Sectional Survey. *Unpublished Manuscript, Centre for AIDS Prevention Studies, S.F., U.S.A.*

Stimmel, A. (1987). AIDS, alcohol and heroin: a particularly deadly combination (editorial). *Advanced in Alcohol and Substances Abuse*, **6**:1–5.

Strans, B., Berenyi, M.R., Huang, J.M. *et al.* (1971). Delayed hypersensitivity in alcoholic cirrhosis. *Ann. J. Dig. Dis.*, **16**:509–16.

Statistics from the World Health Organisation 1993 *AIDS*, **7**:287–8.

Temple, M.T., Leigh, B.C. and Schafer, J. (1993). Unsafe sexual behaviour and alcohol use at the event level: results of a national survey. *Journal of AIDS*, **6**:393–401.

Trocki, K.F. and Leigh, B.C. (1991). Alcohol consumption and unsafe sex: A comparison of heterosexuals and homosexual men. *Journal of Acquired Immune Deficiency Syndrome*, **4**:981–986.

van Griensven, G.J.P., De Vroome, E.M.M., De Wolf, F., Grundsmit, J., Roos, M. and Coutinho, R. (1990). Risk factors for progression of Human Immunodeficiency Virus (HIV) infection among seroconverted and seropositive homosexual men. *Am. J. Epidemiol.*, **132**:203–10.

Valdisserri, R.O., Lyter, D., Leviton, L.C. *et al.* (1988). Variables influencing condom use in a cohort of gay and bisexual men. *American Journal of Public Health*, **78**:801–805.

Weatherburn, P. and Project SIGMA (1992). Alcohol use and unsafe sexual behaviour: Any connection? In P. Aggleton, P.M. Davies and G. Hart 'AIDS: Rights, Risk and Reason,' Falmer Press, London.

Weatherburn, P., Davies, P.M., Hickson, F.C.I., Hunt, A.J., McManus, T.J. and Coxon, A.P.M. (1993). No connection between alcohol use and unsafe sex among gay and bisexual men. *AIDS*, **7**:115–119.

Willoughby, B., Schechter, M.T., Craib, K.J.P. *et al.* (June 1991). Characteristics of risk takers among seronegative men in a gay cohort. *Presented at VII International Conference on AIDS, Florence, Italy.*

Zielinski, M.A. and Bocker, C. (November 1989). Drugs, alcohol and risky sex among gay and bisexual men in a low-incidence area for AIDS. *Presented at Annual Meeting of the American Public Health Association, Boston, U.S.A.*

Zon, L. and Groopman, J. (1988). Haematological manifestations of the human immune deficiency virus. *Seminar Haematol*, **25**:208–18.

7 Alcohol and the Brain: Neuropathology and Imaging Studies

Karl Mann, M.D.

Professor of Psychiatry, University of Tuebingen Medical School, Department of Psychiatry

Our understanding of the specific effects of alcohol on the brain have been revolutionized within the last decade. Controlled neuropathological studies found a reduction in the volume of white matter and a partial degeneration, or even a loss of specific neurons in humans. Using Magnetic Resonance Imaging and CAT-scans, the decrease in volume of white and grey matter was demonstrated *in vivo*. The degree and the time course of brain damage seems to be influenced more by age and gender than by drinking history. There is evidence that female alcoholics develop brain damage more readily than men. When abstinent, an increase in the volume of white and grey matter can be observed. This seems not to be due to the rehydration of brain tissue alone. Controlled studies with positron emission tomography (PET) showed a decrease in the cellular activity in the cortex and the basal ganglia. After abstinence an increase of neuronal activity was found in the cortex, which could represent an increase in synaptic density. Future research will need to deal with the question of whether the central nervous system is capable of partial regeneration. For the study of neuroplasticity, the neurobiological model of alcohol dependence seems to be particularly well suited.

1. INTRODUCTION

All European countries suffer from the sequelae of high alcohol consumption. Individual consumers are apt to different organ damage. The deleterious effects of alcohol on the brain have been known since the last century (Wernicke, 1881, Korsakoff, 1887). Today they can be recognized at the morphological, molecular, and neurochemical levels. Alcohol is rapidly incorporated into biological membranes with consequent changes in ion channel (Roach, 1979), receptor (Charness *et al.*, 1983) and neurotransmitter (Littleton, 1978) functions. At present there is no clear understanding of the inter-relationships between identified morphological, molecular and neurochemical abnormalities and hence a clear understanding of the mechanisms of actions of alcohol on the central nervous system eludes us.

This chapter briefly reviews the classic knowledge of alcohol's damaging effects on the brain. Special emphasis is given to the results of neuroimaging studies and new experimental neuropathologic work, that has been accomplished consecutively. The role of scientists from the European community is emphasized and shortcomings of our research are outlined. Results of electrophysiological and neuropsychological studies are not discussed.

2. NEUROPATHOLOGY IN HUMANS

2.1. Fetal alcohol syndrome (FAS)

Aristotle observed differences in children whose mothers were high consumers of alcohol and of mothers who were not. This was the first description of the fetal alcohol syndrome (FAS), which was "rediscovered" in 1968 by French scientists (Lemoine, *et al.*). As a research paradigm, it has a major impact on our understanding of alcohol's effects on the brain. Clinically the FAS is characterized by:

- growth retardation involving height, weight, and head circumference,
- deficient intellectual and social performance and muscular coordination,
- minor structural anomalies of the face together with more variable involvement of the limbs and the heart.

The basis of this pathology is a cascade of effects that alcohol exerts on the developing cell. Under normal conditions growth factors enhance the growth of cells and their differentiation. Alcohol can diminish these effects (Dow and Riopelle, 1985). A second way of damaging the developing nerve cell is the production of free radicals. They allow calcium to accumulate in the cells (Kukreja and Hess, 1992). The induction of free radical formation is induced by alcohol. The result of both pathogenic processes is a decrease in the overall size of the brain and a diminution in the thickness of the outer layers of the cortex, due to decreases in the total numbers of cells. Impaired nerve cell migration might also play a role in the development of FAS (Miller, 1993).

Clarren *et al.* (1978) studied autopsy specimens of brains from four infants with FAS. Two of them had hydrocephalus. One infant's brain had no corpus callosum and anterior commissure. Two had dilated ventricles, a small cerebellum, and poorly defined pons and medulla. Volk *et al.* (1981) observed impaired maturation of Purkinje cells in rats with FAS. It appears that ethanol can alter both the early phase of brain embryogenesis as well as the later phases of brain growth, including glial cell proliferation and migration. These findings are supported by animal studies. Here again microcephaly is found as well as alterations in the proliferation and migration of neurons and abnormalities of the cerebellum (West and Pierce, 1986; Miller, 1993).

The effects of alcohol on the developing brain are clinically measured by assessing the head circumference. It shows a clear dose dependent effect (Coles *et al.*, 1991). The children of women who stopped drinking at the second trimester had smaller head circumferences than children of women who never drank. The smallest head circumferences were found in women that continued alcohol consumption throughout pregnancy. Some of the above mentioned features were also detected *in vivo* by a magnetic resonance imaging (MRI) study. Mattson *et al.* (in press) found a reduction in the overall brain volume and in the volume of the basal ganglia in four children with FAS. Additionally, one child had an agenesis of the corpus callosum. In another child, the corpus callosum was thinner than normal. A similar effect was found in ten children who did not have the symptoms of FAS, but whose mothers had been drinking excessively during pregnancy. The volumes of their corpus callosum and thalamus were reduced.

2.2. Wernicke's Encephalopathy

The best known features of heavy alcohol consumption in adults are Wernicke's encephalopathy (WE) and Korsakoff' syndrome (KS). WE is directly caused by thiamine deficiency which results from a combination of inadequate dietary intake, reduced gastrointestinal absorption, decreased hepatic storage, and impaired utilization. Only a subset of thiamine-deficient alcoholics develop Wernicke's encephalopathy, perhaps because they have inherited or acquired abnormalities of the thiamine-dependent enzyme transketolase that reduces its affinity for thiamine. Wernicke's encephalopathy is characterized by degenerative changes including gliosis and small hemorrhages in structures surrounding the third ventricle and aqueduct, i.e. the mammillary bodies, hypothalamus, mediodorsal thalamic nucleus, colliculi and midbrain tegmentum. Clinical features associated with the Wernicke-Korsakoff syndrome include memory deficits, ocular signs, ataxia and global confusional states. Most can be related to damaged functional systems in the hypothalamus, midbrain and cerebellum (Peiffer, 1985). In a large neuropathologic study from Scandinavia, 12.5 % of all alcoholics exhibited signs of WE (Torvik *et al.*, 1982).

2.3. Korsakoff 's syndrome

About 80% of alcoholic patients recovering from Wernicke's encephalopathy develop Korsakoff's amnestic syndrome. It is characterized by marked deficits in anterograde and retrograde memory, apathy, an intact sensorium, and relative preservation of other intellectual abilities. Korsakoff's amnestic syndrome may also appear without an antecedent episode of Wernicke's encephalopathy. Acute lesions may be superimposed on chronic lesions, suggesting that subclinical episodes of Wernicke's encephalopathy may culminate in Korsakoff's amnestic syndrome. The memory disorder correlates best with the presence of histopathological lesions in the dorsomedial thalamus. Korsakoff's amnestic syndrome is an infrequent sequela of Wernicke's encephalopahty in nonalcoholics. This observation has led to speculation that ethanol neurotoxicity is an important contributing factor in the memory disorders of alcoholics. Although it is certainly possible that neurotoxic effects of ethanol may worsen the cerebral disorder of thiamine deficiency, it is also clear that Korsakoff's amnestic syndrome can occur in the absence of ethanol. Accounts of thiamine deficiency in prisoners of war include descriptions of some individuals with enduring disorders of mental function. More recent cases provide clearer descriptions of Korsakoff's amnestic syndrome following Wernicke's encephalopathy in nonalcoholics. Quantitative brain morphometry in these uncommon patients will indicate whether ventricular enlargement, shrinkage of cerebral white matter, selective neuronal loss, and simplification of dendritic arbors are specific lesions of ethanol neurotoxicity or previously unrecognized manifestations of thiamine deficiency (Harper, 1993).

2.4. Cerebellar degeneration

Many alcoholic patients develop a chronic cerebellar syndrome related to the degeneration of Purkinje cells in the cerebellar cortex. Quantitative studies revealed a significant loss of cerebellar Purkinje cells by 10%–35% and shrinkage of the cerebellar vermal, molecular and granular cell layers (Torvik and Torp, 1986; Phillips *et al.*, 1987). Evidence for a direct toxic effect of ethanol as the cause is provided by animal models (Riley and Walker, 1978; Volk, 1984). In neuroimaging studies, however, cerebellar ataxia in alcoholics does not correlate with daily, annual, or lifetime consumption of ethanol. As in Wernicke's encephalopathy, thiamine deficiency due to poor nutrition has also been implicated. Cerebellar atrophy has been reported to occur in about 40% of chronic alcoholics (Torvik and Torp, 1986). In our own study of inpatient alcoholics 49% had at least discrete clinical signs of cerebellar atrophy (Mann, 1992).

The diagnosis of alcoholic cerebellar ataxia is based on the clinical history and neurological examination. The ataxia affects the gait most severely. Limb ataxia and dysarthria occur more often than in Wernicke's encephalopathy, whereas nystagmus is rare. CT or MRI scans may show cerebellar cortical atrophy, but a considerable number of alcoholic patients with this finding are not ataxic on examination. Whether these represent subclinical cases in which symptoms will develop subsequently is unclear. It is interesting to note, that impaired cerebellar function improves significantly when abstinence is maintained (Diener *et al.*, 1984).

2.5. Hepatocerebral degeneration

Hepatic encephalopathy develops in many alcoholics with liver disease, and is characterized by altered sensorium, frontal release signs, asterixis, hyperreflexia, extensor plantar responses, and occasional seizures. Whereas some patients progress from stupor to coma and then death, others recover and suffer recurrent episodes. Brains of patients with hepatic encephalopathy show enlargement and proliferation of protoplasmic astrocytes in the basal ganglia, thalamus, red nucleus, pons, and cerebellum, in the absence of neuronal loss or other glial changes.

Patients who do not recover fully after an episode of hepatic encephalopathy go on to develop a progressive syndrome of tremor, choreoathetosis, dysarthria, gait ataxia, and dementia. Hepatocerebral degeneration may progress in a step-wise fashion, with incomplete recovery after each episode of hepatic encephalopathy, or slowly and inexorably, without a discrete episode of encephalopathy. Brain examination reveals astrocytic proliferation, laminar necrosis in the cortex, patchy loss of neurons throughout the cortex, basal ganglia, and cerebellum, and cavitation of the cortico-subcortical junction and superior pole of the putamen (Charness, 1993).

2.6. Marchiafava-Bignami syndrome

Marchiafava-Bignami syndrome is a rare disorder of demyelination or necrosis of the corpus callosum and adjacent subcortical white matter. Harper (1993) describes only one case in 10 years (approximately 10,000 brains). The incidence seems to be higher in France where 17 cases of MFB disease were diagnosed from 8200 necropsies, a prevalence of 0.21% (Hauw *et al.*, 1988). Nine of the cases were associated with pellagra-like changes in the central nervous system. In the same study, the prevalence of WKS was 1.35% which compares with 1.7% and 2.8% from two similar studies (Cravioto *et al.*, 1961; Harper, 1983).

The course may be acute, subacute, or chronic, and is marked by dementia, spasticity, dysarthria, and inability to walk. Patients may lapse into coma and die, survive for many years in a demented condition, or occasionally recover. The disorder was formerly diagnosed only at autopsy, but lesions can now be imaged using CT or MRI.

2.7. Central pontine myelinolysis

Central pontine myelinolysis is a disorder of cerebral white matter that usually affects alcoholics, but also occurs in nonalcoholics with liver disease, including Wilson's disease, malnutrition, anorexia, burns, cancer, Addison's disease, and severe electrolyte disorders, such as thiazide-induced hyponatremia. Central pontine myelinolysis is frequently associated with a rapid correction of hyponatremia; however, the majority of cases occur in alcoholics, suggesting that alcoholism may contribute to the genesis of central pontine myelinolysis in yet undefined ways (Charness, 1993).

The most common macroscopic lesion is a triangular region of pallor in the base of the pons. Approximately 10% of human cases also have symmetric extrapontine lesions, most frequently in the striatum, thalamus, cerebellum, and cerebral white matter. Microscopic examination reveals demyelinated axons with preserved cell bodies except in the center of lesions, which may show cavitation. Myelinolytic lesions can be induced experimentally by rapid correction of chronic hyponatremia.

The lesions of central pontine myelinolysis can be visualized using CT scanning or MRI (e.g. Schroth and Mann, 1989). MRI is more sensitive than CT in imaging the pontine lesions; however, even MRI may be unremarkable early in the course of central pontine myelinolysis. Serial CT or MRI studies indicate that the radiographic lesions may resolve in parallel with patient recovery (Schroth, 1984); thus, the absence of lesions on MRI does not exclude the previous occurence of central pontine myelinolysis.

2.8. Cerebral cortex

Although the majority of the tissue loss from the cerebral hemispheres in alcoholics is accounted for by a reduction in the volume of the cerebral white matter, there is also generally a slight reduction in the volume of the cerebral cortex. This has been demonstrated both pathologically (de la Monte, 1988) and using MRI with quantitative morphometry (Jernigan *et al.*, 1991).

Measurements of cortical thickness have rarely been reported, but Mayes *et al.* (1988) noted a reduction in the frontal region. At the microscopic level several authors have subjectively described a patchy loss of cortical neurones in alcoholics (Courville, 1955; Victor *et al.*, 1971). The first controlled study documenting neuronal loss in alcoholics was done by Harper *et al.* (1987). There was a 22% reduction in the number of neurons in the superior frontal cortex (Brodmann's area 8), but no significant change in the primary motor (area 4), frontal cingulate (area 32) or inferior temporal (areas 20 and 36) cortices (Harper and Kril, 1989). The surviving neurons showed shrinkage in the superior frontal, motor and frontal cingulate cortices (Harper *et al.*, 1987; Harper and Kril, 1989). This finding of cortical damage in alcoholics is consistent with a neuroradiological study (Jernigan *et al.*, 1991). However, it was not confirmed by a recent post mortem study from Denmark (Jensen and Pakkenberg, 1993). These authors counted neurons in a three-dimensional way. Cell numbers did not differ between alcoholics and controls in the frontal, parietal and occipital lobe, nor in hippocampus.

An explanation of these divergent findings may be that there are particular groups of neurons which are more likely to be damaged. An analysis of the pattern of neuronal loss from the superior frontal cortex in alcoholics revealed that large pyramidal neurons, with a somal area greater than 90 μm^2, were selectively lost (Harper and Kril, 1989). This population of large neurons has been recognised as being more vulnerable in both Alzheimer's disease (Terry *et al.*, 1981) and the normal aging process (Terry and Hansen, 1987). There is no evidence to suggest that particular layers of the cerebral cortex are more vulnerable than others (Harper and Kril, 1989). Analysis of cortical neuronal counts in the different alcoholic groups revealed that there is no significant difference between those alcoholics with WKS or cirrhosis of the liver and the uncomplicated alcoholics (Harper and Kril, 1989). This finding suggests that alcohol abuse is responsible for the neuronal loss in the superior frontal cortex and that the additional complication of WKS, although significantly contributing to the brain shrinkage in alcoholics, does not accentuate neuronal loss.

Subpopulations of cortical neurons can now be identified on the basis of their neurochemical content using immunohistochemistry (Beal and Martin, 1986). These techniques have yet to be applied to alcohol-related brain damage. There is some neurochemical and neuropharmacological data to suggest that these techniques might provide useful information (Tran *et al.*, 1981; Freund and Ballinger, 1988a and b). Ultrastructural studies have not been possible using human material. However, Spanish researchers (Ferrer *et al.*, 1986) and Harper and Corbett (1990) have examined and measured the dendritic arbor of cortical neurons in alcoholic subjects using Golgi impregnation techniques. They described a significant reduction in the basal dendritic arbor of layer III pyramidal neurons in both the superior frontal and motor cortices. These studies suggest that even though there is not a significant reduction in numbers of cortical neurons in the motor cortex there are cellular structural abnormalities which could have important functional implications.

3. NEUROPATHOLOGICAL STUDIES IN ANIMAL MODELS

3.1. Alteration of neural cells

Few studies were done in regard to the effect of long term ethanol exposure on the number of neural cells in the hippocampus. The results suggest that ethanol exposure leads to a 10 to 40 percent loss of ventral hippocampal pyramidal cells (Bengoechea and Gonzalo 1991; Cadete-Leite *et al.*, 1989b; Lescaudron and Verna, 1985; Phillips and Cragg, 1983; Walker *et al.*, 1980, 1981). Ethanol exposure also results in a loss of granule cells of the dentate gyrus (Walker *et al.*, 1980b, 1981; Cadete-Leite *et al.*, 1988a,b; Durand *et al.*, 1989) and local circuit interneurons in the hippocampus (Lescaudron *et al.*,

1986) and dentate gyrus (Scheetz *et al.*, 1987a). It is hypothesized that hippocampal pyramidal neurons may be more sensitive to neuronal loss induced by ethanol exposure than
granule cells of the dentate gyrus (Bengoechea and Gonzalo, 1991). It also seems that
pyramidal cells and interneurons located in the ventral portion of the hippocampus are
more sensitive to ethanol exposure than those in the dorsal hippocampus (Lescaudron
and Verna, 1985; Lescaudron *et al.*, 1986). The results of Phillips and Cragg (1983)
suggest that the neuronal loss of pyramidal cells mainly occurred during the withdrawal
period, rather than during ethanol exposure. Loss of granule cells of the dentate gyrus
may also continue through to the withdrawal period (Cadete-Leite, 1988a, 1989a).

The results of Scheetz *et al.* (1987a,b) suggest that there is a genetic susceptibility to
ethanol neurotoxicity. They found that ethanol exposure did not affect the number of
interneurons in the dentate gyrus of ethanol-resistant short-sleep mice, whereas in long-
sleep mice cell frequency was reduced. Neuronal loss results in partial deafferentiation of
surviving neurons. This leads to changes in dendritic morphology which recovers with
time due to sprouting of undamaged afferents (Parnavelas *et al.*, 1974; Cotman and
Nadler, 1978). It is important to know if these mechanisms also appear after ethanol
exposure and if surviving neurons are structurally altered. It has been noted that ethanol
exposure reduces the spine size on dendrites of mouse hippocampal neurons (Phillips
and Cragg, 1983; Lescaudron *et al.*, 1989). It is hypothesised that hippocampal pyramid
cells and dentate gyrus granule cells respond in an opposite manner to ethanol exposure
and withdrawal. After ethanol exposure without withdrawal the dendrites of surviving
hippocampal pyramidal cells exhibit attenuated dendritic branches and/or reduced density
of dendritic spines. These regressive changes revert to near normal or recover completely
during ethanol withdrawal (McMullen *et al.*, 1984; Lescaudron and Verna, 1985; King
et al., 1988; Lescaudron *et al.*, 1989). Conversely, granule cells of the dentate gyrus that
survived ethanol exposure without withdrawal showed compensatory hypertrophy of both
soma and dendrites, which regressed to control level during ethanol withdrawal (Cadete-
Leite *et al.*, 1989a). Scheetz *et al.* (1987b) reported that ethanol exposure reduced the
density of spines and spine synapses in the stratum oriens of the hippocampus in long-
sleep but not in short-sleep mice. It is suggested that ethanol intake limits morphological
recovery from brain damage. The experiments reported yet have examined the effect of
ethanol on reactive synaptogenesis and axonal sprouting after a unilateral lesion in the
entorhinal cortex and found an inhibition of these mechanisms (Lind *et al.*, 1988).
These authors also found that abstinence from ethanol released the supression of axonal
sprouting.

In the cerebellum Tavares and Paula-Barbosa (1982) found that administration of
ethanol for 6 months significantly reduced the number of granule and stellate cells. On
the other hand, significant decreases in the number of basket and Purkinje cells required
12 to 18 months of treatment and the number of Golgi cells was stable even after
18 months of treatment (Tavares *et al.*, 1987a). It must be outlined, however, that the
daily alcohol doses given to the animals were much lower than the consumption in
human alcoholics. The greater vulnerability of granule cells may be due to differences in
the enzymatic properties of the cerebellar cell types. It may be possible that regression of
the other cerebellar neurons ocurred transsynaptically because of parallel fiber regression
and partial deafferentiation. If this is true, the rapidity and extent of regression would

depend on the degree of dependence of parallel fiber innervation. This hypothesis may be supported by the results of some investigations (Tavares *et al.*, 1983b; Phillips, 1985; Tavares *et al.*, 1987b). Conversely, there is evidence that intrinsic neuronal organization or metabolism influences neuronal sensitivity to ethanol (Pentney, 1979, 1982; Tavares *et al.*, 1983; Tavares *et al.*, 1985). Current evidence suggests that rat cerebellar neurons that survive 12 months of ethanol exposure will show some hypertrophy of the dendritic tree (Tavares *et al.*, 1983; 1985; 1987b; Pentney *et al.*, 1989; Pentney, 1991).

3.2. Alteration of glial cells and white matter

Little is known about the affection of glial cells and white matter due to the exposure to ethanol. Sun *et al.*, (1980) reported reductions in myelin isolated from the brains of animals given ethanol chronically. The results of Sedmak *et al.* (1978) point in the same direction. Significant inhibition of cerebral protein breakdown was reported after chronic ethanol exposure (Toth and Lajtha, 1984). Rosengren *et al.* (1985) reported gliosis following chronic ethanol exposure and an increase of DNA without changes of the astroglial marker S-100 protein. Neuronal, astroglial and oligodendroglial cell bodies contain P450IIE1, an enzyme that is active in ethanol oxidation. In the neocortex, olfactory bulb, piriform cortex and thalamic nuclei this enzyme is found in both neuronal and glial cell types. In the cerebellum it is only found in the glial cells. Thus, glial cells may have an active role in metabolizing ethanol in the brain (Hanson *et al.*, 1990).

Astrocytes maintain a certain amount of plasticity in their ability to respond to various injuries and can divide and proliferate throughout life (Kimelberg and Norenberg, 1989). Current research suggests that astroglia also participate in neurotransmission (Teichberg, 1991). For the future it is very important to make more efforts in investigating the role of glial cells in the response of the brain to ethanol.

3.3. Receptor changes

Knowledge about the effects of ethanol on excitatory and inhibitory receptors in the CNS seems to be of great importance for the understanding of ethanol induced brain damage. Available evidence suggests that chronic exposure of animals to ethanol blocks brain glutamate receptors. Consequently, an up-regulation of these receptors is observed. This mechanism might be important in producing an increased susceptibility to excitotoxicity and withdrawal seizures (Dildy and Leslie, 1989; Lovinger *et al.*, 1989, 1990; White *et al.*, 1990).

The GABA receptor complex is structurally altered by ethanol exposure leading to hypofunction and reduction of receptor density on the cell membrane. This implies that neurons normally inhibited via GABA receptors will be disinhibited, contributing to increased neural excitability in ethanol withdrawal (Ticku, 1980; Ticku and Burch, 1980; Morrow *et al.*, 1990; Montpied *et al.*, 1991). Ethanol also alters the expression of the second messenger G-protein (Mochly-Rosen *et al.*, 1988; Pietrzak *et al.*, 1990). Ethanol inhibits the uptake of Ca^{2+} which is an ubiquitous link in stimulus-secretion coupling (Harris and Hood, 1980; Leslie *et al.*, 1983). Ethanol administration leads to a proliferation of voltage dependent calcium channels (Rius *et al.*, 1987). This phenomenon may also be responsible for hyperexcitability and excitotoxicity as well as the increased sensitivity of glutamate receptors and hypofunction of GABA receptors.

4. NEUROIMAGING STUDIES

4.1. Computed Tomography and Magnetic Resonance Imaging Studies

4.1.1. Brain morphology

Since 1978, various CT and MRI studies have demonstrated cortical and subcortical brain damage in alcohol-dependent patients, even when thiamine deficiency was not present (Bergman *et al.*, 1980; Wilkinson and Carlen, 1980; Ron *et al.*, 1982; Jernigan *et al.*, 1991; Mann *et al.*, 1991). These findings did not conform with the mainstream of neuropathologic thinking, as discussed above. Traditionally, brain atrophy in alcoholics was attributed to thiamine deficiency and was restricted mainly to subcortical structures (Victor *et al.*, 1971). Reports on cortical atrophy (Courville, 1955) were questioned as well as the possibility of a direct neurotoxic effect of ethanol (Victor and Adams, 1985).

Against this background *in vivo* neuroimaging techniques, such as computerized tomography (CT) and magnetic resonance imaging (MRI) promised to be a means of clarification. They make it possible to quantify macroscopic structural brain changes and can be used to determine if changes progress with continued drinking or reverse during periods of abstinence. Indeed, a high proportion of subjects showed brain abnormalities even when there had been no reason to suspect the Wernicke-Korsakoff syndrome or other forms of brain damage (Lishman, 1981). In repeated series from Canada, Sweden, Germany, and England it was found that perhaps a half to two-thirds of alcoholics showed diffuse brain changes — enlargement of the ventricles and fissures, and a degree of widening of the cortical sulci (Carlen *et al.*, 1978; Bergman *et al.*, 1980; Ron *et al.*, 1982, Schroth *et al.*, 1985). These were patients attending ordinary treatment facilities, some series even being recruited from heavy drinkers selected from the community (Bergman *et al.*, 1980).

Numerous CT observations of enlarged ventricles in alcoholics (as reviewed by Lishman, 1990) lend credence to the concept that heavy alcohol consumption leads to brain tissue loss, or brain damage. However, CT limited capability for differentiating between white matter and grey matter precludes reliable determination of which tissue type is most affected by chronic alcohol consumption. Furthermore, beam hardening artifact on CT distorts the representation of tissue and fluid material adjacent to bone, making it difficult to obtain accurate estimates of the integrity of cortical sulci, and thus the cortical regions more affected. In contrast, MR images are not distorted by bone; can provide coronal, sagittal, and axial views of the brain; and yield images with better resolution and excellent contrast between white and grey matter (Mann and Bartels, 1992). An additional advantage of MR imaging is that, being free of ionizing radiation, MR scans can be repeated in longitudinal studies without exposing patients to radiation risk.

Many different approaches have been used to assess ventricular or sulcal size on CT or MR images. One approach is to compare images with clinical standards, use a qualitative rating scale, or rank them against one another (Ron *et al.*, 1982; Schroth and Mann, 1989). Another approach involves linear measures of ventricular or sulcal width at various points or tracing ventricular boundaries to calculate area on individual sections (Mann *et al.*, 1991).

Computerized techniques to measure the volume of these CSF-filled spaces, rather than the area of just a single slice, have also been developed and can provide an efficient and reliable approach to image analysis. One such technique involves classifying each pixel as either CSF or tissue for CT scans (Pfefferbaum *et al.*, 1986; Mann *et al.*, 1989) or as CSF and white and grey matter for MRI scans (Schroth *et al.*, 1988). The number of pixels assigned to each compartment in anatomically or geometrically defined regions can be summed mathematically to provide an estimate of the volume of CSF and grey or white matter in that region of interest (ROI). ROIs can include the entire brain, each hemisphere, specific cortical lobes or segments thereof, or subcortical regions such as the diencephalon, caudate nuclei, or lenticular nuclei (Lim and Pfefferbaum, 1989).

Investigators are also exploiting the fine structural resolution in MR images to measure discrete neuroanatomic structures, such as the mammillary bodies (Charness and DeLaPaz, 1987) or the hippocampus (Lim *et al.*, 1990). Thus, MRI offers investigators an opportunity to assess not only global morphological changes, but also alterations in more specific neuroanatomic structures.

Is there a *differential sensitivity of different parts of the brain* to alcohol? This question has entertained many researchers. It is comfounded by the frequent coincidence of several neurological complications of alcoholism, including hepatocerebral degeneration, malnutrition and Wernicke's encephalopathy (WE), head trauma, and others. We do know, however, that even without evidence for WE or Korsakoff's syndrome, a large proportion of alcohol dependent patients exhibit signs of cerebellar atrophy (Lindboe and Loberg, 1988; Mann, 1992). Most post mortem and neuroimaging studies also agree on white matter atrophy and to a lesser extent on damage in the cortex (see chapter 2.8). Many authors describe an overall effect on both hemispheres of the brain often with an accentuation in the prefrontal areas and the diencephalon. In a recent MRI study this specific question was studied. Shear and collegues (1992) found brain shrinkage throughout all peripheral cortical areas studied. Thus, the idea of a "mild, generalized impairment" was strengthened.

4.1.2. Role of intervening variables

Age: Increases in the size of the lateral ventricles and cortical sulci associated with chronic alcohol use were observed *in vivo* using CT (Fox *et al.*, 1976; Bergman *et al.*, 1980; Lishman, 1981; Schroth *et al.*, 1985: Mann *et al.*, 1989), and MRI (Schroth *et al.*, 1988; Chick *et al.*, 1989; Zipursky *et al.*, 1989). MRI studies have confirmed and extended CT studies by showing that with chronic alcohol abuse CSF spaces increase not only subcortically (lateral and third ventricles) but also cortically, with enlarged sulci and subarachnoid spaces affecting all cortices. Furthermore, MRI has shown that increases in CSF volumes are accompanied by reductions in grey (Jernigan *et al.*, 1991; Pfefferbaum *et al.*, 1992) and white (Pfefferbaum *et al.*, 1992) matter volumes, as well as an increase in areas of white matter hyperintensity (Gallucci *et al.*, 1989; Jernigan *et al.*, 1991). The involvement of white matter confirms neuropathological studies, which have reported white matter volume changes seen *in vivo* and may be due to artifacts in specimen preparation and fixation affecting grey matter specifically (grey matter has a higher water content than white matter). It may also be due to the failure to adequately control for the confounding effects of normal age-related changes on grey matter (Jernigan *et al.*, 1990; Lim *et al.*, 1992; Pfefferbaum *et al.*, 1992).

Using an age regression model, Pfefferbaum *et al.* (1988, 1992) have found that CSF volumes exceed age norms to a greater extent in old than young alcoholics. This finding could reflect the cumulative effect of a lifetime of alcohol exposure, the greater vulnerability of the aging brain, or some combination of both. In the first (CT) study (Pfefferbaum *et al.*, 1988), 37 male veteran alcoholics, ranging in age from 26 to 62 years, were studied. In this sample, age and lifetime consumption of alcohol were related; that is, many older alcoholics had been drinking all their lives. Thus, they not only had older brains, but also had experienced the cumulative toxicity of a lifetime of alcohol exposure.

The second (MRI) study (Pfefferbaum *et al.*, 1992) of 49 veteran alcoholics, ranging in age from 23 to 70 years, also found that CSF volumes exceed age norms to a greater extent in old than young alcoholics. In this sample, however, there was no relationship between age, disease duration, or total lifetime intake of ethanol, confirming results described by Mann (1992). The results of these studies are consistent with the proposal that the accelerating association between age and brain damage can be attributed more to the greater vulnerability of the aged brain than to the cumulative effects of a lifetime of exposure of alcohol, a result that was described by European researchers before (Lishman *et al.*, 1981; Mann *et al.*, 1989).

The observed reduction in brain tissue in alcohol-dependent patients is the result of a multifactorial process. A primary candidate is alcohol consumption itself. Direct investigations of the *in vivo* role of alcohol as a neurotoxic or demyelinating agent in humans is of necessity sparse. Animal models provide support (see also Chapter 3.1) for the notion that ethanol is destructive of both white matter (Hansen *et al.*, 1991; Lancaster *et al.*, 1984; Popova and Frumkina, 1985) and grey matter (Pentney and Quackenbush, 1990). However, in humans there is often a surprising lack of association between the amount of alcohol consumed and the amount of cortical shrinkage, as measured by ventricular enlargement on CT or MRI (Lishman, 1990; Mann, 1992). This phenomenon parallels the considerable range in apparent vulnerability to other physiologically devastating effects of alcohol, such as liver damage and cardiovascular disease.

Impaired nutrition is a frequent sequela of chronic alcohol abuse and one that possibly interacts with alcohol exposure to produce liver disease (Lieber, 1989) and pathological changes in the brain (Pratt *et al.*, 1990). Illnesses such as anorexia nervosa involving extreme malnourishment are associated with brain ventricular enlargement, which reverses to some extent with treatment (Krieg *et al.*, 1989). However, alcoholics recruited to research protocols tend not to be severely malnourished at the time of scanning and sometimes even exceed body mass index norms (Agartz *et al.*, 1991), yet they still exhibit brain shrinkage.

Genetic influences: Considerable interest exists in the possibility of a genetic basis for susceptibility to alcohol dependence and/or vulnerability to its deleterious effects. However, neither twin studies nor studies that take family history of alcoholism into account provide much support that the neuroanatomic changes described above would serve as genetic markers that precede disease onset rather than reflect its progression. (Gurling *et al.*, 1984, 1986) have studied monozygotic twins showing discordance for alcoholism and report differences in brain and ventricular volumes, as well as localized brain density measures between the severely dependent and normal drinking cotwins. Twins discordant for less severe levels of alcoholism did not show significant differences. Ron (1983) found no differerence between family-history-positive and family-history-negative alcoholics in the CT neuroanatomic measures, nor did Mann (1992) in his sample of German alcoholics.

Gender: Increasing interest is being paid to the phenomenon of alcoholism among women (Schmidt *et al.*, 1990), its more intense somatic sequelae (Glenn *et al.*, 1989; Haberman and Natarajan, 1989; Jones-Saumty *et al.*, 1981), and mechanisms to account for these sex differences (Frezza *et al.*, 1990). Few *in vivo* brain imaging studies have been reported on women to address the question of whether the brains of alcoholic women are more vulnerable than those of men to the effects of alcohol. This is a complex question in which sex related physiological variables that affect metabolism such as fat/fluid body composition, body/brain size, as well as sex related differences in patterns of alcohol consumption and recognition of alcohol dependence need careful consideration. Jacobson's CT study (1986) examined some of these issues. Its findings are consistent with studies of liver disease (VanThiel and Gavaler, 1988) and neuropsychological functioning (Hochla and Parsons, 1982; Acker *et al.*, 1986) in suggesting that women are more vulnerable than men to the effects of alcohol. In an independent group design Jacobsen found that alcoholic women had similar levels of ventricular enlargement compared to alcoholic men, but after drinking less alcohol for shorter periods. These findings persisted, even after the effects of different body weight and head size were considered. In a prospective test-retest design we reported similar findings (Mann *et al.*, 1992a). Again there was no difference in the amount of brain atrophy between men and women, the men, however, having a significantly longer drinking history. In contrast, a study of a large (n = 400) random sample of men and women from the general population (Bergman *et al.*, 1983) found that women who were classified as "alcohol-dependent", based on their reported alcohol consumption and associated behaviors, were not significantly different in CT measures of ventricular enlargement than those classified as "low-consumers". In contrast, "alcohol-dependent" men had significantly larger ventricles than "low-consumer" men. MRI studies of alcoholic women are underway in several laboratories, but few data have yet been published. One report, based on only 10 alcoholic women, noted that all but 1 subject had ventricular volumes within normal limits of their age (Kroft *et al.*, 1991).

Ethnic variability as a moderating variable in alcoholic brain damage has not been studied systematically so far. The same is true for *the severity of dependency*. Only Melgaard *et al.* (1986) looked at this question. In this Danish study, they were unable to find a correlation between the severity scores of alcoholism and cerebral atrophy. However, they used the Missouri Alcohol Severity Scale, which does not differentiate between the dependence syndrome per se (Edwards and Gross, 1977) and the somatic consequences of heavy consumption. This could be a task for future research.

4.1.3. Reversibility of brain damage

The possibility that abstinence could reverse alcohol-related neuroanatomic brain changes was first demonstrated by Carlen *et al.* (1978) using CT. They confirmed older pneumencephalographic reports that had not been taken serious (e.g. Kircher and Pierson, 1956). Subsequent CT studies of larger samples (Artmann *et al.*, 1981; Mann *et al.*, 1991; Muuronen *et al.*, 1989; Ron, 1983; Schroth *et al.*, 1985) have confirmed reversibility of ventricular enlargement in a proportion of abstinent alcoholics over periods of months to years. Muuronen *et al.* (1989) performed a 5-year follow up of a sample of alcoholic patients initially scanned in 1977–79. Of the 37 patients retested, 16 were classified as abstinent and 21 were still drinking. Ventricular size at follow up was reduced relative to the first assessment in the abstainers but not in the drinkers, implying some reversibility. Ventricles in the abstainers at follow up, however, were still enlarged relative to a nonalcoholic control group.

The reversibility effect is quite small and requires reliable quantitative techniques to be detected. In one study (Zipursky *et al.*, 1989), ventricular volume declined approximately 15 percent during withdrawal. In one of the reports of Carlen *et al.* (1984), long-term reversibility was greater in patients who had their first scan shortly after their last drink, implying that reversibility was mainly accomplished during the initial withdrawal period. Some studies, using MRI (Schroth *et al.*, 1988; Zipursky *et al.*, 1989), have since established that some reversibility does occur within the first few weeks of abstinence. However, one study testing at 36 hours and 10 days after last drink found no change in CT measures (Claus *et al.*, 1987).

The fact that some reduction in brain tissue and increase in CSF volume may be reversible has led to the use of the term "shrinkage", although "atrophy" would be appropriate as well. One hypothesis regarding the reversibility of ventricular and sulcal enlargement with abstinence refers relative brain tissue rehydration during withdrawal. An approach to investigating this hypothesis is to measure the relaxation times of protons from magnetic resonance images of the brain.

4.2. Studies with MRI-relaxation times and MR-spectroscopy

For a given set of acquisition parameters, the signal intensity of an MR image is determined by the spin density and relaxation rates of the protons that generate the image. Some investigators measure relaxation times (T1 and T2) within designated ROIs as the variable of interest. T1 is an exponential time constant measuring the time taken for nuclei to return to equilibrium and realign with the magnetic field, whereas T2 describes signal loss due to interference between nuclei. (T1 and T2 refer to longitudinal and transverse relaxation times, respectively.) T1 is prolonged as the proportion of free to bound water within brain tissue increases (MacDonald *et al.*, 1986). T2 shows similar though slightly less precise function (Bottomley *et al.*, 1984; Fu *et al.*, 1990). Thus, T1 and T2 reflect brain hydration status and offer an approach to assessing the contribution of changes in hydration status to the morphological brain alterations seen in alcoholism (Besson *et al*, 1981; Schroth *et al.*, 1988; Mann *et al.*, 1989; Chick *et al.*, 1989; Mann *et al.*, 1993).

Despite some elegant findings with animal models and the apparent face validity of the relaxation times as a measure of brain hydration, application of this technology to the study of alcohol withdrawal has produced inconsistent results. Since 1981, when Besson *et al.*, reported shorter brain T1s in both grey and white matter in intoxicated alcoholics, which lengthened during withdrawal and abstinence (1 to 6 weeks), there has been a series of studies, many with limited control data, that sampled at different time points and reported conflicting results (Besson *et al.*, 1981, 1989a; Schroth *et al.*, 1988; Smith *et al.*, 1985, 1988). Chick *et al.* (1989) found longer T1s in grey and white matter in the alcoholics measured 2 weeks postwithdrawal, whereas Agartz *et al.* (1991), in a study of comparable design, but using a lower field instrument, found no differences in T1 or T2 between alcoholics and controls. Both studies found correlations between atrophy and T1 (Mander *et al.*, 1989), suggesting that partial voluming (some CSF present in what appears to be a tissue voxel) may contribute to the increased T1 seen in alcoholics. In a recent paper Mann *et al.* (1993) reports a significant drop in CSF volume in a 5-week follow up of abstinent alcoholics. The authors did not observe an increase in T2 times nor in spectroscopically measured T1 times, which would have been predicted if brain tissue rehydration underlay CSF reduction seen with abstinence.

In an autopsy study, Harper *et al.* (1988) concluded that brain shrinkage in alcoholics is not caused by changes in hydration. Drinking status of their sample at time of death, which may have a profound bearing on the state of hydration of the alcoholic's brains, was not reported. In summary, the data on T1 and its relationship to brain hydration are conflicting. Besides possible unreliability of this measure (Bottomley *et al.*, 1987), crucial factors appear to be the time following ethanol withdrawal, adequate tissue sampling to avoid partial voluming effects, and the need for nonalcoholic control values.

MR-spectroscopy: Single voxel (smallest volume of resolution) MRS can detect relative brain tissue concentrations of various endogenous metabolites, especially protons and phosphorus, as well as some exogenous compounds in delimited VOIs (Dager and Steen, 1992). Recent developments in spectroscopic imaging now make it possible to characterize the distribution of these metabolites throughout the brain (Spielman *et al.*, 1992). With proton spectroscopic imaging it is possible to identify peaks representing N-acetyl aspartate (observed primarily in viable neurons), creatine (an energy metabolite), and choline (a precursor to acetylcholine and a constituent of cell membrane synthesis). This technique has only recently been used to assess the constituency of brain tissue in chronic alcoholics (Martin *et al.*, 1995). The spectroscopic visibility of ethanol has also been demonstrated (Hanstock *et al.*, 1990; Mann and Bartels, 1992) and opens the possibility of *in vivo* assessments of acute uptake and distribution of ethanol in the brain.

4.3. Studies of Brain Function with Positron Emission Tomography (PET)

Single photon emission computed tomography (SPECT) and positron emission tomography (PET) are the most common imaging techniques for the assessment of brain function in humans. Both can measure blood flow as indicator of brain function. When neuronal activity increases, regional blood flow rates rise in response to the increased metabolic needs of active neurons. Thus, it is speculated that experimentally observed increases in blood flow rate indicate an increase in neuronal activity. In alcoholics a decrease in blood flow has been detected using SPECT, which is reversible, when abstinence is achieved (Berglund *et al.*, 1987).

Apart from measuring blood flow, PET can be used to quantify the functional activity of neurons by assessing localized brain glucose metabolism. For this purpose, [18]Fluor-labeled 2-deoxy-D-glucose (FDG) or ^{11}C-Glucose are used. Samson *et al.* (1986) studied six abstinent chronic alcoholics without cognitive dysfunction. While the overall metabolic rates in these patients were no lower than those of a matched control group, a significant decline in mesial frontal lobe glucose metabolism was found. Wik and colleagues (1988) found glucose metabolism to be diminished in almost all brain regions in a group of nine alcoholics, compared with controls. Sachs *et al.* (1987) using the [2-^{11}C] deoxyglucose technique, found similar results in 10 alcoholics compared with nonalcoholic controls. These early data were confirmed by more recent studies (Volkow *et al.*, 1992). De Wit *et al.* (1990) described a general decrease in neuronal activity in alcoholic patients. In two PET-studies the FDG method was combined with neuropsychological testing. The decreased glucose metabolism in the frontal cortex correlated with cognitive deficits that are specific for frontal lobe functions (Adams *et al.*, 1993; Wang *et al.*, 1993).

Longitudinal studies with repeated measurements of patients at the beginning and in the course of abstinence revealed an increase and partial normalization of the disturbed glucose metabolism especially in the frontal cortical regions (Volkow *et al.*, 1994). The increase in cellular activity might correspond with an increase in synaptic density and support the idea of a partial regeneration of the CNS under the condition of abstinence. Another application of PET is the detection of specific neurotransmitter receptors in the brain. Given all the changes in sensitivity and density of receptors throughout alcohol dependence, this technique seems to be promising for future research in the field of alcoholism.

5. CONCLUSIONS

Alcohol has detrimental effects on the central nervous system. This is important both for the individual and for society, because it demands better strategies in treatment and prevention. From a scientific perspective *alcohol dependence* can be looked upon as a *neurobiologic model* that provides insight into basic mechanisms. It allows the study of the influence of a defined noxe on the brain, and enables the quantification of regeneration and restitution processes in abstinence. Thus, it has a heuristic potential that goes beyond alcoholism.

6. PROPOSALS FOR FUTURE RESEARCH

Recent advances in our understanding of ethanol's impact on the CNS open a series of new questions. Many research options were outlined in the manuscript. Among those the following suggestions seem to be of special importance:

6.1. Animal experiments

Studies regarding ethanol-induced brain damage differ very much regarding the animals used, the duration of alcohol exposure, the way alcohol is administered and whether periods of withdrawal were included or not. Therefore it is often difficult to compare the results of different studies. It seems necessary to establish more standards for animal research.

Different transmitter systems are involved in the mediation of the CNS-effects of ethanol: The anxiolytic effect, the induction of cognitve deficits, and mood changes are thought to be brought about by the facilitating effect of ethanol on $GABA_A$ receptor function. The neurotransmitter glutamate seems to have prominent effects on neuronal plasticity and by itself may act neurotoxic. This has two major implications for research in the field of alcoholism:

- glutamate/NMDA receptor may be involved in the plastic response underlying the development of tolerance and dependence.

• NMDA receptor up-regulation which develops during ethanol intake, may become
  neurodegenerative during withdrawal.

Tolerance: Many drugs of abuse, independent of their chemical classes and independent of the site of action in the brain, induce tolerance a phenomenon of neuronal plasticity. In all cases tested as yet, the development of tolerance can be blocked with
antagonists of the NMDA receptor. Given that this will be confirmed in further studies it
would be of utmost interest and relevance to test whether the development of tolerance to
ethanol will be suppressed by NMDA-receptor antagonists.

Neurotoxicity: Ethanol is a potent blocker of central glutamate/NMDA receptors. "Up
regulation" of these receptors occurs after chronic ethanol ingestion. After withdrawal of
ethanol the NMDA receptor system is supersensitive as seen in receptor binding studies
and functionally as withdrawal induced seizures. It would be of great interest

• to compare the properties of ethanol vulnerable neurons with ethanol resistant neurons
  with regard to glutamate/NMDA vulnerability and
• to develop neuroprotective strategies to suppress ethanol induced neurotoxicity and
  neurodegeneration.

The results of these studies in animals may help in the search for effective treatment
for humans e.g. by developing new anti-craving drugs, some of which seem to act by
blocking the glutamate/NMDA receptor.

Morphometric and imaging studies in animals could be combined with the above mentioned study on tolerance and neurotoxicity. The nature and degree of brain damage could
be assessed, and the regeneration and/or rehydration process following abstinence could
be studied. This should also include the determination of MR-relaxation times and the
assessment of glucose metabolism using the PET technology. The role of glia cells in the
response of the brain to ethanol would be another target of inquiry.

6.2. Studies in Humans

In a well controlled study in man, the impact of different variables on brain damage and
brain dysfunction should be studied. They include the severity of alcohol dependence,
gender, nutritional factors, etc. (see chapter 4.2). MR volumetry of the relevant brain
regions seems to be promising as well as PET studies of regional cerebral activity and
transmitter systems (i.g. GABA and glutamate/NMDA).

Several clinial trials are underway to reduce alcohol consumption by reducing craving.
Some of the new compounds act by inhibiting excitatory amino acids. This perspective
provides new strategies for research. We are inclined to hypothesize that subjects with a
marked supersensitivity of glutamate receptores (as assessed by PET) respond better to
these drugs than others. In the far future we may even find out, whether the compounds
given preventively are neuroprotective and reduce alcohol induced brain damage.

Acknowledgements

Writing this paper was supported by a grant of the German Minister of Research and
Technology (BMFT, 07 FDA 02). U. Widmann, M.D. from the Institute of Neuropatho-

logy, and W. Schmidt, PhD., from the Institute of Neuropharmacology, University of Tübingen provided valuable help!

References

Acker, C. (1986). Neuropsychological deficits in alcoholics, The relative contributions of gender and drinking history. *Br. J. Addict.*, **81**:395–403.

Adams, K.M., Gilman, S., Koeppe, R.A., Kluin, K.J., Bruneberg, J.A., Dede, D., Berent, S. and Kroll, P.D. (1993). Neuropsychological deficits are correlated with frontal hypometabolism in positron emission tomography studies of older alcoholic patients. *Alcoholism: Clinical and Experimental Research*, **17**:205–210.

Agartz, I., Saaf, J., Wahlund, L.O. and Wetterberg, L. (1991). T1 and T2 relaxation time estimates in the normal human brain. *Radiology*, **181**: 537–543.

Artmann, H., Gall, M.V., Hacker, H. and Herrlich, J. (1981). Reversible enlargement of cerebral spinal fluid spaces in chronic alcoholics. *Am. J. Neuroradiol.*, **2**:23–27.

Beal, M.F. and Martin, J.B. (1986). Neuropeptides in neurological disease. *Ann. Neurol.*, **20**:547–565.

Bengoechea, O. and Gonzalo, L.M. (1991). Effects of alcoholization on the rat hippocampus. *Neurosci Lett*, **123**:112–114.

Beracochea, D., Lescaudron, L., Tako, A., Verna, A. and Jaffard, R. (1987). Build-up and release from proactive interference during chronic ethanol consumption in mice: A behavioral and neuroanatomical study. *Behav Brain Res.*, **25**:63–74.

Berglund, M., Hagstadius, S., Risberg, J., Johanson, T.M., Bliding, A. and Mubrin, Z. (1987). Normalization of regional cerebral blood flow in alcoholics during the first 7 weeks of abstinence. *Acta Psychiatr. Scand.*, **75(2)**:292–208.

Bergman, H., Borg, S., Hindmarsh, T., Idestrom, O.M. and Mutzell, S. (1980). Computed tomography of the brain and neuropsychological assessment of male alcoholic patients and a random sample from the general male population. *Acta Psychiatrica Scandinavica*, **62** (Suppl. 286):47–56.

Bergman, H., Axelsson, G. and Idestrom, C.M. (1983). Alcohol consumption, neuropsychological status and computer-tomographic findings in a random sample of men and women from the general population. *Pharmacol. Biochem. Behav.*, **18**:501–505.

Besson, J.A.O., Glen, A.I.M., Foreman, E.L., MacDonald, A., Smith, F.W., Hutchison, J.M.S., Mallard, J.R. and Ashcroft, G.W. (1981). Nuclear magnetic resonance observations in alcoholic cerebral disorder and the role of vasopressin. *Lancet*, **ii**:923–924.

Besson, J.A.O., Crawford, J.R., Parker, D.M. and Smith, F.W. (1989a). Magnetic resonance imaging in Alzheimer's disease, multi-infarct dementia, alcoholic dementia and Korsakoff's psychosis. *Acta Psychiatr. Scand.*, **80**:451–458.

Bottomley, P.A., Foster, T.H., Argersinger, R.E. and Pfeifer, L.M. (1984). A review of normal tissue hydrogen NMR relaxation times and relaxation mechanisms from 1–100 MHz: Dependence on tissue type, NMR frequency, temperature, species, exicision, and age. *Med. Phys.*, **11**:425–448.

Bottomley, P.A., Hardy, C.J., Argersinger, R.E. and Allen-Moore, G. (1987). A review of 1H nuclear magnetic resonance relaxation in pathology: Are T1 and T2 diagnostic? *Med. Phys.*, **14**:1–37.

Cadete-Leite, A., Tavares, M.A. and Paula-Barbosa, M.M. (1988a). Alcohol withdrawal does not impede hippocampal granule cell progressive loss in chronic alcohol-fed rats. *Neurosci. Lett.*, **86**:45–50.

Cadete-Leite, A., Tavares, M.A., Uylings, H.B. and Paula-Barbosa, M. (1988b). Granule cell loss and dendritic regrowth in the hippocampal dentate gyrus of the rat after chronic alcohol consumption. *Brain Res.*, **473**:1–14.

Cadete-Leite, A., Tavares, M.A., Alves, M.C., Uylings, H.B.M. and Paula-Barbosa, M.M. (1989a). Metric analysis of hippocampal granule cell dendritic trees after alcohol withdrawal in rats. *Alcohol. Clin. Exp., Res.*, **13**:837–840.

Cadete-Leite, A., Tavares, M.A., Pacheco, M.M., Volk, B. and Paula-Barbosa, M.M. (1989b). Hippocampal mossy fiber-CA3 synapse after chronic alcohol consumption and withdrawal. *Alcohol.*, **6**:303–310.

Carlen, P.L., Wortzman, G., Holgate, R.C., Wilkinson, D.A. and Rankin, J.G. (1978). Reversible cerebral atrophy in recently abstinent chronic alcoholics measured by computed tomography scans. *Science*, **200**:1076–1078.

Carlen, P.L., Wilkinson, D.A., Wortzman, G. and Holgate, R. (1984). Partially reversible cerebral atrophy and functional improvement in recently abstinent alcoholics. *Can. J. Neurol. Sci.*, **11**:441–446.

Charness, M.E., Gordon, A.S. and Diamond, I. (1983). Alcohol produces acute and chronic changes in opiate receptors which may correspond to intoxication, tolerance and withdrawal. *Neurology*, **33** (Suppl. 2): p. 175.

Charness, M. (1993). Brain lesions in alcoholics. *Alcoholism. Clin. Exp. Res.*, **17**:2–11.

Charness, M. and DeLaPaz, R. (1987). Mamillary body atrophy in Wernicke's encephalopathy: Antemortem identification using magnetic resonance imaging. *Ann. Neurol.*, **22**:595–600.

Chick, J.D., Smith, M.A., Engleman, H.M., Kean, D.M., Mander, A.J., Douglas, R.H.B. and Best, J.J.K. (1989). Magnetic resonance imaging of the brain in alcoholics: Cerebral atrophy, lifetime alcohol consumption and cognitive deficits. *Alcoholism: Clin. Exp. Res.*, **13**:512–518.

Clarren, S.K., Alvoid, E.C., Sumi, S.M. *et al.* (1978). Brain malformations related to prenatal exposure to ethanol. *J. Pediatr.*, **92**:6467.

Claus, D., Wille, H., Neundörfer, B. and Gmelin, E. (1987). Ist die Zunahme des Hirnvolumens abstinenter Alkoholiker Rehydratationsfolge? *Klinische Wochenschrift*, **65**:185–193.

Coles, C.D., Brown, R.T., Smith, I.E., Platzman, K.A., Erickson, S. and Falek, A. (1991). Effects of prenatal alcohol exposure at school age: I. Physical and cognitive development. *Neurotoxicology and Teratology*, **13(4)**:536–541.

Cotman, C.W. and Nadler, J.V. (1978). Reactive synaptogenesis in the hippocampus. In: Cotman, C.W., (ed). *Neuronal Plasticity*. New York: Raven Press, pp. 227–271.

Cravioto, H., Korein, J. and Silberman, J. (1961). Wernicke's encephalopathy. A clinical and pathological study of 28 autopsied cases. *Arch. Neurol.*, **4**:510–519.

Courville, C.B. (1955). *Effects of Alcohol on the Nervous System of Man*. San Lucas Press, Los Angeles.

Dager, S.R. and Steen, R.G. (1992). Applications of magnetic resonance spectroscopy to the investigation of neuropsychiatric disorders. *Neuropsychopharmacology*, **6,4**: 249–266.

de la Monte, S.M. (1988). Disproportionate atrophy of cerebral white matter in chronic alcoholics. *Arch. Neurol.*, **45**:990–992.

de Wit, H., Metz, J., Wagner, N. and Cooper, M. (1990). Behavioral and subjective effects of ethanol: Relationship to cerebral metabolism using PET. *Alcohol. Clin. Exp. Res.*, **14(3)**:482–489.

Diener, H.C., Dichgans, J., Bacher, M. and Guschlbauer, B. (1984). Improvement of ataxia in alcoholic cerebellar atrophy through alcohol abstinence. *J. Neurol.*, **231**: 258–262.

Dildy, J.E. and Leslie, S.W. (1989). Ethanol inhibits NMDA-induced increases in intracellular CA^{2+} in dissociated brain cells. *Brain Res.*, **499**:383–387.

Dow, K.E. and Riopelle, R.J. (1985). Ethanol neurotoxicity: Effects on neurite formation and neurotrophic factor production *in vitro*. *Science*, **228**:591–593.

Durand, D., Saint-Cyr, J.A., Gurevich, N. and Carlen, P.L. (1989). Ethanol-induced dendritic alterations in hippocampal granule cells. *Brain Res.*, **477**:373–377.

Edwards, G. and Gross, M.M. (1977). Alcohol Dependence: provisional description of a clinical syndrome. *Brit. Med. J.*, **1**:1058–1061.

Ferrer, I., Fabregues, I., Rairiz, J. and Galofre, E. (1986). Decreased numbers of dendritic spines on cortical pyramidal neurons in human chronic alcoholism. *Neuroscience letters*, **69**:115–119.

Fox, J.H., Ramsey, R.G., Huckman, M.S. and Poscke, A.E. (1976). Cerebral ventricular enlargement. Chronic alcoholics examined by computerized tomography. *J. Am. Med. Assoc.*, **236**:365–368.

Freund, G. and Ballinger, W.E. (1988a). Decrease of benzodiazepine receptors in frontal cortex of alcoholics. *Alcohol*, **5**:275–282.

Freund, G. and Ballinger, W.E. (1988b). Loss of cholinergic muscarinic receptors in the frontal cortex of alcohol abusers. *Alcohol Clin. Exp. Res.*, **12**:630–638.

Frezza, M., diPadova, C., Pozzato, G., Terpin, M., Baraona, E. and Lieber, C.S. (1990). High blood alcohol levels in women. *N. Engl. J. Med.*, **322**:95–99.

Fu, Y., Tanaka, K. and Nishimura, S. (1990). Evaluation of brain edema using magnetic resonance proton relaxation times. In: Long, D. (ed.) *Advances in Neurology. Brain Edema*. **52**. New York: Raven Press pp. 165–176.

Gallucci, M., Bozzao, A., Splendiani, A., Masciocchi, C. and Passariello, R. (1989). Wernicke Encephalopathy: MR findings in five patients. *Am. J. Radiol.*, **155**:1309–1314.

Glenn, S.W., Parsons, O.A. and Stevens, L. (1989). Effects of alcohol abuse and familial alcoholism on physical health in men and women. *Health Psychol.*, **8**:325–341.

Gurling, H.M.D., Reveley, M.A. and Murray, R.M. (1984). Increased cerebral ventricular volume in monozygotic twins discordant for alcoholism. *Lancet*, **i**:986–988.

Gurling, H.M.D., Murray, R.M. and Ron, M.A. (1986). Increased brain radiodensity in alcoholism. A co-twin control study. *Arch. Gen. Psychiatry*, **43**:764–767.

Haberman, P.W. and Natarajan, G. (1989). Premature mortality and chronic alcoholism: Medical examiner cases, New Jersey. *Soc. Sci. Med.*, **29**:729–732.

Hansen, L.A., Natelson, B.H., Lemere, C., Niemann, W., DeTeresa, R., Regan, T.J., Masliah, E. and Terry, R.D. (1991). Alcohol-induced brain changes in dogs. *Arch-Neurol.*, **48,9**:939–942.

Hanson, T., Tindberg, N., Ingelman-Sundberg, M. and Kohler, C. (1990). Regional distribution of ethanol-inducible cytochrome P450 IIE1 in the rat central nervous system. *Neuroscience*, **34**:451–463.

Hanstock, C.C., Rothman, D.L., Shulman, R.G., Novotny, E.J., Petroff, O.A.C. and Prichard, J.W. (1990). Measurement of ethanol in the human brain using NMR spectroscopy. *J. Stud. Alcohol.*, **51**:104–107.

Harper, C.G. (1983). The incidence of Wernicke's encephalopathy in Australia: A neuropathological study of 131 cases. *J. Neurol. Neurosurg Psychiatry*, **46**:593–598.

Harper, C., Kril, J. and Daly, J. (1987). Are we drinking our neurones away? *Brit. Med. J., 294*:534–536.

Harper, C.G., Kril, J.J. and Daly, J.M. (1988). Brain shrinkage in alcoholics is not caused by changes in hydration: A pathological study. *J. Neurol. Neurosurg Psychiatry,* **51**:124–127.

Harper, C. and Kril, J. (1989). Patterns of neuronal loss in the cerebral cortex in chronic alcoholic patients. *J. Neurol. Sci.,* **92**:81–89.

Harper, C. and Corbett, D. (1990). Changes in the basal dendrites of cortical pyramidal cells from alcoholic patients — a quantitative Golgi study. *Journal of Neurology, Neurosurgery and Psychiatry,* 53:856–861.

Harper, C. and Kril, J.J., (1993). Neuropathological changes in alcoholics. In National Institute on *Alcohol Abuse and Alcoholism (ed.): Alcohol induced brain damage. Research Monograph,* **22**. pp. 39–69.

Harris, R.A. and Hood, W.F. (1980). Inhibition of synaptosomal calcium uptake by ethanol. *Pharmacol. Exp. Ther.,* 213:562–568.

Hauw, J.-J., De Baecque, C., Hausser-Hauw, C. and Serdaru, M. (1988). Chromatolysis in alcoholic encephalopathies. Pellagra-like changes in 22 cases. *Brain,* 111:843–857, 1988.

Hochla, N.A. and Parsons, O.A. (1982). Premature aging in female alcoholics. A neuropsychological study. *J. Nerv. Ment. Dis.,* **170**:241–245.

Jacobson, R. (1986). The contributions of sex and drinking history to the CT brain scan changes in alcoholics. *Psychol. Med.,* **16**:547–559.

Jensen, G. and Pakkenberg, B. (1993). Are alcoholics drinking their neurons away? *Lancet,* **ii,** 1201–1204.

Jernigan, T.L., Press, G.A. and Hesselink, J.R. (1990). Methods for measuring brain morphologic features on magnetic resonance images: Validation and normal aging. *Arch Neurol.,* **47**:27–32.

Jernigan, T.L., Butters, N., DiTraglia, G., Schafer, K., Smith, T., Irwin, M., Grant, I., Schuckit, M., Cermak, L.S. (1991). Reduced cerebral gray matter observed in alcoholics using magnetic resonance imaging. Alcoholism: *Clinical and Experimental Research,* **15**:418–427.

Jones-Saumty, D.J., Fabian, M.S. and Parsons, O.A. (1981). Medical status and cognitive functioning in alcoholic women. *Alcoholism,* **5**:372–377.

Kimelberg, H.K. and Norenberg, M.D. (1989). Astrocytes. *Scientific American*: 44–52, 1989.

King, M.A., Hunter, B.E. and Walker, D.W. (1988). Alterations and recovery of dendritic spine density in rat hippocampus following long-term ethanol ingestion. *Brain Res.,* **459**:381–385.

Kircher, J. and Pierson, C. (1956). Les atrophies cérébrales dans les toxicomanies: role de la Pneumo-encépholgrahie. Essaies therapeutiques. *Maroc. Med.,* **35**:668–670.

Korsakoff, S.S. (1887). Disturbance of psychic function in alcoholic paralysis and its relation to the disturbance of the psychic sphere in multiple neuritis of non-alcoholic origin. Vestn. Klin. Sudebnoi Psychiatr. *Nevropatol.,* 4,2.

Krieg, J.-C., Lauer, C. and Pirke, K.-M. (1989). Structural brain abnormalities in patients with bulimia nervosa. *Psychiatry Res.,* 27:39–489.

Kroft, C.L., Gescuk, B., Woods, B.T., Mello, N.K.,Weiss, R.D. and Mendelson, J.H. (1991). Brain ventricular size in female alcoholics — An MRI study. *Alcohol.,* **8**:31–34.

Kukreya, R.C. and Hess, M.L. (1992). The oxygen free radical system: From equations through membrane-protein interactions to cardiovascular injury and protection. *Cardiovascular Research,* 26:641–655.

Lancaster, F.E., Philips, S.M., Patsalos, P.N. and Wiggins, R.C. (1984). Brain myelination in the offspring of ethanol-treated rats: In utero versus lactational exposure by cross-fostering offspring of control pairfed, and ethanol treated dams. *Brain Res.,* **309**:209–216.

Lemoine, P., Harousseau, H., Borleyru, J.P. and Menuet, J.C. (1968). Les enfants de parents alcooliques: Anomalies observées à propos de 127 cas. *Ouest Medical,* **21**:476–482.

Lescaudron, L. and Verna, A. (1985). Effects of chronic ethanol consumption on pyramidal neurons of the mouse dorsal and ventral hippocampus: A quantitative histological analysis. *Exp. Brain Res.,* **58**:362–367.

Lescaudron, L., Seguela, P., Geffard, M. and Verna A. (1986). Effects of long-term in the mouse hippocampus: A quantitative immunocytochemical study. *Drug Alcohol Depend.,* **18**:377–384.

Lescaudron, L., Jaffard, R. and Verna, A. (1989). Modifications in number and morphology of dendritic spines resulting from chronic ethanol consumption and withdrawal: A Golgi study in the mouse anterior and posterior hippocampus. *Exp. Neurol.,* **106**:156–163.

Leslie, S.W., Barr, E., Chandler, J. and Farrar, R.P. (1983). Inhibition of fast- and slow-phase depolarization-dependent synaptosomal calcium uptake by ethanol. *J. Pharmacol. Exp Ther.,* **225**:571–575.

Lieber, C.S. (1989). Alcohol and nutrition: An overview. *Alcohol Health and Research World,* **13**:197–205.

Lim, K.O. and Pfefferbaum, A. (1989). Segmentation of MR brain images into cerebrospinal fluid spaces, white and gray matter. *J. Comput. Assist. Tomogr.,* **13**:588–593.

Lim, K.O., Zipursky, R.B., Murphy, G.M. and Pfefferbaum, A., (1992). *In vivo* quantification of the limbic system using MRI: Effects of normal aging. *Psychiatry Res. Neuroimaging,* **35**:15–26.

Lim, K.O., Zipursky, R.B., Watts, M.C. and Pfefferbaum, A. (1990). Decreased gray matter in normal aging: An *in vivo* MR study. *J. Gerontol.,* **47**:B26–B30.

Lind, M., Goodlett, R. and West, J.R. (1988). Time course and reversibility of ethanol's suppressive effects on axon sprouting in the dentate gyrus of the adult rat. Alcoholism: *Clin. Exp. Res.,* **12**:433–439.

Lindboe, C.F. and Loberg, E.M. (1988). The frequency of brain lesions in alcoholics. *J. Neurol. Sci.,* **88**: 107–113.

Lishman, W.A. (1981). Cerebral disorder in alcoholism. Syndromes of impairment. *Brain,* **104**:1–20, 1981.

Lishman, W.A. (1990). Alcohol and the brain. *Br. J. Psychiatry,* **156**:635–644.

Littleton, J. (1978). Alcohol and neurotransmitters. *Clinics in Endocrinology and Metabolism,* **7**:369–384.

Lovinger, D.M., White, G. and Weight, F.F., (1989). Ethanol inhibits NMDA-activated ion current in hippocampal neurons. *Science,* **243**:1721–1724.

Lovinger, D.M., White, G., and Weight, F.F. (1990). NMDA receptor-mediated synaptic excitation selectively inhibited by ethanol in hippocampal slice from adult rat. *J..Neurosci.,* **10**:1372–1379.

MacDonald, H.L., Bell, B.A., Smith, M.A., Kean, D.M., Tocher, J.L., Douglas, R.H.B., Miller, J.D. and Best, J.J.K. (1986). Correlation of human NMR T1 values measured *in vivo* and brain water content. *Br. J. Radiol.,* **59**:355–357.

Mander, A.J., Young, A., Chick, J.D., Ridgway, J. and Best, J.J.K. (1989). NMR T1 relaxation time of the brain during alcohol withdrawal and its lack of relationship wiht symptom severity. *British Journal of Addiction,* **84**:669–672.

Mann, K., Opitz, H., Petersen, D., Schroth, G. and Heimann, H. (1989). Intracranial CSF-volumetry in chronic alcholics: studies with MRI and CT. *Psychiatry Research,* **29**:277–279.

Mann, K., Schroth, G., Stetter, F., Schied, H., Bartels, M., Batra, A. and Heimann, H. (1991). Thiaminmangel und Hirnatrophie bei Alkoholabhängigen. *Nervenarzt.,* **62**:177–181.

Mann, K. (1992). Alkohol und Gehirn — über strukturelle und funktionelle Veränderungen nach erfolgreicher Therapie. Springer Heidelberg, Berlin, New York.

Mann, K., Batra, A., Günther, A. and Schroth, G. (1992a). Do women develop alcoholic brain damage more readily than men? Alcoholism: *Clin. Exp. Res.,* **16**:1052–1056.

Mann, K. and Bartels, M. (1992). The Impact of Magnetic Resonance Imaging and Magnetic Resonance Spectroscopy on Psychiatry. *Fortschr. Neurol. Psychiat.,* **60**:308–314.

Mann, K., Dengler, W., Nägele, T., Klose, U. and Schroth, G. (1993). Liquorvolumetrie und spektroskopische T1-Bestimmung — eine prospektive MR-Verlaufsstudie an Alkoholikern. In: Baumann P. (ed.) *Biologische Psychiatrie der Gegenwart.* Springer, Wien, New York, pp. 547–550.

Mann, K., Dengler, W., Klose, U., Naegele, T. and Mundle, G. (1994). MR-Spectroscopy in Alcoholic Brain Damage: No Evidence for Water Shift in Abstinence (abstract), *Alcoholism, Clinical and Experimental Research,* **2**:430.

Martin, P.R., Gibbs, S.J., Nimmerrichter, A., Riddle, W.R., Welch, L.W. and Willcott, M.R. (1995). Brain Proton Magnetic Resonance Spectroscopy Studies in Recently Abstinent Alcoholics. *Alcoholism: Clin. Exp. Res.* **19**:1078–1082.

Mayes, A.R., Meudell, P.R., Mann, D. and Pickering, A. (1988). Locations of the lesions in Korsakoff's syndrome: neuropathological data on two patients. *Cortex,* **24**:367–388.

Mattson, S.N., Riley, E.P., Jernigan, T.L., Garcia, A., Kaneko, W.M. and Ehlers, C.L. (in press). A decrease in the size of the basal ganglia following prenatal alcohol exposure. *Neurotoxicology and Teratology*

McMullen, P., Saint-Cyr, J.A. and Carlen, P.L. (1984). Morphological alterations in the rat CA1 hippocampal pyramidal cell dendrites resulting from chronic ethanol consumption and withdrawal. *J. Comp. Neurol.,* **225**:111–118.

Melgaard, B., Danielsen, U.T., Sörensen, H. and Ahlgren, P. (1986). The Severity of Alcoholism and its Relation to Intellectual Impairment and Cerebral Atrophy. *British Journal of Addiction,* **81**:77–80.

Miller, M.W. (1993). Migration of cortical neurons is altered by gestational exposure to ethanol. *Alcoholism: Clinical and Experimental Research,* **17(2)**:304–314.

Mochly-Rosen, D., Chang, E.H., Cheever, L., Kim, M., Diamond, I. and Gordon, A.S. (1988). Chronic ethanol causes heterologous desensitization of receptors by reducing alphas messenger RNA. *Nature,* **333**:848–850.

Montpied, P., Morrow, A.L., Karanian, J.W., Ginns, E.I., Martin, B.M. and Paul, S.M. (1991). Prolonged ethanol inhalation decreases gamma-aminobutyric acidA receptor alpha subunit mRNAs in the rat cerebral cortex. *Mol. Pharmacol.,* **39**:157–163.

Morrow, A.L., Montpied, P., Lingford-Hughes, A. and Paul, S.M. (1990). Chronic ethanol and pentobarbital administration in the rat: Effects on GABA$_A$ receptor function and expression in brain. *Alcohol,* **7**:237–244.

Muuronen, A., Bergman, H., Hindmarsh, T. and Telakivi, T. (1989). Influence of improved drinking habits on brain atrophy and cognitive performance in alcoholic patients: A 5-year follow-up study. *Alcohol Clin. Exp. Res.,* **13**:137–141.

Parnavelas, J.G., Lynch, G., Brecha, N., Cotman, C.W. and Globus, A. (1974). Spine loss and regrowth in hippocampus following deafferentiation. *Nature,* **248**:71–73.

Pentney, R.J. (1979). Ethanol related changes in rat cerebellar Purkinje cells. *Anat. Rec.,* **193**: 649.

Pentney, R.J. (1982). Quantitative analysis of ethanol effects on Purkinje cell dendritic tree. *Brain Res.,* **249**:397–401.

Pentney, R.J., Quackenbush, L.J. and O'Neill, M. (1989). Length changes in dendritic networks of cerebellar Purkinje cells of old rats after chronic ethanol treatment. *Alcohol Clin. Exp. Res., 13*:413–419.

Pentney, R. and Quackenbush, L.J. (1990). Dendritic hypertrophy in Purkinje neurons of old Fischer 344 rats after long-term ethanol treatment. *Alcohol Clin. Exp. Res., 14*:878–886.

Pentney, R.J. (1991). Remodeling of neuronal dendritic networks with aging and alcohol. *Alcohol Alcohol, 1*:393–397.

Pfefferbaum, A., Zatz, L. and Jernigan, T.L. (1986). Computer-interactive method for quantifying cerebrospinal fluid and tissue in brain CT scans: Effects of aging. *J. Comput. Assist. Tomogr., 10*:571–578.

Pfefferbaum, A., Rosenbloom, M.J., Crusan, K. and Jernigan, T.L. (1988). Brain CT changes in alcoholics. The effects of age and alcohol consumption. *Alcohol Clin. Exp. Res., 12*:81–87.

Pfefferbaum, A., Lim, K.O. and Rosenblum, M.A. (1992). Structural imaging of the brain in chronic alcoholism, in: Zakhari, S., Witt, E. (eds.), Imaging in Alcohol Research. Rockville, MD, Department of Health and Human Services pp. 99–120.

Peiffer, J. (1985). Zur Frage atrophisierender Vorgänge im Gehirn chronischer Alkoholiker. *Nervenarzt., 56*:649–657.

Phillips, S.C. and Cragg, B.G. (1983). Chronic consumption of alcohol by adult mice: Effect on hippocampal cells and synapses. *Exp. Neurol., 80*:218–226.

Phillips, S.C. (1985). Qualitative and quantitative changes of mouse cerebellar synapses after chronic alcohol consumption and withdrawal. *Exp. Neurol., 88*:748–756.

Pietrzak, E.R., Wilce, P.A. and Shanley, B.C. (1990). Effect of chronic ethanol consumption on phosphoinositol turnover and adenylate cyclase activity in rat brain. *Neurochem. Int., 17*:593–598.

Popova, E.N. and Frumkina, L.E. (1985). Changes in neurons and interneural connections of the higher sections of the motor system in the progeny of alcoholized male and female rats. *Neurosci. Behav. Physiol., 15*:476–479.

Pratt, O.E., Rooprai, H.K., Shaw, G.K. and Thomson, A.D. (1990). The genesis of alcoholic brain tissue injury. *Alcohol Alcohol, 25*:217–230.

Rius, R.A., Bergamashi, S., DiFonso, F., Govonis, S. and Trabucchi, M. (1987). Acute ethanol effect on calcium antagonist binding in rat brain. *Brain Res., 402*: 359–361.

Roach, M.K. (1979). Changes in the activity of Na+K+-ATPase during acute and chronic administration of ethanol, in: Majchrowicz, E., Noble, E.P. (eds.) Biochemistry and pharmacology of ethanol. New York, Plenum Press, pp. 67–80.

Ron, M.A., Acker, W., Shaw, G.K. and Lishman, W.A. (1982). Computerized tomography of the brain in chronic alcoholism. A survey and follow-up study. *Brain, 105*:479–514.

Ron, M.A. (1983). The alcoholic brain: CT and psychological findings. *Psychol. Med., (Monogr Suppl) 3*:1–33.

Rosengren, L.E., Wronski, A., Briving, C. and Haglid, K.G. (1985). Long lasting changes in gerbil brain after chronic ethanol exposure: A quantitative study of the glial cell marker S-100 and DNA. *Alcohol Clin. Exp. Res., 9*:109–113.

Sachs, H., Russell, J.A.G., Christman, D.R. and Cook, B. (1987). Alteration of regional cerebral glucose metabolic rate in non-Korsakoff chronic alcoholism. *Arch. Neurol., 44*:1242–1251.

Sadler, R.H., Sommer, M.A., Forno, L.S. and Smith, M.E. (1991). Induction of anti-myelin antibodies in EAE and their possible role in demyelination. *J. Neurosci. Res., 30*:616–624.

Samson, Y., Baron, J.C., Feline, A., Bories, J. and Crouzel, C. (1986). Local cerebral glucose utilization in chronic alcoholics: A positron tomographic study. *J. Neurol. Neurosurg. Psychiatry, 49*:1165–1170.

Shear, P.K., Jernigan, T.L., Butters, N., Cermak, L.S. (1992). MRI examinations of regional brain volumes in chronic alcoholics (abstract). *31st Annual Meeting of American College of Neuropsychopharmacology* (Abstract), p. 55.

Scheetz, A.J., Markham, J.A. and Fifkova, E. (1987a). Changes in the frequency of basket cells in the dentate fascia following chronic ethanol administration in mice. *Brain Res., 403*:151–154.

Scheetz, A.J., Markham, J.A. and Fifkova, E. (1987b). The effect of chronic ethanol consumption on the fine structure of the CA1 stratum oriens in short-sleep and long-sleep mice. Short-term and long-term exposure. *Brain Res., 409*:329–334.

Schmidt, C., Klee, L. and Ames, G. (1990). Review and analysis of literature on indicators of women's drinking problems. *Br. J. Addict., 85*:179–192.

Schroth, G. (1984). Clinical and CT confirmed recovery from central pontine myelinolysis. *Neuroradiology, 26*:149–151.

Schroth, G., Remmes, U. and Schupmann, A. (1985). Computertomographie Verlaufsuntersuchung von Hirnvolumen-schwankungen vor und nach Alkoholentzugsbehandlung. *Fortschritte der Röntgenstrahlkunde, 142*:363–369.

Schroth, G., Naegele, T., Klose, U., Mann, K. and Petersen, D. (1988). Reversible brain shrinkage in abstinent alcoholics, measured by MRI. *Neuroradiology, 30*:121–126.

Schroth, G. and Mann, K. (1989). Computertomographie und Kernspintomographie in der klinischen Diagnostik und Erforschung der Alkoholkrankheit. In: Schied, H.W., Heimann, H., Mayer, K. (eds.) *Der Chronische Alkoholismus*. Gustav Fischer, Stuttgart. pp. 121–140.

Sedmak, P.A., Sedmak, D., Fritz, J.I. and Peterson, G.R. (1978). Myelination in chronically-alcoholic mice. *Experientia*, **34**:1059–1060.

Shear, P.K., Jernigan, T.L., Butters, N. and Cermak, L.S. (1992). MRI examinations of regional brain volumes in chronic alcoholics (Abstract). 31st Annual Meeting of American College of Neuropsychopharmacology (Abstract), p. 55.

Smith, M.A., Chick, J., Kean, D.M., Douglas, R.H.B., Singer, A., Kendell, R. and Best, J.J.K. (1985). Brain water in chronic alcoholic patients measured by magnetic resonance imaging. *Lancet*, **i**:1273–1274.

Smith, M.A., Chick, J.D., Engleman, H.M., Kean, D.M., Mander, A.J. and Douglas, R.H.B. (1988). Brain hydration during alcohol withdrawal in alcoholics measured by magnetic resonance imaging. Drug *Alcohol Depend.*, **21**:25–28.

Spielmann, D., Pauly, J., Macovski, A., Glover, G. and Enzman, D. (1992). Lipid-suppressed single- and multiple-slice proton spectroscopic imaging of human brain. *J. Magnetic Resonance Imaging*, **2**:253–262.

Sun, G.Y., Danopoulos, V. and Sun, A.Y. (1980). The effect of chronic ethanol administration on myelin lipids. In: Galanter, M., (ed.), Currents in Alcoholism. *Recent Advances* I. Vol. 7. New York, Grune and Stratton, pp. 83–91.

Tavares, M.A. and Paula-Barbosa, M.M. (1982). Alcohol-induced granule cell loss in the cerebellar cortex of the adult rat. *Exp. Neurol.*, **78**:574–582.

Tavares, M.A. and Paula-Barbosa, M.M. (1983b). Lipofuscin granules in Purkinje cells after long-term alcohol consumption in rats. *Alcohol Clin. Exp. Res.*, **7**:302–306.

Tavares, M.A., Paula-Barbosa, M.M., Barroca, J. and Volk, B. (1985). Lipofuscin granules in cerebellar interneurons after long-term alcohol consumption in the adult rat. *Anat. Embryol.*, **171**:61–69.

Tavares, M.A., Paula-Barbosa, M.M. and Cadete-Leite, A. (1987a). Chronic alcohol consumption reduces the cortical layer volumes and the number of neurons of the rat cerebellar cortex. *Alcohol Clin. Exp. Res.*, **11**:315–319.

Tavares, M.A., Paula-Barbosa, M.M. and Verwer, R.W.H. (1987b). Synapses of the cerebellar cortex molecular layer after chronic alcohol consumption. *Alcohol*, **4**:109–116.

Teichberg, V.I. (1991). Glial glutamate receptors: likely actors in brain signaling. *FASEB*, **5**:3086–3091.

Terry, R.D., Peck, A., DeTeresa, R., Schechter, R. and Horoupian, D.S. (1981). Some morphological aspects of the brain in senile dementia of the Alzheimer type. *Ann. Neurol.*, **10**:184–192.

Terry, R.D. and Hansen, L.A. (1987). Neocortical cell counts in normal human adult aging. *Ann. Neurol.*, **21**:530–539.

Ticku, M.K. (1980). The effects of acute and chronic ethanol administration and its withdrawal on GABA receptor binding in rat brain. *Br. J. Pharmacol.*, **70**:403–410.

Ticku, M.K. and Burch, T.P. (1980). Alterations in gamma-aminobutyric acid receptor sensitivity following acute and chronic ethanol treatment. *J. Neurochem.*, **34**:417–423.

Torvik, A., Lindboe C.F. and Rodge S. (1982). Brain lesions in alcoholics. *J. Neurol. Sci.*, **56**:233–248.

Torvik, A. and Torp, S. (1986). The prevalence of alcoholic cerebellar atrophy. A morphometric and histological study of autopsy material. *J. Neurol. Sci.*, **75**: 43–51.

Toth, E. and Lajtha, A. (1984). Effect of chronic ethanol administration on brain protein breakdown in mice *in vivo*. *Subst Alcohol Actions/Misuse*, **5**:175–183.

Tran, V.T., Snyder, S.H., Major, L.F. and Hawley, R.J. (1981). GABA receptors are increased in brains of alcoholics. *Ann. Neurol.*, **9**:289–292.

VanThiel, D.H. and Gavaler, J.S. (1988). Ethanol metabolism and hepatotoxocity: Does sex make a difference? In: Galanter, M., (ed.), *Recent Developments in Alcoholism*. New York: Plenum Press, pp. 291–304.

Victor, M, Adams, R.E. and Collins, G.H. (1971). *The Wernicke-Korsakoff Syndrome*. Philadelphia, Davis.

Victor, M and Adams, R.E. (1985). The alcoholic dementias. In: Vinken, P.J., Bruyn, G.W., Klawans, H.L., (eds)., *Handbook of Clinical Neurology*, North Holland, Amsterdam, Vol. 2:335–352.

Volk, B., Maletz, J., Tiedemann, M., Mall, G., Klein, C. and Berlet, H.H. (1981). Impaired maturation of purkinje cells in the fetal alcohol syndrome of the rat. *Acta Neuropathol.*, **54**:19–29.

Volk, B. (1984). Cerebellar histogenesis and synaptic maturation follwing pre- and postnatal alcohol administration. *Acta Neuropathol. (Berlin)*, **63**:57–65.

Volkow, N.D., Hitzemann, R., Wang, G.J., Fowler, J.S., Burr, G., Pascani, K., Dewey, S.L. and Wolf, A.P. (1992). Decreased brain metabolism in neurologically intact healthy alcoholics. *Am. J. Psychiatry*, **149**:1016–1022.

Volkow, N.D., Wang, G.J., Hitzeman, R., Fowler, J.S., Overall, J.E., Burr, G. and Wolf, A.P. (1994). Recovery of brain glucose metabolism in detoxified alcoholics. *Am. J. Psychiatry*, **151**:178–183.

Walker, D.W., Barnes, D.E., Zornetzer, S.F., Hunter, B.E. and Kubanis, P. (1980). Neuronal loss in hippocampus induced by prolonged ethanol consumption in rats. *Science*, **209**:711–713.

Walker, D.W., Hunter, B.E. and Abraham, W.C. (1981). Neuroanatomical and functional deficits subsequent to chronic ethanol administration in animals. *Alcohol Clin. Exp. Res.*, **5**:267–282.

Wang, G.J., Volkow, N.D., Roque, C.T., Cestaro, V.L., Hitzemann, R.J., Cantos, E.L., Levy, A.V. and Hwan, A.P. (1993). Functional importance of ventricular enlargement and cortical atrophy in healthy subjects and alcoholics as asessed with PET, MR imaging, and neuropsychological testing. *Radiology,* **186**: 59–65.

Wernicke, C. (1881). *Lehrbuch der Gehirnkrankheiten für Ärzte und Studierende*. Fischer, Kassel, Berlin.

West, J.R. and Pierce, D.R. (1986). Perinatal alcohol exposure and neuronal damage. In: West, J.R. ed. Alcohol and *Brain Development*. New York: Oxford University Press. pp. 120–157.

White, G., Lovinger, D.M. and Weight, F.F. (1990). Ethanol inhibits NMDA-activated current but does not alter GABA-acitvated current in an isolated mammalian neuron. *Brain Res.,* **507**:332–336.

Wik, G., Borg, S., Sjogren, I., Wiesel, F.-A., Blomqvist, G., Borg, J., Greitz, T., Nyback, H., Sedvall, G., Stone-Elander, S. and Widen, L. (1988). PET determination of regional cerebral glucose metabolism in alcohol-dependent men and healthy controls using ^{11}C-glucose. *Acta Psychiatr. Scand.,* **78**:234–241.

Wilkinson, D.A. and Carlen, P.L. (1980). Relationship of neuropsychological test performance to brain morphology in amnesic and non-amnesic chronic alcoholics. *Acta Psychiatrica Scandinavica,* **62**:664–666.

Zipursky, R.B., Lim, K.O. and Pfefferbaum, A. (1989). MRI study of brain changes with short-term abstinence from alcohol. *Alcoholism: Clinical and Experimental Research,* **13**:664–666.

8 Musculo-Skeletal Problems in Alcohol Abuse

Alvaro Urbano-Márquez M.D., Ph.D. and
Joaquim Fernández-Solà M.D., Ph.D.

Muscle Research Group and Alcohol Unit, Internal Medicine Department, Hospital Clínic. Faculty of Medicine, University of Barcelona. Villarroel 170, 08036. Barcelona, Spain., Telephone (93) 4.54.60.00. Extension 2240., FAX: (93) 4.51.52.72

Ethanol consumption may produce acute or chronic changes in striated skeletal muscle regardless of other causes such as malnutrition or peripheral neuropathy. The presentation of acute myopathy is sporadic and the prevalence of chronic myopathy varies from 40–60% in an alcoholic population. Women are more sensitive to the toxic effects of ethanol on skeletal muscle. The physiopathological mechanisms which determine the muscle damage induced by ethanol are still not completely understood. However, ethanol is toxic to striated muscle in a dose-dependent manner.

In experimental and human models, the direct effect of ethanol may cause striated muscle damage by alterations in membrane fluidity, channels, pumps and ionic transients, depression of muscle contractility, protein synthesis or mitochondrial or hormonal function.

Muscle pain, swelling and weakness are the main features of acute myopathy. In chronic myopathy, proximal progressive weakness and atrophy are more prominent. There are more subclinical cases, which can be detected from evaluating muscle weakness by myometry. Skeletal involvement is related to other systemic diseases, mainly cardiac, liver and peripheral nerve damage in alcoholic patients. Myocytolysis is the most prominent feature in alcoholic myopathy. Other frequent muscle changes are type II fiber atrophy, regeneration of fibers, internal nuclei, moth-eaten fibers and subsarcolemmical deposition. The diagnosis of alcoholic myopathy requires a characteristic clinical pattern and careful exclusion of other causes of myopathy due to the lack of a specific histological pattern.

Ethanol abstinence is the only effective treatment for alcoholic myopathy. Acute myopathy usually resolves rapidly with abstinence, whereas the recovery of chronic myopathy may be only partial with persistent weakness or irreversible muscle changes. Future trends in alcoholic myopathy are directed to the study of the mechanisms of ethanol-induced cell necrosis and the biochemical or genetic causes of functional cell impairment.

1. INTRODUCTION

Although the generally deleterious effects of excessive alcohol consumption have been recognized for millennia (Mendelson and Nello, 1992), the link between "ardent spirits" and muscular weakness was first described in 1822 by James Jackson of Harvard, who suggested that muscle weakness might recover after abstention. During the same century, the deleterious effects of ethanol on cardiac muscle were described by Bollinger (1884) and Steel (1893), and subsequently recognized by many authors.

Modern recognition of skeletal muscle disease as a complication of alcohol abuse dates from a series of papers from Scandinavia in which Hed (1955), Fahlgren (1957), Ekbom (1964) and coworkers described two clinically different disorders, acute and chronic alcoholic myopathy. These authors also found minor electromyographic and/or muscle histologic abnormalities in asymptomatic alcoholics, suggesting that subclinical muscle disorders were common in these patients. Perkoff (1967) confirmed these findings on subclinical alcoholic myopathy, detectable only by laboratory analysis or electrophysiological studies. Later, Song and Rubin (1972) described the development of muscle damage by ethanol ingestion in human volunteers independently of the action of other pathogenic factors.

In our first studies on human skeletal muscle myopathy we reported a 43% incidence of alcoholic myopathy in chronic alcoholics and a dose-related effect with ethanol (Grau *et al.*, 1983; Urbano-Márquez *et al.*, 1985). Later, the clinical, functional and histological incidence of alcoholic myopathy was studied in a different series of patients, reporting a 42% incidence of muscle weakness, and a 46% incidence of histological changes (Urbano-Márquez *et al.*, 1984, 1985 and 1989). In a prospective study, we showed that ethanol is the most frequent cause of acute rhabdomyolysis (Fernández-Solà *et al.*, 1988). Recently, we studied a series of 50 women in which the incidence of alcoholic cardiomyopathy and skeletal myopathy was similar to a comparable group of men, but requiring lower dose to achieve this damage (Estruch *et al.*, 1991).

2. EPIDEMIOLOGICAL ASPECTS

Ethanol ingestion is still a great health problem in Western industrialized countries. About 10% of adults in Europe and North America drink an excessive quantity of alcohol, with the increased alcohol intake observed in adolescents being of ever greater concern (Eckhardt *et al.*, 1981). Although the incidence of alcoholic muscle damage is not precisely known, the effects of high ethanol intake on cardiac and striated muscle are increasingly recognized (Rubin, 1979; Urbano-Márquez *et al.*, 1989). At least 50% of chronic alcoholics have some type of clinical or subclinical myopathy (Worden, 1976). The differences found in the incidence of myopathy in different series depends on the criteria used to define alcoholic muscle damage; whether acute, chronic or acute episodes in alcoholic patients with chronic myopathy (Martin *et al.*, 1985). Moreover, a progressive increase has been observed in the incidence of myopathy if histological criteria are used instead of clinical or functional criteria (Urbano-Márquez *et al.*, 1984 and 1985).

Acute myopathy. The incidence of acute myopathy is sporadic (Hallera and Knochel, 1984), probably involving 0.5% of the general alcoholic population (Preedy and Peters, 1990) and 1–2% percent of chronic alcoholic patients (Myerson and Lafair, 1970; Pedro-Botet *et al.*, 1986). Acute alcoholic myopathy predominantly effects men from 40–60 years of age (Grau *et al.*, 1983) and is usually related to acute alcoholic intoxication or alcohol withdrawal (Kahn and Meyer, 1970; Hällgren *et al.*, 1980; Gabow *et al.*, 1982; Martin *et al.*, 1982).

Acute myopathy in patients with chronic myopathy. Acute myopathy seems to be more frequent in patients with chronic alcoholic myopathy (Martin *et al.*, 1985). Between 30–46% of patients with chronic alcoholic myopathy report previous episodes of acute symptoms, mostly in the form of muscle pains and cramps in the calves, acute generalized muscle weakness and grossly dark urine, presumably as a reflection of myoglobinuria (Grau *et al.*, 1983; Fernández-Solà *et al.*, 1988).

Chronic myopathy. The incidence of chronic alcoholic myopathy is stable and similar in males and females (Haller *et al.*, 1984; Urbano-Márquez *et al.*, 1985). The estimated prevalence of chronic myopathy depends on the parameter used for diagnosis, since there are many subclinical cases, most of which are undetected. Using clinical parameters for detection, 30% of patients reported proximal muscle weakness or myalgia (Grau *et al.*, 1983; Urbano-Márquez *et al.*, 1989). Around a third of them presented elevated serum creatine kinase (Fernández-Solà *et al.*, 1988). Functional evaluation of muscle weakness with myometric measurements showed muscle weakness (measured by deltoid myometry) in around 42% of patients as compared to controls (Urbano-Márquez *et al.*, 1989). With histological parameters, Martin *et al.* (1982) described a subclinical myopathy involving almost 40% of chronic alcoholic patients. Type-II fiber atrophy has been found in 33% to 60% of chronic alcoholic patients (Martin *et al.*, 1982). In our experience, the incidence of optic microscopic changes in muscle is around 46% of patients (Grau *et al.*, 1983; Urbano-Márquez *et al.*, 1984 and 1985). With ultrastructural microscopy study, almost all alcoholic patients presented different muscle changes.

There are few studies of alcoholic myopathy in women (Slavin *et al.*, 1983). In our experience, the incidence of muscle damage in women seems as frequent as in men. We studied a series of 50 alcoholic women in which 50% presented muscle weakness measured by deltoid myometry and histological criteria of myopathy suggesting increased sensitivity to alcohol damage at a muscular level (Estruch *et al.*, 1991). There are no clinical studies to know the differential sensitivity to alcoholic muscle disease in old and young patients since most of the patients included in clinical studies are middle-aged people (20–45 years)

In alcoholic patients who present with systemic organ damage related to ethanol other than myopathy, the incidence of myopathy seems to be higher than in patients without other manifestations of alcoholic organ damage. Thus, Martin *et al.* (1985) described an incidence of chronic myopathy in 98 out of 151 chronic alcoholic patients. In our experience, in chronic alcoholic patients with dilated cardiomyopathy, the incidence of muscle weakness measured by myometry was 58% as compared to a matched control group and the incidence of histological alcoholic myopathy was 82% (Fernández-Solà, 1984; Urbano-Márquez *et al.*, 1989). These data are clearly higher compared to alcoholic patients without other organ damage. In a prospective study, we corroborated the clinical and histological correlation between skeletal and cardiac damage in chronic alcoholism (Fernández-Solà *et al.*, 1984). Moreover, in our experience, chronic alcoholic patients with cirrhosis show a high incidence of myopathy, ranging from 22% (Martin *et al.*, 1982) to 65% (Estruch *et al.*, 1992).

Although the potential reversibility of muscle damage seems to be almost complete with respect to type-II fiber atrophy (Slavin *et al.*, 1983), other muscle changes such as myocytolysis can not be reversed. Thus, in a 5-year follow-up study with muscle re-biopsy, we studied the potential reversibility of alcoholic myopathy and we were able to corroborate the possible persistence of muscle changes in 5 out of 13 patients despite cessation of alcohol intake. Furthermore, patients who persist in ethanol ingestion may develop muscle changes, or histological muscle damage may progress in intensity (Estruch *et al.*, 1993; Urbano-Márquez *et al.*, 1993).

3. PHYSIOPATHOLOGICAL ASPECTS

The physiopathological mechanisms which determine the ethanol-induced muscle damage are still not completely understood (Haller and Knochel, 1984; Sontag *et al.*, 1991). Many possible target effects of ethanol in the cell make the pathogenesis of alco-holic myopathy difficult to study. Although some muscle changes have been experimen-tally induced in striated muscle (Preedy *et al.*, 1989), there is, unfortunately, no adequate experimental model in which the clinical signs and symptoms of chronic myopathy can be reproduced by ethanol ingestion (Rubin, 1979). Furthermore, in some experimental models in rats (Edmonds *et al.*, 1987), ethanol did not induce muscle changes. Thus, myocytolysis, inflammation, diffuse fibrosis and myoglobinuria have not been reported in animals including primates fed with ethanol.

   The main pathogenic agents believed to be involved in alcoholic myopathy are: 1) ethanol itself, 2) acetaldehyde, 3) mineral, ionic and vitamin deficiencies and 4) malnutrition.

3.1. Direct effect of ethanol

There is no good experimental model for studying the chronic effects of ethanol in tissues in cell culture systems, mainly because of the time limitation for ethanol exposure. Similarly, experimental animal models are different from the human model because of the limitations of administering ethanol to animals. In acute experimental models in, rats (Haller and Drachman, 1980) and in human volunteers (Song and Rubin, 1972), increased creatine kinase and ultrastructural muscle changes were shown to be in direct proportion to the level of blood alcohol, thus reinforcing the hypothesis that alcoholic myopathy preceeds ethanol toxicity (Haller and Knochel, 1984; Urbano-Márquez *et al.*, 1989). Haller (1985) reported a selective vulnerability of type-I fibers, manifested as later type I predominance in regenerating fibers in the rat. Chronic alcoholic myopathy may be related to the lifetime dose of ethanol (Urbano-Márquez *et al.*, 1989), similarly to alcohol induced liver damage (Lelbavh, 1975) in a process independent of malnutrition or vitamin deficiencies. The type of alcohol consumed is not important in the development of alcoholic myopathy (Urbano-Márquez *et al.*, 1989).

   Clinical observations suggest that the dose of ethanol is important in determining muscle injury in acute alcoholic myopathy (Grau *et al.*, 1983; Haller and Knochel, 1984). Thus, alcoholics develop rhabdomyolysis during binge drinking. In severe and subclinical forms of acute alcoholic myopathy, serum creatine kinase levels increase in relation to acute periods of active drinking and fall to normal range during abstinence. The related food deprivation that typically accompanies binge drinking may thus promote the development of levels of ethanol that are toxic to skeletal muscle (Nygren, 1967). Moreover, chronic alcoholics who binge drink have an increased risk of developing acute muscle damage.

At present, the main known mechanisms of ethanol induced alterations in skeletal muscle function are:

3.1.1. *Alterations in muscle membrane fluidity, membrane channels, pumps and ionic transients*

Characteristics of the cell membrane together with the activity of various ion pumps result in the establishment of electrical properties which are essential to the function of these cells and regulate the response of these cells to extracellular signals (Neher, 1952; Lewis *et al.*, 1990). Recent studies suggest that ethanol may alter the lipid structure causing alterations in fluidity that may induce functional changes in the membrane proteins responsible for the maintenance of the internal milieu of the cell (Hoek *et al.*, 1988).

The toxic effects of ethanol presumably derive from the physical properties of the ethanol molecule, which determine its interaction with individual cell structures and enzyme systems. Ethanol alters the configuration and fluidity of isolated cell membranes (Israel *et al.*, 1970; Hoek *et al.*, 1988), presumably by entering the hydrophobic lipid membrane core, and has been shown to inhibit Na^+/K^+-ATPase in membrane preparations from various tissues. With chronic ethanol exposure, activity of Na^+/K^+-ATPase increases in many tissues including skeletal muscle (Israel *et al.*, 1970). As a result, a secondary disruption of transduction systems involving phosphoinositides and diacylglycerol develop. The presence of ethanol interferes with a number of cell functions which involve the transport and binding of calcium. The membrane G- protein system may also be altered by ethanol, producing a decrease of membrane fluidity for Ca^{2+} and other ions (Hoek *et al.*, 1988).

These membrane effects of ethanol provide support for the notion that ethanol may damage cells by altering membrane transport or permeability (Katz, 1982). This hypothesis is supported by the finding of intracellular edema as an early ultrastructural feature and more directly by the observation that skeletal muscle of alcoholics with acute myopathy contains distinct alterations in ion composition including a striking increase in Na^+ and Cl^- (Knochel *et al.*, 1978). Whether these electrolyte derangements are related to a primary abnormality of muscle membrane permeability or transport or are secondary to other cellular effects of ethanol is not known. Membrane permeability is increased by acute alcohol exposure and reduced by chronic alcohol exposure (tolerance effect) (Vanderkooi, 1979; Hoek *et al.*, 1988). *In vitro*, ethanol acutely and reversibly depresses skeletal muscle contractibility by calcium-dependent and also by calcium-independent mechanisms (Danzinger *et al.*, 1991). The first involves a decrease in sarcolemmal Ca^{2+} entry and changes in sarcoplasmic reticulum, decreasing the entrance and increasing the passive leak of Ca^{2+} (Thomas *et al.*, 1989).

In a chronic model of ethanol effect, the Na^+/K^+-ATPase activity seems to increase, suggesting a tolerance effect or a up-regulation of channel receptors (Akera *et al.*, 1973). In cultured skeletal muscle fibers exposed to ethanol, an up-regulation of Na^+ and Ca^{2+} voltage-dependent channels can be demonstrated (Brodie and Sampson, 1990), producing an increase in Ca^{2+} entry in chronic alcoholism. Thomas *et al.* (1989) and DuBell *et al.* (1991) demonstrated an inhibition of Ca^{2+} transients in cardiac myocytes induced by ethanol in voltage-dependent Ca^{2+} channels. We have also reproduced a similar effect in rat skeletal myoblasts incubated with ethanol, observing a dose-dependent decrease in the Ca^{2+} level (Cofan *et al.*, 1995). This decrease in intracellular Ca^{2+} concentration may be partially responsible for alcohol-induced damage to muscle cells.

In addition to Ca^{2+} changes, experimental studies *in vitro* demonstrated the inhibition of muscle contractibility induced by acute ethanol incubation (200 mM) by Ca^{2+}-independent mechanisms (Sonntag *et al.*, 1991). Ethanol may interfere with actin-myosin coupling probably because of the inhibition of Ca^{2+} binding to troponin (Thomas *et al.*, 1989; DuBell *et al.*, 1991). Therefore, the result of ethanol exposure may be a loss of Ca^{2+} storage in the sarcoplasmatic reticulum, a decrease in Ca^{2+} release after depolarization, and reduced muscle contractibility (Sonntag *et al.*, 1991). This hypothesis is consistent with experiments demonstrating that Ca^{2+} partially reverses the ethanol-induced decrease in contraction of the longitudinal muscle. Chronic exposure to ethanol inhibits troponin synthesis and Ca^{2+} binding to troponin C (Preedy and Peters, 1989). Ethanol also may interact with a subunit of the gated calcium channel either by increasing the size of the channel or by altering its conformation possibly via changes in membrane fluidity.

3.1.2. Disturbances in protein synthesis

Recent experimental studies in rats (Preedy and Peters, 1988 and 1989; Preedy *et al.*, 1988) have indicated that rates of protein synthesis are decreased by 15–30% in skeletal muscle exposed to ethanol (Preedy and Peters, 1992). Protein catabolism is not significantly affected by ethanol.

In these studies, protein synthesis was inhibited predominantly in type II (anaerobic, fast twitch) muscle fibers (Preedy *et al.*, 1988 and 1992; Martin *et al.*, 1985). The mechanisms responsible for the inhibition of protein synthesis are unclear. Ethanol reduces protein synthesis by decreasing RNA content in acute experimental alcoholic myopathy in rats (Marway *et al.*, 1990). In a recent study, type-II atrophy of chronic alcoholic patients with myopathy correlated with reductions in muscle protein and serum carnosinase activities (Wassif *et al.*, 1993). The protein composition also correlated with RNA composition. Ethanol may also have direct effects on gene transcription, RNA processing and transport, or on translational processes. Alternatively, the effects of ethanol on gene expression may be secondary to perturbations in cellular processes, such as mitochondrial or membrane activity (Sonntag *et al.*, 1991). Studies using high concentrations of ethanol (0.21–0.84 M) in reticulocytes have suggested additional actions of ethanol on the regulation of protein synthesis (Wu, 1981). Ethanol may inhibit polypeptide synthesis by both activation and inhibitory compound within the cell and by suppression of ternary complex formation (Wu, 1981; Sonntag *et al.*, 1991).

The decrease in protein synthesis is not always reversed with discontinuing ethanol intake as observed in the other effects of ethanol (Sonntag *et al.*, 1991). However, other experimental studies performed in rats by Edmonds *et al.* (1987) did not confirm significant differences in muscle weight or the number or size of type I, IIa or IIb muscle fibers.

3.1.3. Disruption of mitochondrial function

In alcoholics, liver mitochondria displays striking electron-microscopic alterations (including swelling and abnormal cristae) which in animals and humans could be attributed to alcohol itself rather than to other factors (Lieber, 1968 and 1988). It has been proposed that the functional changes in mitochondria may be related to membrane alterations (Waring *et al.*, 1981).

Some authors have suggested the possibility that muscle mitochondria, the organelles which synthesize ATP by oxidative phosphorylation, are morphologically altered in alcoholic myopathy and after ethanol administration in rodents, dogs and monkeys or human beings (Song and Rubin, 1972; Vased *et al.*, 1975; Sarna *et al.*, 1976; Alexander *et al.*, 1977; Rubin, 1979). Chronic ethanol consumption inhibits mitochondrial protein synthesis *in vivo* and *in vitro* (Rubin, 1979). Such changes correlate with decreased function of mitochondria including decreased respiratory rates with a variety of substrates (Pachinger *et al.*, 1975). However, further studies by our group showed a maintenance in the functional respiratory characteristics of skeletal muscle mitochondria and sarcoplasmic-reticular membranes after chronic ethanol treatment in both animal (Cardellach *et al.*, 1991) and human models (Cardellach *et al.*, 1992).

3.1.4. Changes in carbohydrate-glycogen-lipid metabolism

The oxidation of ethanol by skeletal muscle is minimal because of the absence of alcohol-dehydrogenase. Therefore, alterations in the metabolic processes in muscle are either due directly to the effects of ethanol or are secondary to metabolic derangements elsewhere. Changes in redox potential in chronic alcoholism may interfere with the gluconeogenic process (Williamson *et al.*, 1969; Cook *et al.*, 1992). Trounce *et al.* (1990) described a glycolytic deficiency in addition to type-II selective fiber atrophy and mitochondrial failure in a chronic (10 weeks) experimental rat model of skeletal myopathy.

The muscle glycogen metabolism of alcoholics is disturbed (Perkoff *et al.*, 1967; Cook *et al.*, 1992). There is a reduced lactic acid response to ischemic forearm exercise in heavy drinkers (Perkoff *et al.*, 1966; Haller and Knochel, 1984). An inhibitory effect on phosphorylase kinase at low level ethanol concentration is evident (Cussó *et al.*, 1989). Ethanol may induce a transient disorder of muscle glycolysis and produces a subnormal pattern of lactic acid production corroborated by ischemic exercise in patients with symptomatic and subclinical alcoholic myopathy (Perkoff *et al.*, 1966; Cook *et al.*, 1992). A transitory defect in phosphorylase activity has been reported in alcoholic myopathy, thus producing a clinical picture resembling McArdle disease (Cussó *et al.*, 1989).

Selective atrophy of type IIB fibers suggesting a reduced capacity in the anaerobic glycolytic pathway in the proximal muscle in heavy drinkers has been reported (Peters *et al.*, 1985; Preedy and Peters, 1988). Such a reduction may be secondary to the loss of type-II fiber by an unknown mechanism, or alternatively, such a reduction in glucose metabolism might lead to a metabolically induced atrophy (Kiessling *et al.*, 1975). The specific relevance of these changes to acute or chronic alcoholic myopathy is uncertain. The reporting of reduced lactate production with ischemic exercise in other acute illnesses suggests that this may be a non-specific finding (Perkoff *et al.*, 1967; Haller and Knochel, 1984).

Ethanol may also produce changes in the lipid composition of muscle cells (Hoek *et al.*, 1988; Lieber *et al.*, 1988). Short term ethanol exposure produces changes in lipid membrane composition and renders the membrane more fluid. On the contrary, chronic ethanol exposure reduces its fluidity, a situation supposed to be adaptive (Polokoff *et al.*, 1985). The main phospholipid acting as a target for ethanol in the membrane seems to be phosphatidyl-inositol (IP3) (Hoek *et al.*, 1988). There is also an impaired fatty-acid oxidation of the muscle induced by ethanol mitochondrial damage (Rubin, 1979; Hudgson, 1984). The increase of lipid deposition in skeletal and cardiac muscle may be, in part, because of a decrease of fatty acid oxidation (Song and Rubin, 1972; Rubin, 1979; Ward and Peters, 1992). A transitory defect in carnitine has been suggested in chronic alcoholism, although its relevance has not been corroborated (Haller and Knochel, 1984). The abnormality of triglyceride metabolism in skeletal muscle reported by Sunnasy *et al.* (1983) may explain triglyceride deposition in skeletal muscle cells (Hudgson, 1984).

3.1.5. Hormonal influences due to ethanol

Insulin-like factors (IGFs) have been shown to have a role in the differentiation of muscle in the newborn mouse (Jennische *et al.*, 1987) and the regeneration of muscle damage induced by hypoxia or snake venom (Jennische *et al.*, 1987). Because of their important anabolic effects on tissue, a decline in the plasma levels of these hormones may contribute to a reduction in protein synthesis in response to ethanol (Sonntag *et al.*, 1991). Recent reports suggest that plasma levels of IGF-1 may decrease in both animals and humans in response to chronic ethanol, but not in acute ethanol exposure (Jennische *et al.*, 1987) or in the presence of cirrhosis (Salemo *et al.*, 1987). However, these reports were unable to conclude that alcohol specifically influences the secretion of this hormone.

Ethanol administration also reduces plasma growth hormone levels by a mechanism mediated by hypothalamus (Sonntag *et al.*, 1987). These changes in growth hormone are assumed to be responsible for the decrease of IGF-1 levels observed in alcoholism. However, these effects are only related to high doses of ethanol, which can not be maintained in a chronic model of alcoholism (Sonntag and Boyd, 1989) Testosterone stimulates the formation of muscle mass in skeletal muscle. Plasma levels of testosterone decline in response to acute or chronic ethanol administration both in animals and humans (Cicero, 1981; Sonntag *et al.*, 1991). Many of these effects on testosterone appear to be related to a direct effect of ethanol on steroid biosynthesis. However, there have been no studies on the effects of ethanol on androgen receptors in target tissues, specifically skeletal muscle (Sonntag *et al.*, 1991).

3.2. Acetaldehyde

Skeletal muscle cells do not contain the enzyme alcohol-dehydrogenase, thus ethanol is not directly metabolized by skeletal muscle (Haller and Knochel 1984; Hoek *et al.*, 1988). Consequently, the only concentration of acetaldehyde in muscle comes from the hepatic metabolism. Acetaldehyde is oxidized to acetate virtually as rapidly as it produced. Thus, because of the low plasma concentration of acetaldehyde (50 micromolar/L or less), the potential toxic effect of acetaldehyde in muscle cells is low. However, some authors suggest that such low levels of acetaldehyde may induce cellular effects in skeletal muscle *in vitro* and thus, may be relevant in the development of muscle disease in alcoholism (Rubin, 1979; Martin *et al.*, 1982; Haller and Knochel, 1984).

Acetaldehyde decreases ATP cellular levels, causing an energy problem for the cell (Sonntag *et al.*, 1991). Additionally, it may interfere with enzyme activities, possibly due to binding to critical functional groups (Lieber, 1988). In isolated plasma membranes, acetaldehyde (as ethanol itself) inhibits the Na^+, K^+-ATP-ase activity in a dose-dependent manner (Wiiliams *et al.*, 1975; Rubin, 1979; Preedy *et al.*, 1992). Removal of acetaldehyde reverses the inhibition.

Acetaldehyde may act similarly to ethanol, interfering with a number of cell functions. For instance, the transport and binding of Ca^{2+} may be affected and therefore cAMP and adenylate cyclase activity decreases as a result of acute ethanol exposure (Rubin, 1979; Hoek, 1988; Katz, 1982). Acetaldehyde interferes with muscle protein synthesis at a mitochondrial level (Matsukazi and Lieber, 1977). In blood, up to 50 micromolar/L acetaldehyde is achieved in alcoholic patients. Such a concentration experimentally inhibits the association of actin to myosin *in vitro* (Rubin, 1979). Exposure to high levels of acetaldehyde may, in turn, affect mitochondrial function, especially after long-term alcohol consumption (Matsuzaki and Lieber, 1977). However, damage to some cell functions requires high level concentrations and long term exposure to acetaldehyde, a situation not achieved in human alcoholism.

Acetate, which is produced during ethanol metabolism, may reach the muscle cells where the most of this is oxidized and substitutes for other normal oxidative fuels such as carbohydrate. It is unknown whether acetate oxidation plays a role in the reduced muscle lactate production and glucose uptake which accompanies alcohol consumption (Juhlin-Dannfelt *et al.*, 1977). Acetaldehyde, in turn, may cause tissue injury predominantly in the liver through the formation of adduct with proteins, resulting in antibody formation, enzyme inactivation, decreased DNA repair, and alterations in mitochondria, microtubules and plasma membranes (Lieber, 1968). These effects are not so clear at a skeletal muscle level (Hoek, 1988).

3.3. Peroxidation

Free radical injury to muscle may develop depending of three different factors: radicals, nonenzymatic compounds and peroxidases (Sonntag *et al.*, 1991). Experimental muscle peroxidation damage in rats mainly involves older animals (Zerba *et al.*, 1990). Peroxidation may unspecifically contribute to the increase in secondary or delayed muscle injury (Ward and Preedy, 1992), although a clear protagonist in direct muscle damage has yet to be identified (Lieber, 1968). Reductions in imidazole dipeptide content (anserine 18%, carnosine 50%), considered to be antioxidant and/or intracellular buffering agents are not mediating factors in the development of chronic experimental (Ward and Preedy, 1992) and human (Wassif *et al.*, 1993) alcoholic myopathy. Ferritin provides the iron necessary to inhibit lipid peroxidation. Experimentally, iron exposure accentuates the ethanol-induced changes in lipid peroxidation and the glutathione status as demonstrated in the liver, but not in skeletal muscle cells (Lieber, 1988; Valenzuela *et al.*, 1983).

3.4. Disorders in mineral, vitamin or electrolyte balance

Most of these disorders produce only an acute experimental myopathy similar to acute alcoholic skeletal myopathy. The interest in discussing their pathogenesis lies in their temporal relationship with alcohol intake.

3.4.1. Potassium depletion

Potassium depletion may be associated with a syndrome of acute and rapidly evolving muscle injury which closely mimics acute alcoholic myopathy (Haller and Knochel, 1984). Additionally, hypokalaemia is a frequent finding in individuals withdrawing from alcohol because of vomiting and/or diarrhea. Several cases of acute myopathy associated to potassium deficiency have been described in such patients (Martin *et al.*, 1971; Rubenstein and Wainapel, 1977). Serum creatine kinase activity is characteristically elevated in this situation and muscle biopsy shows necrosis associated to vacuolar changes. However, it is unlikely that potassium depletion represents the major cause of acute muscle injury in alcoholism (Adler *et al.*, 1985).

Different authors (Perkoff, 1971; Fernández-Solà *et al.*, 1988; Urbano-Márquez *et al.*, 1989) found no relationship between serum potassium and creatine kinase levels in acute alcoholic myopathy. Further, muscle potassium has been reported to be normal in many patients with acute alcoholic myopathy, even in the presence of mild hypokalaemia (Anderson *et al.*, 1980). Finally, in experimental acute alcoholic myopathy with rhabdomyolysis, muscle injury may occur in the absence of potassium depletion (Haller and Drachman, 1980).

3.4.2. Phosphate depletion

This is another recognized cause of acute myopathy, which may be relevant to the development of alcoholic myopathy. Alcohol has been directly implicated in the development of phosphate depletion in animals fed with alcohol (Blachley, 1980).

A selective phosphate depletion in dogs reproduces many of the electrochemical muscle abnormalities shown in alcoholic patients, but does not cause muscle necrosis (Fuller *et al.*, 1976). Hyper or hyponutrition in hypophosphatemic dogs easily induces frank rhabdomyolysis (Knochel *et al.*, 1978) which reverses with normalization of phosphate levels. An association between the occurrence of hypophosphatemia and the development of acute myopathy in chronic alcoholics has been recognized, demonstrating that, even with normal serum phosphate levels, such patients had low levels of total phosphate in muscle (Knochel *et al.*, 1975; Anderson *et al.*, 1980).

Phosphate depletion commonly occurs in chronic malnourished alcoholic patients, and renourishing without phosphate supplementation may produce acute hypophosphatemic myopathy. However, clinical studies suggest that both severe and subclinical acute myopathy may occur without hypophosphatemia (Haller and Knochel, 1984; Urbano-Márquez *et al.*, 1989). The exact contribution of low muscle phosphate in chronic muscle injury has yet to be established since the exact muscle phosphate content in these situations has not been measured.

3.4.3. Magnesium deficiency

Acute necrotizing myopathy may occur inducing dietary hypomagnesemia (Jones *et al.*, 1969). Hypomagnesemia frequently occurs during ethanol withdrawal. Hypomagnesemia is also a common situation in chronic alcoholism because of low dietary intake, reduced gastrointestinal absorption due to gastrointestinal disease or cirrhosis or enhanced renal excretion as a direct effect of ethanol (Haller and Knochel, 1984). Low levels of Mg^{2+}

may be present in muscle even in the presence of normal plasma Mg^{2+} (Jones *et al.*, 1969; Anderson *et al.*, 1980).

Magnesium deficiency may cause muscle weakness in man. EMG findings in such patients are suggestive of myopathy (Shils, 1969). However, clinical studies have found no association between serum Mg^{2+} and alcoholic myopathy. Thus, the relationship between reduced muscle Mg^{2+} and the occurrence of acute and chronic myopathy still remains unclear.

3.4.4. Calcium depletion

Chronic hypocalcemia may cause unspecific muscle damage as seen in patients with osteomalacia (Young *et al.*, 1978), and may contribute to the increase in muscle damage in alcoholic myopathy. However, the development of alcoholic myopathy has been demonstrated to be independent of serum Ca^{2+} values at both clinical (Urbano-Márquez *et al.*, 1989) and experimental (Adler *et al.*, 1985) levels. Vitamin D deficiency does not play a role in hypocalcemic-induced muscle damage (Hickish *et al.*, 1989).

3.4.5. Selenium depletion

Selenium acts as a marker of gluthatione peroxidase and beta carotene. Its deficiency is also related to alpha-tocopherol in free-radical mediated damage and organ injury in chronic alcoholic patients (Preedy and Peters, 1990; Ward and Peters, 1992). Preedy and Peters (1990) also reported a decrease in selenium levels and plasma tocopherol in chronic alcoholics with myopathy, suggesting that it may influence the pathogenesis of alcohol damage on skeletal muscle through decreasing the protein synthesis rate. An epidemic of cardiomyopathy was described in China (Keshan disease), involving a geographical area with a population which had a nutritional deficiency of selenium. Although cardiomyopathy was relevant, no skeletal muscle changes were described (Thuong *et al.*, 1986).

3.4.6. Cobalt toxicity

Cobalt is the metal which was implicated in the development of epidemic cardiomyopathy in Quebec (Canada) when it was added to beer to decrease the foamy effect. However, no clear relationship with alcoholic myopathy was demonstrated by Sullivan *et al.* (1968)

3.4.7. Vitamin deficicencies

Vitamin A levels are usually low in alcoholics even in the early phases. Ethanol administration to animals has been shown to decrease hepatic vitamin A levels, but no clear influence has been reported in skeletal muscle cells (Sato and Lieber, 1982). Retinol and retinoid acid may serve as substrates in lipid peroxidation induced by ethanol (Lieber, 1968; Leo *et al.*, 1984). However, dietary supplementation with vitamin A does not produce any improvement at neither the hepatic or muscular level in rats (Leo *et al.*, 1982).

Thiamine may be deficient if malabsorption is present in chronic alcoholism. Most patients with alcoholic myopathy, develop the disease without thiamine deficiency

(Rubin, 1979; Grau *et al.*, 1983; Urbano-Márquez *et al.*, 1985). Thus, this deficiency is not crucial for muscle damage development in either animal and human models. Pyridoxine metabolism may be interfered by ethanol, but it is clearly independent of the production of muscle damage (Lieber, 1968). Tocopherol (Vitamin E) is a reducing agent which can be decreased by ethanol intake and its deficiency may play a role in acute alcohol myopathy (Ward and Peters, 1992).

3.5. Disorders in nutrition

At one time, alcoholic myopathy was incorrectly attributed to poor nutrition or general weakness of patients (Rubin, 1979; Urbano-Márquez *et al.*, 1989; Mendelson and Mello, 1992). A possible effect of malnutrition (Klinkerfuss, 1967; Perkoff, 1971) or B1–B6 vitamin-deficiency (Hed *et al.*, 1962) has been suggested in different series.

Although malnutrition has been reported to affect around 20% of the chronic alcoholics in some series (Martin *et al.*, 1975) involving proportionally more women, in our experience, full malnutrition is not present in more than 2% of chronic alcoholic patients (Urbano-Márquez *et al.*, 1989) and similarly affects both sexes (Estruch *et al.*, 1991). In a retrospective study of 250 chronic alcoholic men, 10% presented energy malnutrition, 15% protein malnutrition and 2% both (Nicolás *et al.*, 1993). Malnutrition may, by itself, cause type-II fiber atrophy, but it is not related to the development of acute or chronic alcoholic myopathy since many cases develop in the absence of clear malnutrition criteria at clinical and experimental levels. Different clinical series have demonstrated the independence of malnutrition or vitamin deficiency in the development of alcoholic myopathy (Lieber, 1968; Urbano-Márquez *et al.*, 1989; Wassif *et al.*, 1993).

4. HISTOLOGICAL ASPECTS

There is no specific pattern of alcohol muscle damage at neither optical or ultrastructural levels (Urbano-Márquez *et al.*, 1984 and 1985). Thus, the diagnosis of alcoholic myopathy requires a characteristic clinical pattern and careful exclusion of other causes of myopathy.

4.1. Optic microscopy

The prevalence of the different histological muscle changes in alcoholic patients varies in different series from 46% in asymptomatic chronic alcoholic patients (Urbano-Márquez *et al.*, 1989) to 82% in patients with cardiomyopathy (Fernández-Solà *et al.*, 1994).

The most frequent changes are:

Myocytolysis. This is a necessary finding for many authors to define true alcoholic myopathy (Oh, 1972). It may be preceded by intracellular edema and hypercontracted fibers culminating with degeneration and myofilament dissolution (ghost fibers) with or without phagocytosis. In our experience it is a characteristic finding usually involving around 5–10% of the fibers in around 50% of the cases (Grau *et al.*, 1983; Urbano-Márquez *et al.*, 1989). We observed slight necrosis in 37% of the cases and moderate necrosis in 21% of the cases amongst patients with alcoholic myopathy (Fernández-Solà *et al.*, 1994). Fiber regeneration is a frequent phenomenon after myocytolysis. These fibers appear basophilic on H&E staining.

Atrophy. For some authors this is the most frequent finding in alcoholic myopathy (Slavin *et al.*, 1983; Preedy *et al.*, 1989; Salisbury *et al.*, 1992). The muscle cells of these patients show a wide variability in size, mainly affecting type-II B fibers. Some authors use only this criteria to define alcoholic myopathy (Slavin *et al.*, 1983; Hidgson, 1984 Martin *et al.*, 1985; Edmonds *et al.*, 1987) although there is no consensus on this point (Oh, 1972; Urbano-Márquez *et al.*, 1989; Salisbury *et al.*, 1992) since type-II fiber atrophy may be observed in many different muscle diseases such as malnutrition, steroid treatment, disuse or neuropathy (Dubowitz and Brooke, 1973). Globally it is present in 30% to 50% of all chronic alcoholic patients (Grau *et al.*, 1983; Wassif *et al.*, 1993). A correlation has been proposed between type-II atrophy and reductions in serum protein, muscle protein composition and RNA content (Ward and Preedy 1992; Wassif *et al.*, 1993). This finding appears to be more frequent in alcoholic patients with coexisting malnutrition, neuropathy (Urbano-Márquez *et al.*, 1985; Mills *et al.*, 1986) or other organ damage as well as in patients with a severe degree of myopathy with extensive myocytolysis.

In a morphometrical study of 100 non-selected chronic alcoholic patients, 33% showed type-II fiber atrophy. On exclusion of patients with polyneuropathy, only 15% showed type-II fiber atrophy. When we considered patients with alcoholic myopathy, 45% showed type-II fiber atrophy. In this group, if patients with coexisting neuropathy are excluded, only 25% have type-II fiber atrophy. Type-II atrophy was related to the toxic effects of ethanol, the coexistence of polineuropathy or nutritional problems.

Internal nuclei may be present in up to 10% of the fibers, but it is also an unspecific change, which is not always present in alcoholic myopathy.

Moth-eaten fibers, is an expression of the glycolytic disarray of fibers being evident in NADH staining. In our experience, its prevalence is around 15% (Grau *et al.*, 1983) to 25% (Fernández-Solà *et al.*, 1994). Subsarcolemmical deposition, which is probably due to mitochondrial material accumulated at this level, is evident in NADH and trichome staining. In our experience it is present in 50% of the cases (Grau *et al.*, 1983; Urbano-Márquez *et al.*, 1985; Fernández-Solà *et al.*, 1994).

Inflammation. Interstitial inflammatory infiltrate by lymphocytes, monocytes or macrophage is an unusual finding only occasionally seen in alcoholic myopathy (Grau *et al.*, 1983; Urbano-Márquez *et al.*, 1985). We observed interstitial muscle infiltrate in less than 5% of the chronic alcoholic patients with skeletal myopathy (Grau *et al.*, 1983; Fernández-Solà *et al.*, 1994). The presence of macrophage with phagocytic phenomenon may follow the necrosis of fibers. It is also an unusual phenomenon in alcoholic myopathy. In our experience it is present in 2–5% of the cases (Grau *et al.*, 1983; Fernández-Solà *et al.*, 1994).

Type-I fiber predominance has been referred to in experimental alcoholic myopathy (Haller and Knochel, 1984). In our experience it is quite a frequent phenomenon, involving around 10%–20% of cases (Grau *et al.*, 1983). Interstitial fibrosis, usually reflects a previous necrotic phenomenon. It is unusual in alcoholic myopathy. Fat deposition in endomysia may be present in about 50% of cases. In our experience presence of fat in the endomysium may only be observed in few cases, around 5%.

Other unusual findings reported are: changes similar to "central core disease" and tubular aggregates. We have observed a peculiar case of alcoholic myopathy with tubular aggregates similar to that reported by Chi and Munsat (Chui *et al.*, 1975). Any combination of these histological findings may be present in different patients (Knochel *et al.*, 1975; Grau *et al.*, 1983; Haller and Knochel, 1984).

4.2. Ultrastructural studies

There is no specific change in alcohol muscle damage at an ultrastructural level. However, almost all chronic alcoholic patients show muscle damage at a ultrastructural level regardless of the presence of clinical symptoms or changes in optic microscopy (Hanid *et al.*, 1981; Grau *et al.*, 1983; Urbano-Márquez *et al.*, 1984).

The main reported changes are:

1. Intracellular edema. This may be an early change, preceding myocytolysis.
2. Glycogen and lipid droplets deposited in the intermyofibrillary space.
3. Destruction of myofilaments.
4. Dilatation of sarcoplasmic reticulum.
5. Hypercontracted fibers and
6. Mitochondrial changes (enlargement, vacuolization, cristae disorganization, and formation of myelin bodies) (Klinkerfuss *et al.*, 1967; Song and Rubin, 1972; Martinez *et al.*, 1979).

Ultrastructural muscle changes may precede the development of light microscopy muscle changes or muscle symptoms (Urbano-Márquez *et al.*, 1984). In a series of 19 patients with chronic alcoholism all the patients presented ultrastructural muscle changes, such as mitochondrial alterations, sarcoplasmic reticulum disturbances, lipid and glycogen deposition, and necrotic changes in myofibrilles, with the presence of Rod bodies. However, patients with optical microscopic changes in muscle presented a greater number of necrotic and mitochondrial changes in muscle fibers.

5. CLINICAL MANIFESTATIONS

There are two different clinical pictures of alcoholic myopathy: Acute and chronic (Grau *et al.*, 1983; Haller and Knochel, 1984; Preedy and Peters, 1990). The latter, may be sub-clinical or symptomatic (with clinical manifestations).

5.1. Acute myopathy

Acute myopathy is a syndrome of acute myocytolysis which occurs in binge drinking alcoholics (Kahn and Meyer, 1970; Perkoff, 1971; Haller and Knochel, 1984). It may be asymptomatic, thus detectable only with a transient raise of creatine-kinase or with frank rhabdomyolysis (Fahlgren *et al.*, 1957; Hed *et al.*, 1962; Haller, 1985; Fernández-Solà *et al.*, 1988).

The main clinical manifestations are:

1. Muscle pain (myalgia) of abrupt onset, usually located in the proximal areas of the limbs (shoulder or gird). Typically more prominent in the legs (calves).
2. Muscle swelling, developing over several hours in the same muscle areas affected by pain. Sometimes the affected area has a pseudothrombophlebitic aspect (Prasad *et al.*, 1974).
3. Weakness, of progressive onset on the first or second day predominating in the legs being noticeable, for example, in a difficulty to going upstairs.

All these symptoms may recur after acute ingestion of ethanol (Kopyt *et al.*, 1984; Urbano-Márquez *et al.*, 1989).

There are occasional descriptions of severe cases of acute necrotizing myopathy with widespread muscle involvement, involving pectoral, pharyngeal, sternocleidomastoid, and to a lesser degree the diaphragm in addition to limb muscles (Hed *et al.*, 1955; Haller and Knochel, 1984). Clinical symptoms are usually accompanied by a transient rise in creatine kinase of about eight times the basal level (Hälgren *et al.*, 1980; Gabow *et al.*, 1982). The most serious complications of acute alcoholic myopathy are myoglobinuria-induced acute-tubular necrosis and renal failure (Rowland, 1972). However, this situation is limited in most cases and only requires clinical support until resolution (Haller and Knochel, 1984).

Electromyographic (EMG) findings are common in acute myopathy (Oh, 1976) presenting short potentials of motor unit, interferential pattern, polyphasia and spontaneous fibrillation due to abnormal irritability of muscle fibers. Worden (1976) described the phenomenon of "Burst suppression" where acute alcoholic ingestion causes an inability to maintain the motor unit potentials during muscle contraction. There is a good relationship between EMG and histological findings, thus EMG can be used to detect muscle involvement in acute alcoholic myopathy (Seneviratne, 1975; Grau *et al.*, 1983). Occasionally, acute alcoholic myopathy coexists with hypophosphatemia and hypokalaemia, alcoholic abstinence or convulsions, which may potentiate the deleterious effect of ethanol on skeletal muscle, and should be conveniently solved (Grau *et al.*, 1983; Haller and Knochel, 1984). In our experience, 33% of the patients with chronic alcoholic myopathy also presented acute symptoms of myopathy (Grau *et al.*, 1983; Urbano-Márquez *et al.*, 1984 and 1989).

5.2. Chronic myopathy

This is the most frequent and well-known picture of alcoholic muscle disease. It is an evolving syndrome of predominantly proximal weakness and muscle atrophy complicated by prolonged alcohol abuse (Grau *et al.*, 1983; Urbano-Márquez *et al.*, 1985 and 1989). Women are equally affected as men, with around 42% of the patients showing clinical weakness and 46% demonstrating histologic evidence of myopathy (Estruch *et al.*, 1991).

Typical symptomatic cases present a gradual (in weeks or months) weakness affecting predominantly the hip and shoulder girdles. Patients report weakness of hip or knee extension. The upper and lower limbs are equally affected. Muscle weakness produces some changes in the patients, decreasing laboral capacity and the possibilities of performing physical exercises and their lifestyle. Proximal muscle atrophy is characteristic and, in some cases, is profound. Other occasional symptoms are local swelling, myalgia, fasciculation and myotonic or myasthenic phenomena, which are exceptional findings in our experience. This picture may coexist with other toxic effects of ethanol such as cirrhosis and alcoholic dilated cardiomyopathy.

Symptoms and laboratory evidence of acute muscle injury are not seen in patients with chronic myopathy. The increase in muscle enzymes, creatine kinase or myoglobin is not constant, and is reported in 10–30% of the cases (Haller and Knochel, 1984). Electrophysiological changes in chronic myopathy are present only in 10–50% of the patients (Oh, 1976; Worden, 1976), with short-duration and short-amplitude motor unit potentials, and diphasic or polyphasic potentials.

Subclinical chronic myopathy is a frequent condition of patients with chronic ethanol ingestion in which only a decrease in muscle strength with or without electromyographic or histological muscle changes are present, but without clinical symptoms (Grau *et al.*, 1983). Some of these patients have some degree of muscle atrophy but with normal levels of serum muscle enzymes. This subclinical chronic alcoholic myopathy may be more common than previously suspected, since most cases remain undetected (Haller and Knochel, 1984). In our experience, 46% of the chronic alcoholic patients have skeletal myopathy and 20% present an asymptomatic form, shown only by performing other diagnostic procedures such as myometry, or muscle biopsy (Urbano-Márquez *et al.*, 1985). There is a good correlation between clinical and histological findings in chronic alcoholics, thus most alcoholic patients reporting muscle symptoms show histologic evidence of muscle damage (Fernárdez-Solà *et al.*, 1994).

The relationship between acute and chronic myopathy has yet to be established. According to some authors (Ekbom, 1964; Haller and Knochel, 1984), patients with chronic myopathy typically have no history of acute myopathy and patients with acute myopathy have no apparent predisposition to developing chronic disorders. However, other authors describe some kind of overlapping between acute and chronic myopathy (Perkoff *et al.*, 1967; Rubin, 1979). Some patients with chronic myopathy report previous muscle pains, cramps in the calves, episodes of acute generalized weakness and grossly dark urine (probably reflecting myoglobinuria) (Hed *et al.*, 1962; Kopyt *et al.*, 1984). In our experience, we have reported a 33% incidence of acute symptoms in patients with chronic myopathy (Grau *et al.*, 1983; Urbano-Márquez *et al.*, 1989). In addition, patients with chronic muscle weakness reported acute myopathic episodes more frequently than patients without chronic myopathy. This data supports the idea of overlapping cases and the potential of chronic myopathy to present acute muscle symptoms.

One important aspect to comment upon is the implication that ethanol-induced skeletal muscle damage may have on lifestyle of the patients. Sometimes, this skeletal muscle involvement induces occupational changes. In most cases, muscle weakness produces a change in the patients' way of life because they have less strength to move heavy objects or to perform moderate exercise and thereby decreasing manual dexterity and normal activity. More interesting is the relationship that skeletal muscle damage has on cardiac and respiratory muscle involvement. As we later comment, skeletal muscle damage is a good marker to detect alcoholic cardiomyopathy, a condition which implies a severe prognosis and high mortality in most cases of chronic alcoholic patients. Therefore, there is reason to believe that skeletal muscle damage may relate to intercostal and diaphragmatic involvement, which may cause a decrease in the respiratory function of these patients.

6. MYOPATHY-CARDIOMYOPATHY RELATIONSHIP IN ALCOHOLIC MUSCLE DISEASE

Since skeletal and cardiac muscle are alike in many aspects and are equally affected by the toxic effects of ethanol in a dose-dependent manner (Grau *et al.*, 1983; Urbano-Márquez *et al.*, 1989), there is reason to consider that a correlation may exist between cardiac and skeletal muscle damage in chronic alcoholism (Song and Rubin, 1972; Rubin, 1979).

This possible correlation was previously suggested at a clinical level by some authors (Seneviratne, 1975; Lynch, 1976). In our experience, there is a clear correlation between skeletal and cardiac myopathy in chronic alcoholism at both clinical (Urbano-Márquez *et al.*, 1989) and histological levels (Fernández-Solà *et al.*, 1994). In a prospective study of a group of chronic alcoholic males with dilated cardiomyopathy, the muscle strength of patients with cardiomyopathy was significantly lower than that of alcoholics with normal cardiac function and that of patients with nonalcoholic dilated cardiomyopathy. Moreover, 82% of the alcoholic patients with cardiomyopathy showed histological findings of skeletal myopathy, as compared to 35% of the alcoholics with normal cardiac function. The extent of cardiac dysfunction amongst alcoholics with cardiomyopathy correlates with the severity of clinical myopathy and muscle strength. Patients with more severe degrees of cellular hypertrophy and interstitial fibrosis of the myocardium exhibit a greater decrease in deltoid muscle strength and more severe histological myopathy (Fernández-Solà *et al.*, 1994). The correlation between cardiac and skeletal muscle damage at both clinical and histological levels, reinforces the hypothesis that ethanol exerts similar toxic effects on both types of striated muscle. The relationship between muscle and cardiac damage seems to be similar in women as we demonstrated in a prospective study of 50 women, in which half showed histological evidence of myopathy and a third of them functional evidence of cardiomyopathy. Women, however, are more sensitive to the cardiotoxic effects of ethanol (Estruch *et al.*, 1991).

7. PROGNOSIS-REVERSIBILITY

In 1822, James Jackson of Harvard reported that the muscle weakness found in chronic alcoholics may recover after abstention. Since then, the reversibility of ethanol myopathy has been generally accepted, although some authors remain uncertain. Despite the high prevalence of this disorder, the natural history of alcoholic myopathy remain unknown (Haller and Knochel, 1984).

Acute myopathy is usually reversible in days or weeks when alcohol abuse is discontinued, except in cases of fatal rhabdomyolysis and myoglobinuria (Nygren *et al.*, 1967; Gabow *et al.*, 1982). Fatal cases are exceptional and are related to the development of acute renal failure (Hed *et al.*, 1955). Most cases of acute alcoholic myopathy can be resolved with good clinical support and renal failure is rare. We have not observed any fatal cases (Grau *et al.*, 1984; Urbano-Márquez *et al.*, 1984 and 1989; Fernández-Solà *et al.*, 1988).

Chronic myopathy usually resolves in most cases within a period of 2–12 months. Some authors refer to a universal reversibility of chronic alcohol myopathy (Martin *et al.*, 1985). Type II atrophy recovery has been shown occur after months of abstinence (Rosow *et al.*, 1976; Slavin *et al.*, 1983; Martin *et al.*, 1985). In some patients, some degree of muscle atrophy and weakness persists for years (Ekbom *et al.*, 1964; Rosow *et al.*, 1976).

In a five-year follow-up study of 40 chronic alcoholic patients, we studied the influence of alcohol ingestion in terms of clinical symptoms, muscle strength and histological parameters (Urbano-Márquez *et al.*, 1993). Thus, none of 23 patients abstaining from ethanol reported either muscle weakness or episodes of acute muscle symptoms. In fact, most of the abstaining patients who had muscle weakness in the baseline study reported a subjective improvement in muscle strength. However, almost half (11 out of 23) did not obtain the same muscle strength (mean minus 2 standard deviation) of a matched control group. Of 17 actively drinking alcoholics, 15 (88%) reported muscle weakness and presented a decrease in muscle strength on comparing the baseline study with the final assessment. The histological studies of these patients showed a complete regression of the myopathy in 9 of the 23 patients from the abstaining group (39%), although 5 (22%) had a persistent mild myopathy. In the group of patients with persistent alcohol intake, none showed a histological regression of myopathy. Of the eight chronic alcoholic patients without histological myopathy in the baseline study who relapsed, mild myopathy was present in five muscle-biopsy specimens. In this study, complete ethanol abstinence was the only independent variable in the improvement of muscle strength and age appeared to play no part. However, in some cases, muscle lesion did not entirely recover.

8. RESEARCH PROPOSALS

Future research in the study of alcoholic myopathy in humans should be directed at both the components which are involved: 1) fiber necrosis and 2) functional impairment of the muscle cells. Potential targets at the cellular level include excitation-contraction coupling, contractile proteins, mitochondria and energy metabolism. The mechanisms by which these may be affected include the formation of adducts, perturbation of signalling pathways and modifications of membrane lipid structure. A particularly interesting field to be studied is the genetic modifications that may be produced by long-term ethanol exposure, and how altered gene expression contributes to functional aberrations at the cellular level. These procedures should be evaluated by measurements of excitation-contraction coupling in human muscle cells, analysis of signal transduction pathways and protein phosphorylation, by measuring mRNA levels and protein expression patterns. The influence of ethanol on the regulation of these components by hormones and growth factors should also be investigated.

References

Adler, A.J., Fillipone, E.J. and Berlyne, G.M. (1985). Effect of chronic alcohol intake on muscle composition and metabolic balance of calcium and phosphate in rats. *Am. Physiol. Soc.*, (I):584–588.

Akera, T., Reeh, R.H., Marquis, W.J., Tobin, T. and Brody, T.M. (1973). Lack of relationship between brain (Na$^+$+K$^+$)-activated adenosine triphosphatase and the development of tolerance to ethanol in rats. *J. Pharmacol. Exp. Ther.*, **185**:594–601.

Alexander, C.S., Sekhri, K.K. and Nagasawa, H.T. (1977). Alcoholic cardiomyopathy in mice: electron microscopic observations. *J. Moll. Cell Cardiol.*, **9**:247–254.

Altura, B.M., Altura, B.T. and Gebrewold, A. (1990). Comparative effects of ethanol, acetaldehyde and acetate on arterioles and venules in skeletal muscle: direct in situ studies on the microcirculation and their possible relationships to alcoholic myopathy. *Microcir. Endoth. Lymphatics*, **6**:108–126.

Anderson, R., Cohen, M., Haller, R.G. *et al.* (1980). Skeletal muscle phosphorus and magnesium deficiency in alcoholic myopathy. *Mineral Elect. Metab.*, **4**:106–112.

Blachley, J.D., Ferguson, E.R., Carter, N.W. *et al.* (1980). Chronic alcohol ingestion induces phosphorous deficiency and myopathy in the dog. *Trans. Assoc. Am. Phys.*, **93**:116–122.

Bollinger, O. (1984). Ueber die Haufigkeit und Ursachen der idiopathischen Herzhypertrophie in Munchen. *Dtsh. Med. Wochenschr.*, **10**:180.

Brodie, C. and Sampson, S.R. (1990). Effects of ethanol on voltage-sensitive Na+ channels in cultured skeletal muscle: up-regulation as a result of chronic treatment. *J. Pharmacol. Exper. Ther.*, **255**, 3:1195–1201.

Cardellach, F., Taraschi, T.F., Ellingson, J.S., Stubbs, C.D., Rubin, E. and Hoek, J.B. (1991). Maintenance of structural and functional characteristics of skeletal-muscle mitochondria and sarcoplasmic-reticular membranes after chronic ethanol treatment. *Biochem. J.*, **274**:565–573.

Cardellach, F., Galofré, J., Grau, J.M., Casademont, J., Hoek, J.B., Rubin, E. and Urbano-Márquez, A. (1992). Oxidative metabolism in skeletal muscle mitochondria from patients with chronic alcoholism is normal. *Ann. Neurol.*, **31**:515–518.

Chui, L.A., Neustein, H. and Munsat, T.L. (1975). Tubular aggregates in subclinical alcoholic myopathy. *Neurology*, **25**:405–412.

Cicero, T.J. (1981). Neuroendocrinological effects of alcohol. *Ann. Rev. Med.*, **32**:123–142.

Cook, E.B., Adebiyi, L.A.Y., Preedy, V.R., Peters, T.J. and Palmer, T.N. (1992). Chronic effects of ethanol on muscle metabolism in the rat. *Biochem. Biophys. Acta.*, **1180**:207–214.

Cussó, R., Vernet, M., Cadefau, J. and Urbano-Márquez, A. (1989). Effects of ethanol and acetaldehyde on the enzymes of glycogen metabolism. *Alcohol and Alcoholism*, **24**:291–297.

Danzinger, R., Sakai, M., Capogrossi, M.C. *et al.* (1991). Ethanol acutely and reversibly suppresses excitation-contraction coupling in cardiac myocytes. *Cir. Res.*, **68**:1660–1666.

DuBell, W.H., Boyet, M.R., Spurgeon, H.A., Talo, A., Stern, M.D. and Lakkatta, E.G. (1991). The cytosolic calcium transient modulates the action potential of rat ventricular myocytes. *J. Physiol.*, **436**:347–369.

Dubowitz, V. and Brooke, M.H. (1973). Muscle Biopsy: A Modern Approach. WB Saunders Co, Philadelphia.

Eckhardt, M.J., Harford, T.C., Kaleber, C.T. *et al.* (1981). Health hazards associated with alcohol consumption. *JAMA*, **246**:648–666.

Edmonds, B.T., Pendergast, D.R., Arabadjis, P.G., Hardacker, J.W., Chan, A.W.K. and York, J.L. (1987). Muscle fiber composition and length-tension relationships in rats chronically exposed to alcohol. *Alcohol*, **4**:485–491.

Ekbom, K., Hed, R., Kustein, L. and Astrom, K.E. (1964). Muscle affectations in chronic alcoholism. *Arch. Neurol.*, **10**:449–458.

Estruch, R., Fernández-Solà, J., Paré, C., Nicolás, J.M., Rubin, E. and Urbano-Márquez, A. (1991). Effects of chronic alcoholism on skeletal and cardiac muscle in women. *Alcohol and Alcoholism*, **26**:240 (abst).

Estruch E., Fernández-Solà J., Junqué A., Monforte R. Paré C., Rubin E. and Urbano-Márquez A. (1992). Relationship between cardiomyopathy and liver disease in chronic alcoholism. *Alcohol and Alcoholism*, **27**(suppl 1):**63** (abst).

Estruch, R., Fernández-Solà, J., Villegas, E., Paré, C., Junqué, A. and Urbano-Márquez, A. (1993). Reversibility of alcoholic cardiomyopathy with ethanol abstinence. *Alcohol and Alcoholism*, **28**:244 (abst).

Fahlgren, H., Hed, R. and Lundmark, C. (1957). Myonecrosis and myoglobinuria in alcohol and barbiturate intoxication. *Acta. Med. Scand.*, **158**:405–412.

Fernández-Solà, J., Grau, J.M., Pedro-Botet, J., Casademont, J., Estruch, R., Company X. and Urbano-Márquez, A. (1988). Rabdomiólisis no traumática: análisis clínico y morfológico de 53 casos. *Med. Clin. (Bar)*, **90**:199–202.

Fernández-Solà, J., Estruch, R., Grau, J.M., Paré, C., Urbano-Márquez, A. and Rubin, E. (1994). The relation of alcoholic myopathy to cardiomyopathy. *Ann. Intern. Med.*, **120**:529–536.

Fuller, T.J., Carter, N.W., Barcenas, C. *et al.* (1976). Reversible changes of muscle cell in experimental phosphorus deficiency. *J. Clin. Invest.*, 1019–1024.

Gabow, P.A., Kaehny, W.D. and Kelleher, S.P. (1982). The spectrum of rhabdomyolysis. *Medicine (Balt)* 1982; **61**:141–152.

Grau, J.M. and Urbano-Márquez, A. (1983). Alcohol y sistema muscular esquelético. *Med. Clin. (Bar)*, **80,12**:545–549.

Haller, R.G. and Drachman, D.B. (1980). Alcoholic rhabdomyolysis: an experimental model in the rat. *Science*, **208**:412–415.

Haller, R.G. and Knochel, J.P. (1984). Skeletal muscle disease in alcoholism. *Med. Clin. N. Am.*, **68**:91–103.

Haller, R.G. (1985). Experimental acute alcoholic myopathy. A histochemical study. *Muscle and Nerve*, **8**:195–203.

Hällgren, R., Lundin, L., Roxin, L.E. *et al.* (1980). Serum and urinary myoglobin in alcoholics. *Acta. Med. Scand.*, **208**:33–39.

Hanid, A., Slavin, G., Mair, W. *et al.* (1981). Fiber type changes in striated muscle of alcoholics. *J. Clin. Pathol.*, **34**:991–995.

Hed, R., Larsson, H. and Wahlgren, F. (1955). Acute myoglobinuria. Report of a case with fatal outcome. *Acta. Med. Scand.*, **152**:459–463.

Hed, R., Lundmark, C., Fahlgre, H. and Orell, S. (1962). Acute muscular syndrome in chronic alcoholism. *Acta. Med. Scand.*, **171**:585–599.

Hickish, T., Colstom, K.W., Bland, J.M. and Maxwell, J.D. (1989). Vitamin D deficiency and muscle strength in male alcoholics. *Clin. Sci.*, **77**:171–176.

142   *Alvaro Urbano-Márquez and Joaquim Fernández-Solà*

Hoek, J.B., Taraschi, T.F. and Rubin, E. (1988). Functional implications of the ethanol with biologic membranes: Actions of ethanol on hormonal signal transduction systems. *Seminars in Liver Disease*, **8**:36–46.

Hudgson, P. (1984). Alcoholic myopathy. *Br. Med. J.*, **288**:584–585.

Israel, Y., Kalant, H., LeBlanc, E., Bernstein, J.C. and Solozar, I. (1970). Changes in cation transport and (Na-K) activated adenosine triphosphatase produced by chronic administration of ethanol. *J. Pharmacol. Exp. Ther.*, **174**:330–336.

Israel, Y. (1970). Cellular effects of alcohol: a review. *J. Stud. Alcohol.*, **31**:293–316.

Jackson, J. (1982). On peculiar diseases resulting from the use of ardent spirits. *N. Engl. J. Med. Surg.*, **21**:351–353.

Jennische, E. and Hansen, H.A. (1987). Transient expression of insulin-like growth factor-1 immunoreactivity in skeletal muscle cells during postnatal development in the rat. *Acta. Physiol. Scand.*, **131**:619–622.

Jennische, E., Skottmer, A. and Hansson, H.A. (1987). Satellite cells express the trophic factor IGF-1 in regenerating skeletal muscle. *Acta. Physiol. Scand.*, **129**:9–16.

Jones, J.E., Shane, S.R., Jacobs, W.H. *et al.* (1969). Magnesium balance studies in chronic alcoholism. *Ann. NY Acad. Sci.*, **162**:934–945.

Juhlin-Dannfelt, A., Ahlborg, G., Hagenfeldt, L. *et al.* (1977). Influence of ethanol on splachnic and skeletal muscle substrate turnover during prolonged exercise in man. *Am. J. Physiol.*, **233 (3)**: E195–E202.

Kahn, L.B. and Meyer, J.S. (1970). Acute myopathy in chronic alcoholism. *Am. J. Clin. Pathol.*, **53**:516–530.

Katz, A. (1982). M. Effects of ethanol on ion transport in muscle membranes. *Fed. Proc.*, **41**:2456–2459.

Kiessling, K.H., Pilström, L., Bylund, A.C. *et al.* (1975). Effects of chronic ethanol abuse on structure and enzyme activities of skeletal muscle in man. Scand. *J. Clin. Lab. Invest.*, **35**:601–607.

Klinkerfuss, G., Bleisch, V., Dioso, M.M. and Perkoff, G.T. (1967). A spectrum of myopathy associated with alcoholism. II. Light and electron microscopic observations. *Ann. Intern. Med.*, **67**:493–510.

Knochel, J.P., Bilbrey, G.L., Fuller, T.J. *et al.* (1975). The muscle cell in chronic alcoholism: the role of possible phosphate depletion in alcoholic myopathy. *Ann. NY Acad. Sci.*, **252**:274–286.

Knochel, J.P., Barcenas, C., Cotton, J.R., Fuller, T.J., Haller, R. and Carter, N.W. (1978). Hypophosphatemia and rhabdomyolysis. *J. Clin. Invest.*, **62**:1240–1246.

Kopyt, N., Myers, A., Mandel, S. and Shachter, N. (1984). Recurrent rhabdomyolysis as a manifestation of alcoholic myopathy. *Arch. Intern. Med.*, **144**:821–823.

Lelbavh, W.K. (1975). Cirrhosis in the alcoholic and its relation to the volume of alcohol abuse. *Ann. NY Acad. Sci.*, **252**:85–105.

Leo, M.A., Arai, M., Sato, M. and Lieber, C.S. (1982). Hepatotoxicity of moderate vitamin A and ethanol in rat. *Gastroenterology*, **82**:194–205.

Leo, M.A., Iida, S. and Lieber, C.S. (1984). Retinoid acid metabolism by a system reconstituted with cytochrome P-450. *Arch. Biochem. Biophys.*, **234**:305–312.

Lewis, D., Lechleiter, J.D., Kim, D., Nanavati, C. and Claphan, D.E. (1990). Intracellular regulation of ion channels in cell membranes. *Mayo. Clin. Pro.*, **65**:1127–1143.

Lieber, Ch. S. (1968). Metabolic effects produced by alcohol in the liver and other tissues. *Adv. Intern. Med.*, **14**:151–199.

Lieber, C.S. (1988). Biomedical and molecular basis of alcohol-induced injury to liver and other tissues. *N. Engl. J. Med.*, **219,25**:1639–1650.

Lynch, P.G. (1976). Acute cardiomyopathy with rhabdomyolysis in chronic alcoholism. *Br. Med. J.*, **1**:44–46.

Marway, J.S., Preedy, V.R. and Peters, T.J. (1990). Experimental alcoholic skeletal muscle myopathy is characterized by a rapid and sustained decrease in muscle RNA content. *Alcohol and Alcoholism*, **25,4**:401–406.

Martin, J.B., Craig, J.W., Eckel, R.E. *et al.* (1971). Hypokalemic myopathy in chronic alcoholism. *Neurology*, **21**:1160–1168.

Martin, F.C., Slavin, G. and Levi, A.J. (1982). Alcoholic muscle disease. *Br. Med. Bul.*, **38**:53–56.

Martin, F., Ward, K., Slavin, G., Levi, J. and Peters, T.J. (1985). Alcoholic skeletal myopathy, a clinical and pathological study. *Quart. J. Med.*, **218**:233–251.

Martin, F.C. and Peters, T.J. (1985). Assessment *in vitro* and *in vivo* of muscle degradation in chronic skeletal muscle myopathy of alcoholism. *Clin. Sci.*, **68**:693–700.

Martínez, A.J., Hoohmand, H. and Faris, A.A. (1973). Acute alcoholic myopathy. Enzyme histochemistry and electron microscopic findings. *J. Neurol. Sci.*, **20**:245–252.

Matsukazi, S. and Lieber, C.S. (1977). Increased susceptibility of hepatic mitochondria to the toxicity of acetaldehyde after chronic ethanol consumption. *Biochem. Biophys. Res. Commun.*, **75**:1059–1065.

Mendelson, J.H. and Mello, N.K. (1992). Medical diagnosis and treatment of alcoholism. Mc Graw-Hill Inc Pub, New York: 263–287.

Mills, K.R., Ward, K., Martin, F. and Peters, T.J. (1986). Peripheral neuropathy and myopathy in chronic alcoholism. *Alcohol and Alcoholism*, **21**:357–362.

Myerson, R.M. and Lafair, J.S. (1970). Alcoholic muscle disease. *Med. Clin. N. Am.*, **54**:723–730.

Neher, E. (1992). Ion channels for communication between and within cells. *Science*, **152**:498–502.

Nicolás, J.M., Estruch, R., Antúnez, E., Sacanella, E. and Urbano-Márquez, A. (1993). Nutritional status in chronic alcoholic men from the middle socioeconomic class and its relation to ethanol intake. *Alcohol and Alcoholism*, **28**:551–558.

Nygren, A. (1967). Serum creatine phosphokinase in chronic alcoholism. *Acta. Med. Scand.*, **182**:383–397.

Oh, S.J. (1972). Alcoholic myopathy A critical review. *J. Med. Sci.*, 1972; **9**:79–95.

Oh, S.J. (1976). Alcoholic myopathy. Electrophysiological study. *Electromyogr. Clin. Neuropsicol.*, **16**:205–218.

Pachinger, O., Mao, J., Fauvel J.M. *et al.* (1975). Mitochondrial and function and excitation-contraction coupling in the development of alcoholic cardiomyopathy. *Recent Adv. Stud. Cardiac. Struct. Metab.*, **5**:423–429.

Pedro-Botet, J., Grau, J.M., Casademont, J., Estruch, E., Fernández-Solà, J., Urbano-Ispizua, A., Mont, L. and Urbano-Márquez, A. (1986). Prevalencia del alcoholismo crónico y patología asociada al mismo en los enfermos ingresados en el departamento de Medicina Interna de un hospital general. *Med. Clin. (Bar)*, **87**:101–103.

Perkoff, G.T., Hardy, P. and Velez-García, E. (1966). Reversible acute muscular syndrome associated with alcoholism. *N. Engl. J. Med.*, **274**:1277–1285.

Perkoff G.T., Dioso M.M., Bleisch V. *et al.* (1967). A spectrum of myopathy associated with alcoholism I. Clinical and laboratory features. *Ann. Intern. Med.*, **67**:481–492.

Perkoff, G.T. (1971). Alcoholic myopathy. *Ann. Rev. Med.*, **22**:125–132.

Peters, T.J., Martin, F.C. and Ward, K. (1985). Chronic alcoholic skeletal myopathy-common and reversible. *Alcohol*, **2**:485–489.

Polokoff, M.A., Simon, T.J., Harris, R.A., Simon, F.R. and Iwashashi, M. (1985). Chronic ethanol increases liver plasma membrane fluidity. *Biochemistry*, **24**:3114–3120.

Prasad, P., Tabatnick, B. and Kotler, M.N. (1974). Recurrent acute alcoholic myopathy simulating deep vein thrombosis in association with cardiomyopathy and parasystolic ventricular tachycardia. *Hopkins Med. J.*, **134**:226–232.

Preedy, V.R. and Peters, T.J. (1988). Acute effects of ethanol on protein synthesis in different muscle protein fractions of the rat. *Clin. Sci.*, **74**:461–466.

Preedy, V.R. and Peters, T.J. (1988). The effect of chronic ethanol ingestion on protein metabolism in Type I and Type II fibre rich skeletal muscle of the rat. *Biochem. J.*, **254**:631–639.

Preedy, V.R., Duane and P., Peters, T.J. (1988). Comparison of the acute effects of ethanol on liver and skeletal muscle protein synthesis in the rat. *Alcohol Alcohol*, **23**:155–161.

Preedy, V.R., Bateman, C.J., Salisbury, J.R., Price, A.B. and Peters, T.J. (1989). Ethanol-induced skeletal muscle myopathy: Biochemical and histochemical measurements on type I and type II fibre-rich muscles in the young rat. *Alcohol and Alcoholism*, **24**:533–539.

Preedy, V.R. and Peters, T.J. (1989). The effect of chronic ethanol ingestion on synthesis and degradation of soluble protein fractions of skeletal muscle from inmature and mature rats. *Biochem. J.*, **259**:261–266.

Preedy, V.R. and Peters, T.J. (1990). Alcohol and skeletal muscle disease. *Alcohol and Alcoholism*, **25**:177–187.

Preedy, V.R. and Peters, T.J. (1992). Effects of chronic ethanol consumption and pair feeding on rates of protein synthesis and nucleic acid composition in rat tibia. *Alcohol and Alcoholism*, **27**:29–37.

Preedy, V.R., Keating, J.W. and Peters, T.J. (1992). The acute effects of ethanol and acetaldehyde on rates of protein synthesis in type I and type II fibre-rich skeletal muscles of the rat. *Alcohol and Alcoholism*, **27**:241–251.

Puszkin, S. and Rubin, E. (1975). Adenosine diphosphate effect on contractibility of human muscle actomyosin: inhibition by ethanol and acetaldehyde. *Science*, **188**:1319–1320.

Rossow, J.E., Keeton, R.G. and Hewlett, R.H. (1976). Chronic proximal muscular weakness in alcoholics. *S. Afr. Med. J.*, **50**:2095–2098.

Rowland, R.P. and Penn, A.S. (1972). Myoglobinuria *Med. Clin. N. Am.*, **50**:1233–1256.

Rubenstein, A.E. and Wainapel, S.F. (1977). Acute hypokalemic myopathy in alcoholism. A clinical study. *Arh. Neurol.*, **34**:553–555.

Rubenstein, A.E. and Wainapel, S.F. (1977). Acute hypokalemic myopathy in alcoholism. A histological and histochemical study. *Dis. Nerv. Syst.*, **38**:287–289.

Rubin, E. (1979). Alcoholic myopathy in heart and skeletal muscle. *N. Engl. J. Med.*, 1979; **301**:28–33.

Salemo, F., Locatelli, V. and Müller, E.E. (1987). Growth hormone hyper-responsiveness to growth hormone releasing hormone in patients with severe liver cirrhosis. *Clin. Endocrinol.*, **27**:183–190.

Salisbury, J.R., Preedy, V.R., Rose, P.E., Deverell, M.H. and Peters, T.J. (1992). Ethanol-induced chronic myopathy in the young rat: a light and electron microscopic study in type I or type II fibre-rich skeletal muscles. *Alcohol and Alcoholism*, **27,5**:493–500.

Sarna, J.S., Ikeda, S., Fisher, R. *et al.* (1976). Biochemical and contractile properties of heart muscle after prolonged alcohol administration. *J. Mol. Cell. Cardiol.*, **8**:951–972.

Sato, M. and Lieber, C.S. (1982). Hepatic vitamin A depletion in alcoholic liver injury. *N. Engl. J. Med.*, **307**:597–601.

Seneviratne, B.B. (1975). Acute cardiomyopathy with rhabdomyolysis in chronic alcoholism. *Br. Med. J.*, **4**:378–380.

Shils, M.E. (1969). Experimental human magnesium depletion. *Medicine (Balt)*, **48**:61–85.

Slavin, G., Martin, F., Ward, P., Levi, J. and Peters, T. (1983). Chronic alcohol excess is associated with selective but reversible injury to type 2B muscle fibres. *J. Clin. Pathol.*; **36**:772–777.

Song, S.K. and Rubin, E. (1972). Ethanol produces muscle damage in human volunteers. *Science*, **21**:327–328.

Sonntag, W.E. and Boyd, R.L. (1989). Diminished insulin-like growth factor-1 levels after chronic ethanol: Relationship to pulsatile growth hormone release. *Alcohol Clin. Exp. Res.*, **13**:3–11.

Sonntag, W.E., Boyd, R.L., D'Costa, A. and Breese, C.R. (1991). Influence of ethanol on functional and biochemical characteristics of skeletal muscle. Drug and Alcohol Abuse Reviews, **2**:403–423.

Steell, G. (1893). Heart failure as a result of chronic alcoholism. *Med. Chron.*, **18**:1.

Sullivan, J., Parker, M. and Carson, S.B. (1968). Tissue cobalt content in "beer drinkers myocardiopathy". *J. Lab. Clin. Med.*, **71**:893.

Sunnasy, D., Cairns, S.R., Martin, F., Slavin, G. and Peters, T.J. (1983). Chronic alcoholic skeletal myopathy: a clinical, histological and biochemical assessment of muscle lipids. *J. Clin. Pathol.*, **36**:778–784.

Thomas, A.P., Sass, E.J., Tun-Kirchmann, T.T. and Rubin, E. (1989). Ethanol inhibits electrically-induced calcium transients in isolated rat cardiac myocytes. *J. Moll. Cell. Cardiol.*, **21**:555–560.

Thuong, T., Anzepy, Ph., Blondean, M. and Richard, Ch. (1986). Baisse du taux serique de sélenium chez les alcoholiques chroniques avec or sans cardiomyopathie dilatée. *Presse Med.*, **15**:693–696.

Trouce, I., Byrne, E. and Dennett, X. (1990). Biochemical and morphological studies of skeletal muscle in experimental chronic alcohol myopathy. *Acta. Neurol. Scand.*, **82**:386–391.

Urbano-Márquez, A., Estruch, R., Grau, J.M., Casademont, J., Pedro-Botet, J. and Rozman, C. (1984) Estudio ultrastructural muscular de los pacientes enólicos crónicos con y sin miopatía. *Med. Clin. (Bar)*, **84**:647–650.

Urbano-Márquez, A., Estruch, R., Grau, J.M. *et al.* (1985). On alcoholic myopathy. *Ann. Neurol.*, **17**:418.

Urbano-Márquez, A., Estruch, R., Grau, J.M., Casademont, J., Sala, M. and Fernández-Huerta, J.M. (1985). Patología muscular en pacientes con ingesta cránica de alcohol. *Med. Clin. (Bar)*, **84**:643–646.

Urbano-Márquez, A., Estruch, R., Navarro-López, F., Grau, J.M., Mont, L. and Rubin, E. (1989). The effects of alcoholism on skeletal and cardiac muscle. *N. Engl. J. Med.*, **320**:409–411.

Urbano-Márquez, A., Estruch, R., Sacanalla, E., Fernández-Solà, J., Nicolás, J.M. and Antúnez, E. (1993). Partial reversibility of alcoholic myopathy with ethanol abstinence: a five-year follow-up study. *Alcohol and Alcoholism*, **28**:251 (abst).

Valenzuela, A., Fernández, V. and Videla, L.A. (1983). Hepatic and biliary levels of glutathione and lipid peroxides following iron overload in the rat: effect of simultaneous ethanol administration. *Toxicol. Appl. Pharmacol.*, **70**:87–95.

Vanderkooi, J.M. (1979). Effects of ethanol on membranes: a fluorescent probe study. *Alcohol. Clin. Exp. Res.*, **3**:60–63.

Vased, S.C., Chaksrvarti, R.N., Subrahmanyam, D. *et al.* (1975). Myocardial lesions induced by prolonged alcohol feeding in rhesus monkeys. *Cardiovasc. Res.*, 1975, **9**:134–140.

Ward, R.J. and Peters, T.J. (1992). The antioxidant status of patients with either alcohol-induced liver damage or myopathy. *Alcohol and Alcoholism*, **27**:359–365.

Ward, R.J. and Preedy, V.R. (1992). Imidazole dipeptides in experimental alcohol-induced myopathy. *Alcohol and Alcoholism*, **27,6**:633–639.

Waring, A.J., Rottenberg, H., Ohnishi, T. and Rubin, E. (1981). Membranes and phospholipids of liver mitochondria from chronic alcoholic rats are resistant to membrane disordering by alcohol. *Proc. Natl. Acad. Sci. USA*, **78**:2582–2586.

Wassif, W., Preedy, V.R., Summers, B., Duane, P., Leigh, N. and Peters, T.J. (1993). The relation between muscle fibre atrophy factor, plasma carnosinase activities and muscle RNA and protein composition in chronic alcoholic myopathy. *Alcohol and Alcoholism*, **28**:325–331.

Williams, J.W., Tada, M., Katz, A.M. *et al.* (1975). Effect of ethanol and acetaldehyde on the (Na^+-K^+)-activated adenosine-triphosphatase activity of cardiac plasma membranes. *Biochem. Pharmacol.*, **24**:27–32.

Williamson, J.R., Scholz, R., Thurman, R.G. *et al.* (1969). Transport of reducing equivalents across the mitochondrial membrane of rat liver. In: Papa, S., Targer, J.M., Quagliariello, E. and Slater, E.C. (Eds). The energy level and metabolic control in mitochondria. Adriatica Editrice, Bari (Italy): 411–429.

Worden, R.E. (1976). Pattern of muscle and nerve pathology in alcoholism. *Ann. NY Acad. Sci.*, **273**:351–359.

Wu, J.M. (1981). Control of protein synthesis in rabbit reticulocytes: inhibition of polypeptide synthesis by ethanol. *J. Biol. Chem.*, **256**:4164–4167.

Young, A., Brenton, D.P. and Edwards, R.H.T. (1978). Analysis of muscle weakness in osteomalacia. *Clin. Sci. Mol. Med.*, **54**:31P.

Zerba, E., Komorowski, T.E. and Faulkner, J.A. (1990). Free radical injury to skeletal muscles of young, adult and old mice. *Am. J. Physiol.*, **27**:C429–C435.

9 Alcohol and the Pancreas

H. Sarles, J.P. Bernard and C.D. Johnson

INSERM, U 315, 46 boulevard de la Gaye, 13009 MARSEILLE cédex 09

Knowledge of the relationships between alcohol consumption and pancreatic pathology is progressing rapidly, partly because experimental and basic research is now based on a precise knowledge of the pathology and epidemiology of alcohol-induced pancreatic diseases. There is probably no link between overall alcohol consumption and pancreatic cancer but a possible link with beer drinking and a probable protective effect of wine consumption. Acute pancreatitis caused by alcohol is usually a complication of chronic pancreatitis. The possibility of complete healing after alcohol withdrawal is possible but has not been demonstrated. Nevertheless, different alcohol-induced changes with obstruction to flow due to chronic lesions very probably play a part in the onset of acute lesions. Chronic pancreatitis is the main complication of alcohol consumption. It is in reality a calcic lithiasis, very similar to tropical chronic pancreatitis. The main phenomenon seems to be the crystallization of calcium salts due to calcium saturation of pancreatic juice, protein hyperconcentration and decreased biosynthesis and secretion of lithostathine, the secretory crystallization-inhibitor of pancreatic juice.

INTRODUCTION

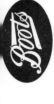

It has been known for a long time that alcohol consumption is associated with a high frequency of pancreatic diseases. The relationship with pancreatic cancer, though possible, is not proven and the two main pancreatic diseases known to be alcohol-associated are acute and chronic pancreatitis. Unfortunately, the definitions of these diseases vary from one paper to another, especially in the North American literature, which often makes the interpretation of the data difficult. Besides, experimental animal models were frequently designed without knowledge of the precise lesions and etiology of the human alcohol-induced pancreatic disease. In this review, we will describe not only experimental studies but also the biology, epidemiology and pathology of the human diseases suspected to be related to alcohol consumption. This is timely as it is now possible to explore pancreatic secretion and function in humans as well as in animals.

I ALCOHOL AND PANCREATIC CANCER

A Epidemiology

Results of case control studies are contradictory. In a review (Raymond and Bouchardy, 1990), a non significant increase in risk of pancreatic carcinoma with alcohol misuse, often limited to one gender, was found in 7 papers, no relation at all in 11 papers, and a negative relation, particularly with wine, in 6 papers. In the more recent literature (1991– 1992), four studies did not show significant correlation between alcohol misuse and pancreatic cancer: In Netherlands, a negative relationship with wine was found (Bueno de Mesquito *et al.,* 1992). A positive correlation was found in only 5 papers which, however, did not distinguish the different types of beverages. Three papers demonstrated a correlation between pancreatic cancer and beer consumption (Durbec *et al.,* 1983; Raymond *et al.,* 1987; Cuzick and Babiker, 1989). In conclusion, it is unlikely that ethanol per se could be a cause of pancreatic cancer. Wine possibly has a protective effect and beer may be correlated with the risk of cancer. Nitrosamines have a strong carcinogenic effect on the pancreas and beer (and whisky) are possible sources of nitrosamines. These points deserve further studies.

B Experimental research

There is little experimental research in this field. In the rat and in the hamster, ethanol caused an enhancing effect on the modulation of pancreatic carcinogenesis by fat (Woutersen *et al.,* 1986). In the rat, given ethanol with a fat rich diet, but not ethanol alone, induced ductal dysplasia (Jalovaara *et al.,* 1986).

Thus, at the present time, there are no strong arguments suggesting that ethanol be a cause of pancreatic cancer.

II MODIFICATIONS INDUCED IN EXPERIMENTAL ANIMALS AND IN HUMANS BY ALCOHOL CONSUMPTION

A The rat model

The acute oral administration of lethal doses of ethanol has no effect on the pancreas (Sarles *et al.,* 1971b). When rats received 20 per cent alcohol freely, protein precipitates were frequently observed in their pancreatic juice. After two years, lesions very similar to those of human alcoholic pancreatitis were observed (Sarles *et al.,* 1971b): fibrosis, destruction of acini and dilatation of ducts covered with a flat epithelium and filled with protein plugs. These lesions are only found in some lobules surrounded by normal parenchyma. Their intensity varies from one animal to another and, as in humans, similar though less frequent lesions are observed in "non alcoholic controls". These alcohol-induced lesions have been confirmed by different authors (Kakaya *et al.,* 1979; Singh, 1987). Temporary occlusion of bile-pancreatic ducts with Ethybloc (R) in alcoholic rats can induce the formation of calcified stones (Pap and Boros, 1989).

The mean protein concentration in pancreatic juice of these "alcoholic rats" was greater than that of controls (Sarles *et al.,* 1971b) and the transit time of newly synthesized proteins from endoplasmic reticulum to zymogen granules was normal, but was increased from zymogen granules to intraacinar lumen (Lechene de la Porte and Sarles, 1974) which suggests a stimulation of acinar cell function.

The pancreatic secretory response to chronic alcohol consumption varies with fat and protein intake (Sarles *et al.,* 1971a), with time (Bode *et al.,* 1986; Grönroos *et al.,* 1988) and with anaesthesia and after surgery. This explains the contradictory results in an abundant literature. Nevertheless, it was generally found that ethanol increases enzyme biosynthesis in well nourished rats (Korsten *et al.,* 1978). It is, however, not clear that secretory studies on the *in vivo-in vitro* model with isolated lobules reflects what happens in the intact animal, nor is it clear whether the effects of a liquid diet are the same as those of more usual food. Chronic alcohol feeding increases the pancreatic protease content if the diet is rich in fat and this effect is more marked in females (Ramo *et al.,* 1986).

Eight months of alcohol feeding decreases the number of muscarinic receptors in the pancreas (Grönroos *et al.,* 1989) which could be a consequence of increased release of acetylcholine (increased cholinergic tone) and could explain increased protein secretion by the pancreas. Choline acetyltransferase is increased in alcohol treated rats and acetylcholine-esterase is decreased (Perec *et al.,* 1979) which also suggests increased cholinergic tone.

In conclusion, in the rat, acute alcohol administration has no effect on the pancreas. Chronic alcohol consumption increases the frequency of spontaneously-occuring pancreatic lesions with formation of non calcified protein plugs in the ducts; in most circumstances, it increases the biosynthesis and secretion of protein, mostly proteases.

B The dog model

Chronic administration to dogs of 2 g/kg ethanol for two years leads to lesions resembling the initial lesions of human chronic pancreatitis: non-calcified intraductal protein precipitates, dilatation of some ducts, flattening of duct epithelium and periductal fibrosis. The secretory response to ethanol varies with the dietary content of fat and protein (Devaux *et al.,* 1990). Environmental conditions may also modify and even reverse the alcohol-induced secretory modifications: when our kennel was covered so that the exercise area which had been previously open to the elements was covered over, there was a gradual conversion of the response to ethanol from inhibition to stimulation (Sarles *et al.,* 1984). This is important in interpretating various studies which are dependant on nutritional and environmental conditions, generally badly defined.

Alcohol-induced modifications of the dog pancreatic secretion are generally held to be neurally mediated. A review of the subject has been recently reported by Sarles and colleagues (1989). As the effects of ethanol are different between dogs unaccustomed to the prolonged consumption of alcohol (non alcoholic dogs), and in dogs receiving regularly alcohol for some months (alcoholic dogs), these two situations will be studied separately.

1 Effects of acute ethanol administration in non-alcoholic dogs

The action of ethanol on pancreatic secretion appears to be more complex that it was originally thought. Intravenous administration of 1 g/kg ethanol inhibits protein and to a lesser extent water and bicarbonate secretion (Bayer *et al.,* 1972; Tiscornia *et al.,* 1973; Noel-Jorand and Sarles, 1983; Robles Diaz *et al.,* 1985). This inhibitory effect is observed on basal, meal stimulated and cholinergic stimulated secretion, but not on cerulein stimulated secretion (Kubota *et al.,* 1983). In contrast, low doses of ethanol (0.40 g/kg) stimulate pancreatic secretion, and this stimulation persists a certain time after blood ethanol levels have returned to normal (Noel-Jorand and Sarles, 1983). Stimulation and inhibition are abolished by atropine, pentolinium and vagotomy. This suggests that in non alcoholic dogs, ethanol triggers two opposite reflexes transmitted by the vagus nerves: stimulation at low ethanol blood levels and inhibition at higher levels. These responses can be demonstrated in the same animals, and appear to be related to changes in blood levels, rather than steady state concentrations (Noel-Jorand and Sarles, 1983).

2 *Effects of acute ethanol administration in alcoholic dogs*

When dogs received 2 g/kg ethanol into the stomach for two years, the inhibitory action of alcohol disappeared. Alcohol-induced stimulation persisted (Tiscornia *et al.,* 1974) and this response was abolished by atropine but not by pentolinium (Sarles *et al.,* 1991). This suggests that the reflexes induced by ethanol in non alcoholic dogs are abolished by chronic alcohol consumption, ethanol acting in this case on the intrapancreatic ganglion-cell i.e. increasing cholinergic tone.

3 *Neural imputs*

There is a considerable evidence for permanent alteration in the neural imput to the pancreas in chronic alcoholic dogs. Chronic alcohol consumption inhibits the early 15 min fluid response to 2 deoxyglucose that is vagally mediated directly to the pancreas. Long term ethanol administration produces histochemical changes indicative of alterations in cholinergic activity in the dog pancreas (Sarles *et al.,* 1991). In conclusion, alcohol has a complex action on pancreatic secretion. Both inhibition and stimulation are neurally mediated. The disappearance in chronic alcoholic dogs of the alcohol-induced inhibition explains how the pancreatic secretion of alcoholic dogs has an increased concentration of protein, at least when dogs have a fat- and protein-rich diet and a free access to open air.

C Alcohol induced modifications of pancreatic secretion in man

In man, as well as in dogs, an intravenous infusion (600 mg/kg) ethanol or an intragastric injection of 40% ethanol reduce volume of secretion and output of bicarbonate, lipase and chymotrypsin (Mott *et al.,* 1972; Panche *et al.,* 1982). This is very similar to that observed in dogs and is attributed to alcohol-induced modifications of cholinergic reflexes. Vagal neuropathy occurs in chronic alcoholics (Duncan *et al.,* 1980) and the above effect does not occur in these patients. Given by mouth, alcohol has only a weak action on pancreatic secretion (Hajnal *et al.,* 1989), but it inhibits the secretory response to a meal (Hajnal *et al.,* 1990).

The biochemical modifications of pancreatic (not duodenal) juice, secondary to alcohol consumption, are:

1 Modifications related to alcohol consumption found in the pancreatic juice of all alcoholics, whether or not they present with chronic pancreatitis.

a) Increased concentration of protein. This is maximal when pancreatic juice is collected shortly after cessation of alcohol consumption. It is is still significantly increased but less so after one week and is not found after 3 weeks abstinence (Sarles *et al.*, 1991). Similarly, protein synthesis is increased as shown by the passage of 75 selenium-methionine into pancreatic juice. In dogs, this could be related to the observed increased cholinergic tone. The assumption that this mechanism operates in alcoholic men is in agreement with the fact that the Na^+ and Cl^- content of the sweat is increased in these patients (Sarles *et al.*, 1963). Protein hyperconcentration increases the viscosity of pancreatic juice and favours calcium-salt nucleation.

b) Decreased secretion of lithostathine. This will be discussed below. It is observed as well in alcoholics without pancreatitis and in the calcic form of hereditary pancreatitis or the topical form of calcifying pancreatitis.

c) Decreased concentration of citrate (Boustière *et al.*, 1985) which is probably related to interference between ethanol metabolism and tricarboxylic-acid cycle. The reduced concentration of citrate should facilitate precipitation of calcium salts.

d) Decreased secretion of bicarbonate (Sahel and Sarles, 1979).

e) Changes in the ratio of protesases to anti-proteases and the ratio of chymotrypsinogen 1/chymotrypsinogen 2 (Rinderknecht *et al.*, 1979) which could facilitate acute lesions.

2 Modifications that are seen with any type of pancreatic lesions and which are probably secondary to transudation of interstitial fluid as a result of lesions of the duct epithelium are an increased concentration of serum protein (Sahel & Sarles, 1979) and calcium (Boustière *et al.*, 1985). This increased calcium concentration increases the precipitation of calcium salts and explains the late formation of calcified stones and the late peripheral calcification of protein calculi.

3 Lactoferrin concentration was found to be increased in the pancreatic and duodenal juice of patients with chronic calcifying pancreatitis, generally alcoholic patients (Clemente *et al.*, 1971; Estevenon *et al.*, 1975). Though contradictory results have been published, this has been recently confirmed (Hayakawa *et al.*, 1993). Its significance is unknown.

III ETHANOL METABOLISM BY THE PANCREAS

The pancreas is able to metabolise ethanol (Gyr *et al.*, 1984; Hamamoto *et al.*, 1990). Pancreatic alcohol dehydrogenase activity is approximately 15% of that seen in the liver (Gyr *et al.*, 1984). Ethanol uptake occurs by simple diffusion. In humans, after orally administered ethanol, pancreatic juice ethanol concentrations were transiently higher than those in blood (Gjorup *et al.*, 1990). The same has been observed in dogs (Robles Diaz *et al.*, 1985). When alcohol blood levels reach 25 mmol (1.15 g/liter), the concentration in pancreatic cells is 16 MM, close to the V_{max} of ethanol oxidation by pancreatic cells (Gyr *et al.*, 1984). Pancreatic alcohol dehydrogenase is increased by alcohol consumption during the first months, but not after 24 months (Sarles *et al.*, 1991). Alcohol consumption increases triglyceride (Gyr, 1989) and collagen biosynthesis (Nakayamaka *et al.*, 1980) by the pancreas (Gyr *et al.*, 1984).

IV ALCOHOLIC ACUTE AND CHRONIC PANCREATITIS DEFINITION

According to the Marseille-Rome classification (Sarles, 1991), acute pancreatitis is defined as a group of lesions generally considered to be reversible: oedema, necrosis, haemorrhagic necrosis and fact necrosis. In contrast, chronic pancreatitis is a group of diseases characterized by the persistence of lesions which generally progress even if their cause is eliminated: irregular sclerosis with destruction and loss of exocrine parenchyma, either focal, segmental or diffuse, associated with varying degrees of dilatation of segments of the duct system. The adjectives "relapsing" or "recurrent" should be avoided. They are commonly used both for the recurrence of reversible acute lesions (secondary to common bile duct stones for instance) and for chronic pancreatitis, the main symptom of which is generally the recurrence of episodes of pain. They should not be used because they correspond to a syndrome and not to a disease.

In several studies, we showed that the epidemiological features of acute and of chronic pancreatitis (gender-ratio, age, frequency of gallstones and alcoholism) were so different that it was extremely improbable that acute pancreatitis, particularly necrosis, could be the cause of chronic pancreatitis (Sarles *et al.*, 1965). Later, we confirmed the findings of Adler that acute experimental haemorrhagic necrosis in the rat healed without sequelae. The exception is the acute lesions caused by intraductal injection of bile salts: In this case, the persistence of patchy chronic lesions is due to duct lesions induced by bile-salts and subsequent duct strictures and not to acinar necrosis (Sarles *et al.*, 1993). Therefore acute pancreatitis, though it is a frequent complication of chronic pancreatitis, is not its cause, except in rare cases of stricture of pancreatic ducts.

V ALCOHOLIC ACUTE PANCREATITIS

A Is alcoholic acute pancreatitis an early manifestation of alcoholic chronic pancreatitis?

There are strong arguments backing this assumption.

a) Acute pancreatitis is observed in chronic alcoholics who have recently increased their consumption of alcohol and is not seen in occasional drinkers (Kager *et al.*, 1972).

b) The follow-up of patients with acute pancreatitis (mostly alcoholics) shows that with the passage of time, almost all cases develop pancreatic stones (Bernades *et al.*, 1983). Gullo *et al.*, (1988) showed that the disease progressed inexorably but less rapidly when patients stop drinking. In contrast, Amman *et al.* (1986) suggested that about one third of the patients who presented with acute alcoholic pancreatitis do not progress towards chronic pancreatitis. However, they diagnosed chronic pancreatitis by the presence of calcified calculi and the fecal chymotrypsin test which are not as precise as the pancreatic function test used by Gullo *et al.* Furthermore, some "healed" patients presented with cysts, slight insufficiency or lesions, which suggests that the definition of resolution and return to normality may have been too broad. As a conclusion, it is probable that in most if not all cases, alcoholic, acute pancreatitis are the first manifestations of chronic alcoholic pancreatitis.

B Pathophysiology of acute alcoholic pancreatitis

a) Chronic alcohol consumption was unable per se to induce acute pancreatitis in the rat, but increased the severity of acute pancreatitis due to other causes, for instance cerulein hyperstimulation (Quon *et al.,* 1992), intraductal injection of bile salts associated with a fat rich diet (Ramo, 1987) or obstruction to the flow of pancreatic juice (Lesko *et al.,* 1989).

b) Reber's group has shown that alcohol in the cat increased the permeability of ducts to macromolecules and the frequency of acute pancreatitis induced by intraductal trypsin injection (Harvey *et al.,* 1988).

c) It has been confirmed that ethanol consumption decreased pancreatic blood flow (Widdinson *et al.,* 1992).

d) The role of free radicals has been suggested. Pretreatments with either superoxide dismutase, catalase or allopurinol ameliorate pancreatic injury (Sanfey *et al.,* 1986; Nordback *et al.,* 1991).

In conclusion, ethanol alone is not able to produce acute pancreatitis, but increases the lesions due to different causes. The mechanism of this aggravation is probably complex. One has to remember that acute alcohol-related pancreatitis is (generally) a complication of chronic pancreatitis. Therefore, obstruction of the flow of pancreatic juice by plugs, stones or strictures should play an important role, as it does in acute pancreatitis complicating cancer. It is possible that acute alcohol consumption aggravates the consequences of duct obstruction due to lesions induced by chronic alcoholism.

VI ALCOHOLIC CHRONIC PANCREATITIS

A Pathology of alcoholic chronic pancreatitis

Previous morphological studies by our group showed that they are two main types of chronic pancreatitis: *obstructive chronic pancreatitis* due to obstruction of the pancreatic duct preexisting to pancreatitis (tumours, scars, congenital anomalies). This is not related to alcohol consumption. And a condition found in approximately 95% of chronic patients with pancreatitis called *calcifying chronic pancreatitis*, with the formation of calcified pancreatic calculi (Payan *et al.,* 1972; Sarles, 1991; Sarles *et al.,* 1992). Morphometric studies and spatial reconstruction of the pancreatic ducts showed that chronic calcifying pancreatitis was in reality a lithiasis: before lesions of ducts and acini could be observed, there is precipitation of a protein and calcium carbonate crystals in the ducts. Chronic alcoholic pancreatitis is a pancreatic lithiasis which resembles kidney lithiasis more than hepatic cirrhosis.

The most characteristic lesions of calcifying chronic pancreatitis that differentiate it from obstructive pancreatitis are: (i) the patchy, lobular distribution of lesions, one lobule or group of lobules presenting with lesions of different intensity from neighbouring lobules; (ii) the presence of protein precipitates or plugs in the ducts and sometimes in the acinar lumen (and later of calculi), (iii) the severity of ductal lesions, with atrophy of epithelium, and dilatation (iiii) inflammatory infiltration of intrapancreatic nerves and ganglia (61, 62). These findings of our group have been confirmed by others (Suda *et al.,*

1990; Singh and Reber, 1990). We recently showed that there were different types of pancreatic lithiasis characterized by different biochemical composition of the calculi, modifications of pancreatic juice and underlying aetiology.

The disease was most frequently called calcic lithiasis or regularly calcified calculi. This disease generally has basically a nutritional origin: alcohol in some countries, malnutrition in others. The "temperate" alcoholic form and the tropical form present with the same lesions and the same modifications in the composition of pancreatic juice (Sarles *et al.*, 1994): Except for some exceptional hereditary cases, calcic lithiasis is a nutritional disease and alcoholic pancreatitis is a calcic pancreatic lithiasis. This evidence led us to study the pancreatic lithogenesis instead of trying to reproduce chronic pancreatitis with repeated acute lesions. This approach led to the discovery of new families of proteins (Sarles *et al.*, 1989).

In the second form of pancreatic lithiasis which will not be discussed in detail, radiolucent or protein lithiasis, the calculi do not initially contain calcium salts, but are composed of degraded forms of lithostathine without affinity for calcium. After a time, the protein core of the calculi may be covered by a shell of calcium salts giving the radiological appearance of a "target". This development is more rapid in alcoholics, but protein lithiasis, which is frequently hereditary is not related either to nutritonal disorders or to alcohol or tobacco. The late peripheral calcification could be due to increased calcium concentration in juice secondary to ductal lesions. The influence of alcoholism on this late calcification could be related to alcohol-induces modifications of pancreatic secretion as described above.

B Epidemiology of alcoholic calcic lithiasis (chronic calcifying pancreatitis)

The clinical onset is generally mainly in men in the 3rd to 5th decade of life. Alcohol is apparently the main cause of chronic calcifying pancreatitis not only in Europe, North America (including Mexico), Japan and temperate countries of South America (such as Chile and Argentina) and of Africa (such as South Africa), but also in some tropical countries such as Brazil, and many countries of Central Africa with the exception of Nigeria and Zaire (Sarles *et al.*, 1989, 1991).

A statistical relationship between ethanol consumption and the risk of developing chronic pancreatitis has been described (Durbec and Sarles, 1978). The best correlation is with the average daily consumption. There is a linear relationship between the daily alcohol consumption from 21–40 g up to 300 g per day and the log of the risk. There is no statistical threshold for toxicity but a continuous spectrum, from very sensitive individuals who will develop chronic pancreatitis with doses of alcohol as low as 1–20 g per day, to the high tolerance of patients who will have to drink more than 200 g per day before they develop the disease and finally those who will not develop chronic calcifying pancreatitis even with the highest tolerable alcohol consumption. The longer the duration of consumption at any level, the greater the risk (Durbec *et al.*, 1980). Neither the type of beverage (wine, beer, whisky, sake, cachaça, etc.) nor the rythm of consumption (regular daily or intermittent at week-ends) affects the risk (Durbec & Sarles, 1978). There is no racial or ethnic susceptibility (Sarles *et al.*, 1979), but females are more susceptible than males (Durbec *et al.*, 1980).

Other risk factors are protein and fat consumption and tobacco smoking. Twenty years ago in Europe, there was a linear relationship between protein intake and the log of the risk as for ethanol. In contrast, there was an U-shaped relationship with fat consumption, low and high fat diets increasing the risk equally in comparison with average fat diets of 80–110 g per day (Durbec *et al.,* 1978). This suggests that average fat diets should be prescribed to patients instead of the usual low-fat diet which apparently increases the risk. The role of different types of fat or protein is not known.

During the last twenty years, the relationship between the risk of developing chronic pancreatitis and fat or protein consumption have changed dramatically in Europe. In France, Germany and Italy, three European countries where dietary intake was restricted during World War II, the diet of patients 20 to 30 years ago was richer in protein and fat than the diet of matched controls. This difference was not observed in the U.S.A. (Mezey *et al.,* 1988). At present, this association is no longer observed in France, Britain, Hungary, Switzerland where nutrition is well balanced, but it is still found in Mexico and Burundi (Sarles *et al.,* 1991) where nutritional standards are poor. This suggests that undernutrition decreases the risk of alcoholic pancreatitis and that after dietary restrictions have ended, chronic pancreatitis was more likely in patients on a high-fat, high protein diet. Another further argument suggests that the risk for alcoholic pancreatitis is decreased by protein malnutrition: in Brazil where alcoholic chronic pancreatitis generally develops in people undernourished compared to European standards, the average daily alcohol-consumption of patients is above 300 g/day, approximately twice that of European patients, and the duration of excessive consumption is shorter (R. Dani, personnal communication).

The effect of tobacco smoking has been investigated by several authors (Yen *et al.,* 1982; Lowenfels *et al.,* 1987). Smoking is significantly related to the risk of developing chronic pancreatitis but not cirrhosis. Moreover, the mean age at clinical onset of pancreatitis is lower amongst smokers (Bourlière *et al.,* 1991). The risks of alcohol, fat, protein and tobacco are additive on a logarithmic basis. This means that the risks due to fat, protein and tobacco multiply the risk due to alcohol and therefore modify the individual susceptibility to alcohol, which is, however, by far the heaviest risk factor (Durbec *et al.,* 1980).

As there is no statistical threshold of risk for any of the factors studied, it is impossible to define idiopathic pancreatitis exactly. Thus, if only alcohol consumption is considered, should a chronic pancreatitis patient who consumes 15 g/day be defined as "idiopathic chronic pancreatitis patient" or a patient with a low ethanol threshold who would not have developed the disease if he had been abstinent? "Idiopathic" cases in abstinents could be due to high-protein high- or low-fat diet or tobacco, either alone or in association.

In England and Wales where the annual per capita consumption of alcohol rose from 4.0 litre in 1960 to 7.7 litre in 1969, the increase in the number of patients with chronic pancreatitis began in 1976 for men and 1980 for women (Johnson and Hostking, 1991). This is in agreement with the duration of alcohol consumption before symptoms develop in France. This increased incidence of alcoholic chronic pancreatitis following an increased consumption of alcohol is observed through out the World. Therefore, it is difficult to have an idea of the real frequency of the disease. Hospital statistics are biased by the degree of competence of physicians. Autopsy statistics over-estimate the frequency as the real frequency of silent cases is not known. In most serious reports, it varies from 2 to 4 per thousand (Sarles *et al.,* 1979).

The large differences observed in individual tolerances suggests the role of a pre-existing factor, possibly genetic. The only marker of heredity is an increased frequency of blood group 0 (Marks *et al.,* 1973; Gullo *et al.,* 1977) in chronic pancreatitis. The results of prevalence studies of HLA antigen and various other markers are contradictory and probably not different between patients and controls (Sarles, 1986).

Another argument for an hereditary predisposition to either alcoholic chronic pancreatitis or liver cirrhosis is that the morphotypes of patients presenting with these diseases are different (Pietri *et al.,* 1991). The coexistence of cirrhosis and chronic alcoholic pancreatitis is not as frequent as could be expected for two diseases that are both related to alcohol consumption. This frequency differs if the diagnosis of cirrhosis is systematically performed by a liver biopsy of pancreatic patients (4.3 to 24.6 per cent of cirrhosis in pancreatic patients) or by clinical and biological methods where it is lower but variable (frequently 2 per cent). This could be due to the fact that cirrhosis is frequently asymptomatic in its first stages and that the average age for the clinical onset of alcoholic cirrhosis is above 60 years but below 40 years for chronic pancreatitis. Less protein in the diet of cirrhotic patients with pancreatitis than in pancreatic patients without cirrhosis could also explain the low incidence of the coexistence (Montalto *et al.,* 1992).

C Lithogenesis in alcoholic lithiasis (alcoholic chronic pancreatitis)

In the early stages of the disease, pancreatic juice contains increased numbers of calcium crystals which are larger than in normal juice, and an increased number of protein precipitates consisting of a peptide called lithostathine H2 (formerly PSP-SI) which is an insoluble residue of a secretory protein called lithostathine S (formerly PSP-S2-5). In the late stages, calculi consist of more than 95% calcium salts, mostly calcium carbonate in the form of calcite, and a small quantity of a degraded form of lithostathine S called lithostathine C. We have, therefore, to explain two phenomena: precipitation of calcium salts, and precipitation of protein (Sarles *et al.,* 1989).

1) Precipitation of calcium

As pancreatic juice is saturated in Ca^{++} (Moore and Verine, 1987; Gérolami *et al.,* 1989), it is surprising that so few people develop pancreatic calculi: the calcium saturation explains the presence in normal pancreatic juice of some tiny calcite crystals. It is therefore necessary to postulate the existence of one or more calcium stabilizers able to prevent the precipitation of calcium.

Many organic and inorganic substances may act as stabilizers of supersaturated pancreatic juice, including Mg^{++}, Zn^{++}, ATP, citrate ion, pyrophosphate and mucopolysaccharides. Moreover the peculiar role of ductal epithelium has been recently underlined. The absorption of bicarbonate and secretion of H^+ ions through this epithelium during the interdigestive period, is able to increase significantly the solubility index of $CaCO_3$ and helps to prevent lithogenesis (Gérolami *et al.,* 1989). Finally fourteen years ago, the discovery of a new protein (PSP) (Pancreatic Stone Protein) (De Caro *et al.,* 1979) involved in stone formation led us to investigate its physiological role and its implication in the pathophysiology of calcic lithiasis.

Pancreatic stone protein, recently renamed lithostathine (Sarles *et al.,* 1990), present both in pancreatic stones and plugs in an insoluble form has a molecular weight of 15000 dalton (lithostathine H2) (Guy *et al.,* 1983). The original molecule, lithostathine S, is secreted in normal pancreatic juice as a group of 4 glycoproteins (17-22000 dalton) (De Caro *et al.,* 1987). It is synthesized as a 144 amino acid single chain in the endoplasmic reticulum of the acinar cells from a specific mRNA for lithostathine (Giorgi *et al.,* 1985). Lithostathine is concentrated with enzymes in zymogen granules (Lechene de la Porte *et al.,* 1986). It is very sensitive to trypsin hydrolysis which produces a long insoluble C-terminal peptide of 133 amino acids (lithostathine H2) and a small glycosylated N terminal undecapeptide (lithostathine H1). A fibrillar protein named pancreatic thread protein (PTP) had been isolated in bovine and human pancreatic juice (Gross *et al.,* 1985a; 1985b). The partial amino acid sequence of PTP strongly suggests that it is similar to lithostathine H2, the trypsin-degraded C-terminal fragment of lithostathine. The role of lithostathine is to inhibit CaCO$_3$-nucleation and crystal growth in pancreatic juice. This biological activity is carried by the N-terminal undecapeptide (Bernard *et al.,* 1992); similar molecules which prevent crystallization of calcium salts were found in saliva (Hay *et al.,* 1979), urine (Nakagawa *et al.,* 1983) and bile (Shimizu *et al.,* 1989).

What is the role of lithostathin in the pathogenesis of chronic pancreatitis? Three separate series of experiments suggest reduced synthesis of lithostathine in chronic calcifying pancreatitis. Firstly, the concentration of lithostathine measured by radial immunodiffusion or ELISA with polyclonal antibodies is significantly decreased in pancreatic juice of patients with calcic lithiasis of different aetiologies (Multigner *et al.,* 1985; Provansal Cheylan *et al.,* 1989). However, some discrepancies remain when lithostathine concentration is estimated by RIA with a specific monoclonal antibody (Schmiegel *et al.,* 1990). The explanation is that the monoclonal antibody used in this method recognizes preferentially minor isoforms and hydrolyzed forms of the protein and therefore is not suitable for quantitative analysis. Recently, using HPLC, we confirmed that lithostathine concentration was significantly decreased in the pancreatic juice of alcoholic and hereditary calcic lithiasis patients and of asymptomatic alcoholics (Bernard *et al.,* 1995).

Secondly, the mRNA levels of lithostathine, chymotrypsin, trypsin and colipase in the pancreas of calcic lithiasis patients and of controls were compared: lithostathine mRNA levels in calcic lithiasis were one third of those in controls, suggesting that gene expression is specifically reduced (Giorgi *et al.,* 1985): The mRNA of the above enzymes and coenzymes were similar.

Thirdly, immunolocalisation studies showed smaller amounts of lithostathine in the endoplasmic reticulum and zymogen granules of acinar cells from calcic lithiasis patients compared to controls (Leçhene de la Porte *et al.,* 1986). This suggests that there is a reduced rate of synthesis and secretion of lithostathine in the pancreas of calcic lithiasis patients. This reduced level of lithostathine in pancreatic juice is likely to enhance calcium carbonate crystal formation and growth.

The exact role of alcohol on calcium precipitation should be considered on three levels: a) indirect by effects on protein concentration: in men as well as in dogs, chronic ethanol consumption increases the total concentration of protein in pancreatic juice and promotes protein precipitation; protein plugs could act as nucleating agents for CaCO$_3$ crystallization. Furthermore, increased protein concentration facilitates the nucleation of calcium salts; b) alcohol consumption significantly reduces citrate concentration in pancreatic juice (36). This decrease of a calcium chelator could facilitate calcium precipitation;

Table 9.1

	Lithostathine biosynthesis	Lithostathine concentration in juice	Calcium salt calculi
Non alcoholic controls	N	N	0
Alcoholic control	?	↘	0
Calcific alcoholic	↘	↘	+
Calcific tropical (1) lithiasis	?	↘ (1)	+
Hypercalcemic	??	?	+
hereditary	?	↘ (1)	+
Proteic lithiasis (2)	?	N (1)	0

[1] Unpublished data. 2 In the late stages of proteic lithiasis, there is peripheral calcification of calculi. Lithostathine concentration in juice is normal but the concentration of calcium as well as serum protein is increased with pancreatic lesions. N = normal

c) two studies have shown that a significant decrease in lithostathine secretion occurs in the pancreatic juice of chronic alcohol-drinkers whether or not they have pancreatitis. This suggests that although a decreased lithostathine secretion is a necessary condition for pancreatic lithogenesis (no case of calcic lithiasis with normal lithostathine levels has been found), this secretory defect alone is not sufficient for the development of the lesion. The defect of lithostathine secretion is not specific alcoholism but is also found in hereditary and idiopathic forms of calcic lithiasis. It is possible that lithostathine biosynthesis could be regulated by different mechanisms including genetic and nutritional effects and possibly by adaptation to ethanol, as found with pancreatic proteases (Table 9.1).

2) Precipitation of protein

The morphological and biochemical studies discussed above showed that the first visible lesion of calcic lithiasis was the presence of protein plugs in pancreatic ducts. Although a small number of protein precipitates can be demonstrated in pancreatic juice from normal subjects, the frequency of these plugs is increased in asymptomatic alcoholics (Guy *et al.*, 1983). The increase in protein concentration observed in alcoholics could therefore play a role in protein precipitation. Moreover biochemical studies on protein plugs have shown that they are mainly composed of the 133 amino acid C-terminal insoluble peptide lithostathine H2. It is logical to assume that hydrolysis of native lithostathine may occur by tryptic cleavage. The precise mechanism of this hydrolysis remain unknown. However, once formed, the fibrils of lithostathine H2 probably increase the cohesion of calculi by attachment of calcic crystals (Mariani *et al.*, 1991).

Finally the role of protein GP-2 which is present in pancreatic plugs must be considered. This glycoprotein is tightly attached to the inner membrane of the secretory granules through a glycosyl-phosphatidyl-inositol linkage. It is released in pancreatic juice after cleavage from the membrane by phospholipase C; it has a tendency to self aggregate at neutral pH and shares a great sequence homology with the Tamm-Horsfall protein, a major component of renal tubular casts (Hoops and Rindler, 1991). The possible relationships between lithostathine and GP2 in protein plugs are actually unknown.

VII CONCLUSION AND PROPOSALS FOR FUTURE RESEARCH

Main problems for the future research, include:

1) relationship between consumption of wine, beer, nitrosamines and pancreatic cancer,
2) long term follow-up of patients presenting their first attack of acute pancreatitis to investigate the possible healing of the lesions if patients abstain,
3) investigation of possible modifications of cholinergic, adrenergic and peptidergic nerves in the pancreas of alcoholics with or without chronic pancreatitis,
4) molecular genetic studies of lithostathine in patients and controls to determine whether the molecular defects are responsible for the sensitivity to ethanol,
5) mechanisms of alcohol-induced modifications of lithostathine biosynthesis and secretion,
6) an explanation of why only some alcoholics develop chronic pancreatitis though all of them have decreased levels of lithostathine: Are there other calcium crystallization-inhibitors in pancreatic juice?
7) what is the role of protein GP2 and of lactoferrine: Is it dependent on alcohol consumption?

Bibliography

Amman, R.N., Buehler, H., Bruehlmann, W., Kehl, O., Muench, R. and Stamm, B. (1986). Acute (non progressive) alcoholic pancreatitis: prospective longitudinal study of 144 patients with recurrent alcoholic pancreatitis. *Pancreas*, **1**:195–203.

Bayer, M., Rudick, J., Lieber, C.S. and Janowitz, H.D. (1972). Inhibitory effects of ethanol on canine exocrine pancreatic secretion. *Gastroenterology*, **63**:619–626.

Bernades, P., Belghitti, J., Athouel, M., Mallardo, M., Breil, P. and Fekete, F. (1983). Histoire naturelle de la pancréatite chronique. *Gastroentérol Clin. Bio.*, **7**:8–13.

Bernard, J.P., Adrich, Z., Montalto, G., De Reggi, M., Sarles, H. and Dagorn, J.C. (1992). Inhibition of nucleation and crystal growth of CaCO₃ by human lithostathine. *Gastroenterology*, **103**:1277–1284.

Bernard, J.P., Barthet, M., Gharib, B., Michel, R., Sahel, J., Lilova, A., Dagorn, J.C. and De Reggi, M. (1995). Quantitation of human lithostathine in pancreatic juice by high performance liquid chromatography. *Gut*, **36**:630–636.

Bode C., Durr, H.K. and Bode, J.C. (1986). Effects of short and long-term alcohol feeding in rats on pancreatic enzyme content and enzyme secretion in isolated lobules *in vitro*. *Int. J. Pancreatol.*, **1**:129–139.

Bourlière, M., Barthet, M., Berthezene, P. and Sarles, H. (1991). Is tobacco a risk factor for chronic pancreatitis and alcoholic cirrhosis? *Gut*, **32**:1392–1395.

Boustière, C., Sarles, H., Lohse, J., Durbec, J.P. and Sahel, J. (1985). Citrate and calcium secretion in the pure human pancreatic juice of alcoholic and non alcoholic men and of chronic pancreatitis patients. *Digestion*, **32**:19.

Bueno De Mesquito, H.B., Maisonneuve, P., Moerman, C.J., Runia, S. and Boyle P. (1992). Lifetime consumption of alcoholic baverages, tea and coffee and exocrine carcinoma of the pancreas: a population-based case-control study in the Netherlands. *Int. J. Cancer*, **50**:514–522.

Clemente, F., Ribeiro, T., Colomb, E., Figarella, C. and Sarles, H. (1971). Comparaison des protéines des sucs pancréatiques humains normaux et pathologiques. Mise en évidence d'une protéine particulière dans la pancréatite chronique calcifiante. *Biochem Biophys Acta*, **251**:456-466.

Cuzick, J. and Babiker, A.G. (1989). Pancreatic cancer, alcohol, diabetes mellitus and gall bladder case. *Int. J. Cancer*, 415–422.

De Caro, A., Bonicel, J., Rouimi, P., De Caro, J., Sarles, H. and Rovery, M. (1987). Complete amino acid sequence of an immunoreactive form of human pancreatic stone protein isolated from pancreatic juice. *Eur. J. Biochem.*, **168**:201–207.

De Caro, A., Lohse, J. and Sarles, H. (1979). Characterization of a protein isolated from pancreatic calculi of men suffering from chronic calcifying pancreatitis. *Biochem. Biophys. Res. Comm.*, **87**:1176–1182.

Devaux, M.A., Lechene De la Porte, P., Johnson, C.D. and Sarles, H. (1990). Structural and functional effects of long-term alcohol administration on the dog exocrine pancreas submitted to two different diets. *Pancreas*, **5**:200–209.

Duncan, G., Johnson, R.H., Lambr, D.G. and Whiteside, E.A. (1980). Evidence of vagal neuropathy in chronic alcoholics. *Lancet*, **ii**:1053–7.

Durbec, J.P., Bidart, J.M. and Sarles, H. (1980). Interaction between alcohol and other foodstuffs. Epidemiological aspects. Les Colloques de l'INSERM, Alcohol and the Gastrointestinal Tract, INSERM, Paris, ed., **95**:35–52.

Durbec, J.P., Chevillotte, G., Bidart, J.M., Berthezene, P. and Sarles, H. (1983). Diet, alcohol, tobacco and risk of cancer of the pancreas: a case-control study. *Br. J. Cancer*, **47**:463–470.

Durbec, J.P. and Sarles, H. (1978). Multicenter survey on the etiology of pancreatic diseases. Relationship between the risk of developing chronic pancreatitis and alcohol, protein and lipid consumption. *Digestion*, **18**:337–350.

Estevenon, J.P., Sarles, H. and Figarella, C. (1975). Lactoferrin in the duodenal juice of patients with chronic calcifying pancreatitis. *Scand. J. Gastroent.*, **10**:327–330.

Gérolami, A., Marteau, C., Matteo, A., Sahel, J., Portugal, H., Pauli, A.M., Pastor, J. and Sarles, H. (1989). Calcium carbonate saturation in human pancreatic juice: possible role of ductal H^+ secretion. *Gastroenterology*, **96**:881–884.

Giorgi, D., Bernard, J.P., De Caro, A., Multigner, L., Lapointe, R., Sarles, H. and Dagorn, J.C. (1985). Pancreatic stone protein. I. Evidence that it is encoded by a pancreatic messenger ribonucleic acid. *Gastroenterology*, **89**:381–386.

Gjorup, I., Dueholm, S., Andersen, B. and Burcharth, F. (1990). Ethanol in pancreatic juice after oral and intravenous administration. *Gut*, **31**:1411–1413.

Grönroos, J.M., Aho, H.J., Meklin, S.S., Hakala, J. and Nevalainen, J.J. (1988). Pancreatic digestive enzymes and ultrastructure after chronic alcohol intake in the rat. *Extr. Pathol.*, **35**:197–208.

Grönroos, J.M., Kaila, T., Aho, H.J. and Nevalainen, T.J. (1989). Decrease in the number of muscarinic receptors in rat pancreas after chronic alcohol intake. *Pharmacol. Toxicol.*, **64**:356.

Gross, J., Brauer, A.W., Bringharst, R.F., Corbe, H.C. and Margolies, M.N. (1985a). An inusual bovine pancreatic protein exhibiting pH dependent globule-fibril transformation and unique amino acid sequence. *Proc. Nat. Acad. Sci.*, **82**:5627–5631.

Gross, J., Carlsson, R.I., Brauer, A.W., Margolies, M.N., Warshaw, A. and Wands, J.R. (1985b). Isolation, characterization and distribution of an unusual pancreatic human secretory protein. *J. Clin. Invest.*, **76**:2215–2216.

Gullo, L., Barbara, L. and Labo, G. (1988). Effects of cessation of alcoholism on the course of pancreatic disfunction in alcoholic pancreatitis. *Gastroenterology*, **95**:1063–1068.

Gullo, L., Costa, P.L. and Labo, G. (1977). Chronic pancreatitis in Italy. Aetiological, clinical and histological observations based on 252 cases. *Rendiconti di Gastroenterologia*, **9**:97–104.

Guy, O., Roblez, Diaz, G., Adrich, Z., Sahel, J. and Sarles, H. (1983). Protein content of precipitates present in pancreatic juice of alcoholic subjects and patients with CCP. *Gastroenterology*, **84**:102–107.

Gyr, K.E., Singer, M.V. and Sarles, H. (1984). *Pancreatitis concepts and classification*. Excerpta Medica, Amsterdam, Internatioanl Congress series, 642.

Hajnal, F., Flores, M.C., Radley, S. and Valenzuela, J.E. (1990). Effects of alcohol and alcoholic beverages on meal-stimulated pancreatic secretion in humans. *Gastroenterology*, **89**:191–196.

Hajnal, F., Flores, M.C. and Valenzuela, J.E. (1989). Effects of alcohol and alcoholic beverages on non stimulated pancreatic secretion in humans. *Pancreas*, **4**:486–491.

Hamamoto, T., Yamada, S. and Hirayama, L. (1990). Non oxydative metabolism of ethanol in the pancreas. Implication in alcoholic damages. *Biochem Pharmacol.*, **39**:241–245.

Harvey, M.H., Cates, M.C. and Reber, H.A. (1988). Possible mechanisms of acute pancreatitis induced by ethanol. *Am. J. Surg.*, **155**:49–55.

Hay, D.I., Moreno, E. and Schlesinger, T.H. (1979). Phosphoprotein inhibitors of calcium phosphage from salivary secretion. *Inorg. Perspect. Biol. Med.*, **2**:271–285.

Hayakawa, T., Takaharu, K., Tokimura, S., Toshiyuki, M., Harada, H., Ochi, K. and Tanaka, J. (1993). Secretory components and lactoferrin in pure pancreatic juice in chronic pancreatitis. *Dig. Dis. Sci.*, **38**:7–11.

Hoops, T.C. and Rindler, M.S. (1991). Isolation of the cDNA encoding glycoprotein 2 (GP2) the major zymogen granule membrane protein: homology to Uromodulin/Tam Horsfall protein. *J. Biol. Chrem.*, **266**:4257–4263.

Jalovaara, P., Romo, J. and Apaja-Sarkkinen, M. (1986). Occurence of pancreatic ductal cell dysplasia in rat fed with a high fat diet and ethanol. *Histol Histopathol.*, **1**:377–82.

Johnson, C.D. and Hostking, S. (1991). National statistics for diet alcohol consumption and chronic pancreatitis in England and Wales 1960–1988. *Gut*, **32**:1401–1405.

Kager, L., Lindberg, S. and Agren, G. (1972). Alcohol consumption and acute pancreatitis. *Scand. J. Gastroentérol.*, **7**:15.

Kakaya, J., Jakabe, T., Koizumi, M., Dataolka, S., Kamei, T. and Oyama, K. (1979). Effect of Long term feeding on the pancreas in rats. *Gastroenterologia Japonica*, **14**:327–335.

Korsten, M.A., Wilson, J.S. and Leiber, C.S. (1978). Interactive effects of dietary protein and ethanol on rat pancreas protein synthesis and enzyme secretion. *Gastroenterology*, **99**:229–236.

Kubota, K., Magee, D.F. and Sarles, H. (1983). Biphasic action of intravenous ethanol on dog exocrine pancreatic secretion. *Dig. Dis. Sci.*, **28**:1116–1120.

Lechene De La Porte, P., De Caro, A., Lafont, H. and Sarles, H. (1986). Immunohistochemical localization of pancreatic stone protein in the human digestive tract. *Pancreas*, **1**:301–308.

Lechene De La Porte, P. and Sarles, H. (1974). Etude par autoradiographie du transit et de l'excrétion des enxymes pancréatiques dans la cellule acineuse de rats alcooliques. *Biol Gastroentérol* (Paris), **7**:61–64.

Lesko, G., Siech, M., Sokolowski, A. and Snormann, H. (1989). Experimental acute pancreatitis in rats after chronic and chronic plus acute ethanol administration in combination with a pancreatic juice oedema. *Int. Surg.*, **74**:77–80.

Lowenfels, A.B., Zwemer, F.L. and Thanghani (1987). Pancreatitis in a native american indian population. *Pancreas*, **2**:694–697.

Mariani, A., Bernard, J.P., Provansal Cheylan, M., Nitsche, S. and Sarles, H. (1991). Differencies of pancreatic stone morphology and content in patient with pancreatic lithiasis. *Dig. Dis. Sci.*, **36**:1509–1516.

Marks, R.H., Banks, S. and Louw, J.H. (1973). Chronic pancreatitis in the Western cape. *Digestion*, **9**:447–453.

Mezey, E., Kolman, C.J., Diehl, A.M., Mitchell, M.C. and Herlong, H.F. (1988). Alcohol and dietary intake in the development of chronic pancreatitis and liver diseases. *Am. J. Clin. Nutr.*, **48**:148–151.

Montalto, G., Cambon, P., Bernard, J.P., Durbec, J.P. and Sarles, H. (1992). Chronic pancreatitis in southern France. Evolution of dietary habits and natural history. Frequency of liver cirrhosis and other histological changes. *Eur. J. Gastroent. & Hepatol.*, **4**:733–738.

Moore, E.W. and Verine, H.J. (1987). Pancreatic calcification and stone formation: a thermodynamic model for calcium in pancreatic juice. *Am. J. Physiol.*, **252**:707–718.

Mott, C., Sarles, H., Tiscornia, O.M. and Gullo, L. (1972). Inhibitory action of alcohol on human exocrine pancreatic secretion. *Am. J. Dis., Dis.*, **17**:902–910.

Multigner, L., Sarles, H., Lombardo, D. and De Caro, A. (1985). Pancreatic stone protein. II. Implication in stone formation during the course of CCP. *Gastroenterology*, **89**:387–391.

Nakagawa, Y., Abram, V., Herby, F.J., Kaiser, E.T. and Coe, S.L. (1983). Purification and characterization of the principal inhibitor of calcium exalate monohydrate crystal growth in human urines. *J. Biol. Chem.*, **258**:12594–12600.

Nakayamaka, K., Yamada, M. and Hirayama, C. (1980). The effects of ethanol on glycyl-prolyl dipeptidyl-aminopeptidase activity in the rat pancreatic and liver. *Biochem. Pharmacol.*, **29**:3210–3211.

Noel Jorand, M.C. and Sarles, H. (1983). Simultaneous mechanisms on exocrine pancreatic secretion initiated by alcohol in the conscious dog. *Dig. Dis. Sci.*, **28**:179–182.

Nordback, I.H., Mac Gowan, S., Potter, J.J. and Cameron, J.L. (1991). The role of acetaldehyde with pathogenesis of acute alcoholic pancreatitis. *Ann. Surg.*, **214**:671–678.

Pap, A. and Boros, L. (1989). Alcohol-induced chronic pancreatitis in rats after temporary occlusion of biliopancreatic ducts with Ethi bloc *Pancreas*, **4**:249–255.

Payan, H., Sarles, H., Demirdjan, M., Gauthier, A.P., Cross, R.C. and Durbec, J.P. (1972). Study of the histological features of chronic pancreatitis by correspondence analysis. Identification of chronic calcifying pancreatitis as an entity. *Biomedecine*, **18**:663–670.

Perec, C.F., Celener, D., Tiscornia, O.M. and Baratti, C. (1979). Effects of chronic ethanol administration on the autonomic innervation of salivary glands and pancreatic heart. *Am. J. Gastroentérol.*, **72**:4–50.

Pietri, H., Rizzo, L., Telechea, J., Bernard, J.P., Berthezene, P. and Sarles, H. (1991). Liver cirrhosis and calcifying chronic pancreatitis are associated with different morphotypes. *Digestion*, **48**:173–178.

Planche, N.E., Palasciano, G., Meullenet, J., Laugier, R. and Sarles, H. (1982). Effect of intragastric alcohol on pancreatic and biliary secretion in man. *Dig. Dis. Sci.*, **27**:449–453.

Provansal Cheylan, M., Mariani, A., Bernard, J.P., Sarles, H. and Dupuy, P. (1989). Pancreatic stone protein: quantification in pancreatic juice by Elisa and comparison with other methods. *Pancreas*, **4**:680–689.

Quon, M.G., Kugelmas, M., Wisner, J.R., Chandrasoma, P and Valenzuela, J.E. (1992). Chronic alcohol consumption intensifies cerulein-induced acute pancreatitis in the rat. *Int. J. Pancreatol.*, **12**:31–39.

Rano, O.J., Jalovaara, P. and Korkonen, L.K. (1986). The effect of rat rich, protein rich and carbohydrate rich diets combined with long-term ethanol ingestion on the pancreatic proteolytic enzymes in rats. *Res. Exp. Med.* (Berl), **186**:343–352.

Ramo, O.T. (1987). Antecedents long term ethanol consumption in combination with different diets alters the severity of experimental acute pancreatitis in rat. *Gut*, **28**:64–69.

Raymond, L. and Bouchardy, C. (1990). Les facteurs de risque du cancer du pancréas d'après les études épidémiologiques ananlytiques. *Bull Cancer*, **77**:47–68.

Raymond, L., Infante, F., Thuyns, A.J, Voirol, M. and Lowenfels, A.B. (1987). Alimentation et cancer du pancréas. *Gastroentérol. Clin. Biol.*, **11**:488–492.

Rinderknecht, H., Renner, I.G. and Carmack, C. (1979). Trypsinogen variants in pancreatic juice of healthy volunteers, chronic alcoholics and patients with pancreatitis and pancreatic cancer. *Gut*, **20**:886–891.

Robles Diaz, G., Devaux, M.A. and Sarles, H. (1985). Effect of acute and oral administration on canine exocrine pancreatic secretion. *Digestion*, **32**:77–85.

Sahel, J. and Sarles, H. (1979). Modifications of pure human pancreatic juice induced by chronic alcohol consumption. *Dig. Dis. Sci.*, **24**:897–905.

Sanfey, H., Sarr, M.G., Bulkey, G.B. and Cameron, J.L. (1986). Oxygen derived free radicals and acute pancreatitis: a review. *Acta Physiol Scand*, **548**:109–118.

Sarles, H., Augustine, P., Laugier, R., Mathew, S. and Dupuy, P. (1994). Pancreatic lesions and modifications of pancreatic juice in tropical chronic pancreatitis (tropical calcic diabetes). *Dig. Dis. Sci.*, **36**:1337–1344.

Sarles, H., Bernard, J.P. and Johnson, C. (1989). Pathogenesis and epidemiology of chronic pancreatitis. *Annual Review of Medicine*, **40**:453–468.

Sarles, H., Camarena, J. and Gomez Santana, C. (1992). Radiolucent and calcified pancreatic lithiasis. Two different diseases. Role of alcohol and heredity. *Scand. J. Gastroentérol.*, **27**:71–76.

Sarles, H., Camarena-Trabous, J., Gomez-Santana, C., Choux, R. and Iovanna, J. (1993). Acute pancreatitis is not a cause of chronic pancreatitis in the absence of residual duct strictures. *Pancreas*, **8**:354–357.

Sarles, H., Cros, R.C., Bidart, J.M. and the International Group for the Study of Pancreatic Diseases (1979). A multicenter inquiry into the etiology of pancreatic diseases. *Digestion*, **19**:110–125.

Sarles, H., Dagorn, J.C., Giorgi, D. and Bernard, J.P. (1990). Renaming pancreatic stone protein as lithostathine. *Gastroenterology*, **99**:900–903.

Sarles, H., Figarella, C. and Clemente, F. (1971a). The interaction of ethanol, dietary lipids and protein on the rat pancreas. I. Pancreatic enzymes. *Digestion*, **4**:13–22.

Sarles, H., Johnson, C.D., Devaux, M.A., Noel Jorand, M.C., Robles Diaz, G. and Schmidt, D. (1984). Influence of environmental conditions on exocrine pancreatic response to intravenous injection of ethanol and 2 deoxyglucose in the dog. *Dig. Dis. Sci.*, **29**:1925.

Sarles, H., Johnson, C.D. and Sauniere, J.F. (1991). *Pancreatitis new data and geographical distribution*. I Vol, Arnett, Blackwell.

Sarles, H., Lebreuil, G., Tasso, F., Figarella, C., Clemente, F., Devaux, M.A., Fagonde, B. and Payan, H. (1971b). Comparison of alcoholic pancreatitis in rat and man *Gut*, **12**:377–388.

Sarles, H., Pastor, J., Pauli, M. and Barthelemy, M. (1963). Determination of pancreatic function. *Gastroenterologia*, **99**:279–300.

Sarles, H., Sarles, J.C., Camatte, R., Muratore, R., Gaini, M., Guien, C., Pastor, J. and Leroy, F. (1965). Observations on 205 confirmed cases of acute pancreatitis recurrent pancreatitis and chronic pancreatitis. *Gut*, **6**:545–559.

Sarles, H. (1992). *Chronic pancreatitis and diabetes*. Bailler's clinical endocrinology and metabolism, **6**:745–775.

Sarles, H. (1991). Definition and classification of pancreatitis. *Pancreas*, **6**:470–474.

Sarles, H. (1986). Etiopathogenesis and definition of chronic pancreatitis. *Dig. Dis. Sci.*, **31**:91S–107S.

Schmiegel, W., Burchert, M. and Kalthoff, H. (1990). Immunochemical characterization and quantitative distribution of pancreatic stone protein in sera and pancreatic secretions in pancreatic disorders. *Gastroenterology*, **99**:1421–1430.

Shimizu, S., Sabray, B., Veis, A., Ostrow, J.D., Rege, R.V. and Dawes, L.G. (1989). Isolation of an acidic protein from cholesterol gallstones which inhibits the precipitation of calcium carbonate *in vitro*. *J. Clin. Invest.*, **84**:1990–1996.

Singh, H. (1987). Alcoholic pancreatitis in rats fed ethanol in a nutritionaly adequate diet. *Int. J. Pancreatol*, **2**:311–324.

Singh, H. (1986). Modification by sex of diet and ethanol effect on rat pancreatic acinar cell metabolism. *Pancreas*, **1**:164–171.

Singh, S.M. and Reber, H.A. (1990). The pathology of chronic pancreatitis. *World J. Surg.*, **14**:2–10.

Suda, K., Mogaki, M., Oyama, T. and Matsumoto, Y. (1990). Histopathologic and immunohistochemical studies on alcoholic pancreatitis and chronic obstructive pancreatitis. *Am. J. Gastroentérol.*, **85**:271–276.

Tiscornia, O., Gullo, L. and Sarles, H. (1973). The inhibition of canine exocrine pancreatic secretion by intravenous ethanol. *Digestion*, **9**:231–240.

Tiscornia, O., Palasciano, G. and Sarles, H. (1974). Effects of chronic ethanol administration on canine exocrine pancreatic secretion. *Digestion*, **11**:172–182.

Widdinson, A.L., Alvarez, C., Scharz, M. and Reber, H.A. (1974). The influence of ethanol on pancreatic blood flow in cats with chronic pancreatitis. *Surgery*, **112**:202–208.

Woutersen, R.A., Vangarderen-Hoetmen, A., Boex, J., Feringa, A.W. and Scherer, E. (1986). Modulation of putative preneoplastic foci of exocrine pancreas of rats and hamsters. I. Interaction of dietary fat and ethanol. *Carcinogenesis*, **7**:1587–93.

Yen, S., Hsieh, C.C. and Mac Mahon, B. (1982). Comparison of alcohol and tobacco and other risk factors for pancreatitis. *Am. J. Epidemiol.*, **116**:407–414.

10 Alcohol and Malignancies

A.J.Tuyns, M.D.

International Agency for Research on Cancer, 150, Cours Albert Thomas, 69008 Lyon, France

Chronic alcohol intake causes damage in the central and peripheral nervous system. It is responsible for diseases of the liver and of the pancreas. Chronic consumption of alcoholic beverages also increases the risk of cancer at most levels of the upper aero-digestive tract. This has been common medical knowledge for several decades. Attempts to produce cancer with alcoholic beverages in laboratory animals, however, have always been unsuccessful, and therefore there has been a persistent belief among scientists that alcoholic beverages could not be carcinogenic to man. Over the last twenty years evidence has nevertheless been accumulating from epidemiological studies which demonstrates unequivocally that many human cancers are related to consumption of alcoholic beverages.

GEOGRAPHY, ALCOHOL CONSUMPTION AND CANCER MORTALITY

The consumption of alcoholic beverages is known to vary considerably throughout Europe, and the pattern of consumption as well as beverages consumed also differ from one country to another. In Mediterranean countries and in Portugal, people drink wine in rather large quantities, while in countries in Central and North-West Europe people mainly drink beer. In many European countries there has been a trend towards an increased consumption, but this seems to have slowed down in recent years. Table 10.1 summarizes the evolution of alcohol consumption in the countries of the EEC, between 1960 and 1985.

When epidemiologists started mapping cancer mortality in Europe, they noticed similar variations for certain cancers. The highest mortality rates for such cancers as buccal, laryngeal and oesophageal cancer were found in South-West Europe: France, Italy, Spain and Portugal, all countries known to be great consumers of alcohol, particularly in the form of wine. This is illustrated in Figure 10.1 for laryngeal cancer in 1975–1976 (Tuyns, 1982).

This map, as most figures and tables in this chapter, refers to males. The level of mortality and of incidence is much lower in females; the difference is almost certainly due to

163

Table 10.1   Alcohol consumption in the Countries of the European Community, in liters of Ethnol per head

	1960	*1965*	*1970*	*1975*	*1980*	*1985*
Belgium	6.4	7.3	8.9	10.1	10.8	10.5
Denmark	4.2	5.0	6.8	9.1	9.1	9.9
France	17.5	17.3	16.2	16.1	14.9	13.3
Germany (F.R.)	6.8	9.3	10.3	11.3	11.4	10.8
Greece	5.2	5.0	5.3	5.3	6.7	6.8
Ireland	3.0	4.5	5.9	7.7	7.3	6.2
Italy	12.1	12.8	13.7	12.8	13.0	11.6
Netherlands	2.6	4.2	5.6	8.7	8.8	8.5
Portugal	10.4	13.9	9.9	13.3	10.0	13.1
Spain	6.6	11.2	12.1	14.1	12.4	11.8
United Kingdom	4.2	4.6	5.1	6.6	7.1	7.1

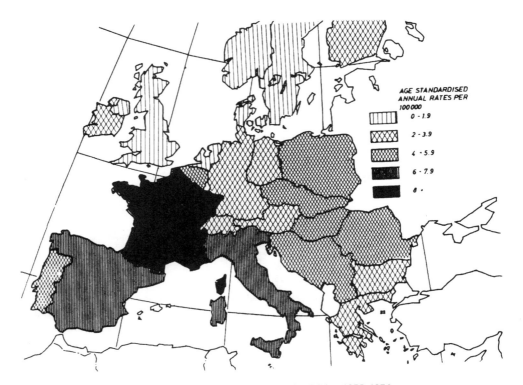

Figure 10.1   Laryngeal Cancer Mortality in European Countries. Males. 1975–1976.

the fact that alcohol consumption is much greater in males, particularly in Southern Europe. The matter is further discussed later. More recent studies in the EEC have confirmed that the contrast between the countries quoted and the rest of Europe still holds true in the mid-seventies (IARC, 1992) as seen in Table 10.2.

Table 10.2 Mortality from seleted cancers in the seventies, in Countries of the European Community

| | *Mouth* | | *Oesophagus* | | *Larynx* | |
	M	F	M	F	M	F
Belgium	2.9	0.7	3.9	1.0	4.6	0.3
Denmark	2.4	1.1	3.1	1.1	1.8	0.3
France	14.4	1.1	14.0	1.1	11.6	0.4
Germany (FR)	3.2	0.7	3.8	0.7	2.4	0.2
Ireland	3.9	1.6	6.1	3.8	2.2	0.6
Italy	6.0	0.9	4.8	0.9	6.7	0.3
Luxemburg	6.4	0.9	6.7	1.4	6.7	0.2
Netherlands	1.9	0.7	3.3	1.2	1.9	0.1
United Kingdom	2.8	1.3	5.7	2.9	1.7	0.4
Average EEC	6.5	1.0	7.1	1.4	5.6	0.3

The similarity of the distributions suggests that these cancers might be related to alcohol consumption. Within some of these countries, there were regions with exceptionnaly high rates. In the French province of Britanny, for example, the overall death rate for oesophageal cancer was found to be 21.4 per 100,000 in males (Tuyns and Massé, 1973), compared to a national average rate of 12.7 — a figure which was itself much higher than the 5 or 6 per 100,000 reported in the UK and in other European countries. These exceptionnally high regional rates had previously been found to be positively and significantly correlated with the mortality from cirrhosis and other neuropsychiatric disorders caused by alcohol (Tuyns, 1970). This observation led to more systematic case-control investigations in two French "départements" first in Ille-et-Vilaine and later in Calvados. The results of these studies will be described below.

The unusual distribution of oesophageal cancer mortality was further confirmed by a systematic examination of regional mortality throughout the EEC countries (IARC, 1992). The map below (Figure 10.2) shows the unequal distribution of oesophageal cancer mortality in the European Community.

CANCER MORTALITY AND CANCER INCIDENCE

Not all patients suffering from these cancers die from their disease and mortality, therefore, under-estimates their importance as a public health problem. Incidence figures provide a better measurement but such data have become available only in a more recent period and are limited in the largest countries to regions operating a cancer registry. These incidence rates for around 1985 are shown in Table 10.3 (IARC, 1992). They confirm the geographic differences previously observed with mortality and show large differences within countries, illustrated by the excessively high rate of oesophageal cancer in Calvados (France) and the differences noted in Italy, between the Center and the South (Latina, Ragusa) and the North of the country where most other Italian Cancer registries are located.

Average values for each country have been calculated on the basis of the existing registries, assuming that the regions mentioned are representative of the entire country — an assumption that is not unreasonable. When the national average incidence rates so calculated

A.J. Tuyns

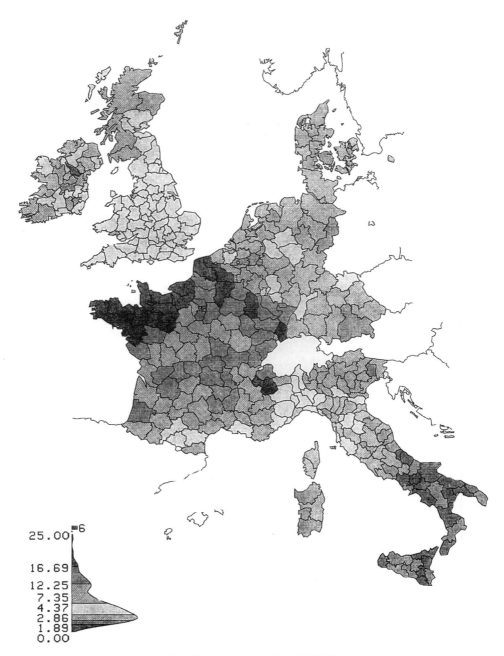

Figure 10.2   Oesophageal Cancer Mortality in Countries of the E.E.C Males.

Table 10.3 Incidence of Mouth, Hypopharynx, Oesophagus, and Larynx cancer in the EEC countries

		Mouth, Oroph.	*Hypophar.*	*Oesophagus*	*Larynx*	*Combined*
DENMARK		3.4	0.7	3.9	5.6	13.5
FRANCE	Bas-Rhin	25.9	15.2	18.7	12.8	72.7
	Calvados	21.9	13.4	26.5	12.5	74.3
	Doubs	17.2	8.6	13.1	12.2	51.1
	Isère	13.3	6.2	9.5	11.6	40.6
	Somme	18.2	10.1	19.3	17.5	65.1
	Tarn	8.0	3.1	7.1	9.4	27.5
Average 6 reg.		18.1	9.9	15.5	12.2	55.6
GERMANY	Saarland	7.2	2.5	6.1	7.9	23.7
IRELAND	Southern	2.1	1.2	4.5	4.0	11.7
ITALY	Florence	3.2	1.0	3.1	14.2	21.6
	Genoa	4.4	1.3	3.8	14.6	24.0
	Latina	3.7	–	1.9	7.5	13.1
	Varese	7.5	2.8	7.6	14.9	32.7
	Parma	4.6	2.1	4.2	13.0	23.8
	Ragusa	1.6	0.1	1.6	7.4	10.7
	Romagna	1.9	0.4	1.9	10.6	14.8
	Torino	5.8	0.8	4.1	14.7	25.4
	Trieste	6.9	2.3	5.6	15.9	30.8
Average 9 reg.		4.7	1.4	4.2	13.3	23.5
NETHERL.	Eindhoven	2.3	0.8	3.2	5.6	12.0
	Maastricht	3.2	1.1	3.7	5.7	13.8
Average 2 reg.		2.7	0.9	3.4	5.6	12.7
PORTUGAL	V.N.de Gaia	5.5	1.7	8.5	10.7	26.4
SPAIN.	Basque C.	8.3	3.3	10.3	20.4	42.3
	Tarragona	3.6	1.4	5.7	10.2	20.9
	Granada	4.6	0.5	4.4	16.2	25.6
	Murcia	3.7	0.8	4.2	15.3	23.9
	Navarra	6.4	1.1	6.6	17.8	31.9
	Zaragoza	3.1	0.8	4.6	16.1	24.5
Average 6 reg		5.2	1.5	6.3	16.4	29.3
UNITED KINGDOM, ENGLAND & WALES						
	Birmingham	2.1	0.9	5.5	4.4	12.8
	Mersey	3.1	1.0	8.2	4.6	16.9
	North-West	3.1	0.7	8.0	5.0	16.8
	Oxford	1.4	0.3	3.5	3.3	8.6
	S.Thames	1.6	0.6	6.7	3.8	12.7
	South-West	1.5	0.5	6.5	3.3	11.9
	Trent	1.9	0.6	7.1	4.4	14.0
	Yorkshire	2.3	0.6	5.8	4.7	13.4
Average 8 reg.		2.1	0.6	6.5	4.2	13.5
SCOTLAND	East Scotl.	2.7	0.3	8.5	5.1	16.6
	North Scotl.	3.3	0.2	9.4	5.6	18.5
	N-E. Scotl.	3.1	0.8	9.0	4.0	16.8
	S-E. Scotl.	2.7	0.9	6.2	4.9	14.7
	West Scotl.	3.4	0.8	9.3	6.2	19.7
Average 5 reg.		3.2	0.8	8.5	5.5	17.9
Average 13 reg.		2.2	0.7	6.8	4.4	14.1

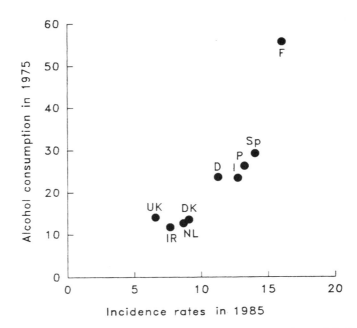

Figure 10.3 Correlation between Alcohol counsumption in 1975 and total incidence of alcohol-related cancers in 1975, in the countries of the CEE. Average alcohol consumption per capita in liters of pure alcohol per year and total yearly incidence rates per 100,000 for mouth, oropharynx, hypopharynx, oesophagus and larynx cancers, around 1985, in countries of the EEC.

are compared to the consumption values in Table 10.1, there is an obvious correspondence between both sets of values. This is shown in Figure 10.3 which shows an almost perfect correlation ($r = 0.91$) between the average national consumption of alcohol in 1975 and the incidence of all alcohol-related cancers in 1985.

As striking as such an observation may be, it can by no means be considered as a proof of the association. Correlation studies of this kind are useful for providing clues or indications but they do not demonstrate the association (Breslow and Enstrom, 1974). Much more sophisticated approaches based on individual observations need to be used in order to conclude the causal basis of an association. Many such studies have been undertaken and have indeed confirmed the association.

COHORT STUDIES ON ALCOHOLICS

Most reported cohort studies have been carried out by alcohologists on the patients who had been treated in their centres for an alcohol problem. They examined thoroughly the survival of these patients and their causes of death. They noticed, as expected, an excess mortality from causes directly related to alcoholism, such as delirium tremens, cirrhosis and even traffic accidents. They also found an excess of deaths attributed to cancer. The excess was limited to certain localisations, particularly mouth, larynx, pharynx, hypophar-

Table 10.4 Cohort studies on "Alcoholics". Mortality ratios: observed vs expected deaths

Author and group studied	Mouth	Pharynx	Oesoph.	Larynx	Liver
Sundby (1967) Norwegian alcoholics	5.0	4.4	4.1	3.1	2
Jensen (1980) Danish brewery workers.	1.4	1.9	2.1	2.0	1.5
Hirayama (1975) Japanese alcohol consumers	3.5	1.5	1.8	1.4	1.2
Hakulinen (1974) Finnish alcoholics	—	5.7	4.1	1.4	2.5
Robinette (1979) US veterans alcoholics		2.2	2.0	1.7	1
Schmidt (1981) Canadian alcoholics		4.2	3.2	4.3	2
Monson (1975) Massachusetts alcoholics		3.2	1.9	3.8	1
Klatsky (1981) Kaiser permanente study		4.0			
Cohort studies on abstinent groups					
Lemon (1980) Mormons in Utah	0.30	0.39	0.37	0.34	0.81
Enstrom (1980) Mormons in Calif.	0.10	0.42	0.45	0.30	0.41

ynx and oesophagus. (Sundby, 1967; Nicholls *et al.*, 1974; Monson and Lyon, 1975; Klatsky *et al.*, 1981). The most extensive and prolonged follow-up studies showing this were those of the Toronto group (Schmidt and De Lint, 1972; Schmidt and Popham, 1981).

Conversely, some authors investigated population groups known to abstain from smoking and drinking alcohol for religious reasons, such as the Mormons in Utah (Enstrom, 1975; Enstrom, 1980) or the 7th Day Adventists (Wynder *et al.*, 1959; Phillips *et al.*, 1980). They observed that such people had less cancers at those same sites in comparison with the local general population. This provided additional evidence of the association. Table 10.4 shows the mortality ratios observed in some of these cohort studies. From the point of view of the epidemiologist, the most remarkable feature about all these studies is the constancy of their results: the cancers in excess were the same: mouth, pharynx, larynx, oesophagus and liver (Tuyns, 1978).

CASE-CONTROL STUDIES

Such studies have been carried out by cancer epidemiologists who wanted to detect risk factors by comparing cancer patients with adequate groups of controls. Studies in the USA showed that for cancer of the mouth and pharynx (Rothman and Keller, 1972; Rothman, 1978) and for cancer of the larynx (Wynder *et al.*, 1976) there is an increased risk related to alcohol as well as to tobacco consumption. In the latter study, however, the authors concluded that the predominant factor was tobacco and that alcohol only enhanced this effect.

In the first European study carried out in Ille-et-Vilaine (France) on oesophageal cancer, a linear relationship was found between risk of developing oesophageal cancer and average daily consumption of alcohol (Tuyns *et al.*, 1977) as can be seen in Table 10.5.

Table 10.5 Relative/Risks of oesophageal cancer in males in relation to average daily consumption of alcohol

Average consumption (g. pure ethnol per day)	Crude	Relative Risks Adjusted for tabacco consumption
0–20	1.0	1.0
21–40	1.4	1.2
41–60	3.6	3.4
61–80	6.8	6.1
81–100	8.1	6.6
101 & +	19.7	18.3

In the same population and at the same period of time, a similar observation was made for patients with ascitic cirrhosis (Péquignot *et al.,* 1977). For oesophageal cancer, there was an increased risk with amount smoked. After adjustment for smoking, however, the risks related to alcohol consumption did not change substantially. By combining alcohol and tobacco consumption, the risks observed were much higher, as can be seen in Table 10.6. The values suggested a multiplicative effect.

These results were later confirmed by a study in Calvados with a larger number of patients — enough to examine separately the role of tobacco and of alcohol, among non-drinkers and among non-smokers respectively. A dose-response was observed for alcohol in the absence of smoking — a strong argument in favour of an independent role of alcohol (Tuyns, 1983). It was further shown that the relative risk for a given level of consumption was almost identical for males and for females (Table 10.7); a similar observation was made in Italy (La Vecchia *et al.,* 1989). Thus the very high gender-ratio of about 20 to 1 in Normandy is not due to some greater susceptibility of males but it simply reflects the much greater intake by males as compared to females.

Table 10.6 Relative risks of oesophageal cancer in relation to both alcohol and tobacco consumption

Average Consumption (g ethanol per day)	Average Tobacco Consumption (g. tobacco per day)		
	0–9	10–19	20 & +
0–40	1.0	3.4	5.1
41–80	7.3	8.4	12.3
81 & +	18.0	19.9	44.4

Table 10.7 Risks of developing an Oesophageal cancer among non-smokers, in relation to average daily consumption of alcohol in g., in Calvados

Average Consumption (g. ethanol per day)	Males		Females	
	No of cases	Relat. risk	No of cases	Relat. risk
0–40	7	1.0	25	1.0
41–80	15	3.8	8	5.6
81–120	9	10.2	3	11.0
121 & +	8	101.0	—	—

Several other studies have since been published in European countries. In one such study on laryngeal and hypoharyngeal cancer, incorporating population groups in France, Italy, Spain and Switzerland (Tuyns *et al.*, 1988), it was shown that the multiplicative scheme also applied to larynx and to hypopharynx, although cancer of the lower larynx was predominantly related to smoking and hypopharynx to drinking. In a more recent study on oral and oro-pharyngeal cancer (Boffetta *et al.*, 1992), tobacco was shown to be more strongly associated with soft palate lesions, while patients with cancer of floor of mouth and oral tongue had higher relative risks for alcohol drinking than subjects with cancer at other sites.

CIRRHOSIS, PRIMARY LIVER CANCER AND ALCOHOL

Primary liver cancer seems to develop only in a liver damaged by some chronic infection or intoxication. It is often, but not always, accompanied by the lesions of cirrhosis. The disease is highly prevalent in many developing countries and it is almost certainly related to chronic infection by the hepatitis B virus and/or intoxication by aflatoxin.

In most European countries, excessive consumption of alcohol is the most widespread cause of cirrhosis; the proportion of cases attributable to the disease may reach very high values. In France, it has been estimated that 93% of cirrhoses are probably due to alcohol (Péquignot *et al.*, 1978). In one of the largest autopsy studies ever published (Miyaji, 1976) 65% of the cases with primary liver cancer were associated with cirrhosis. In West European countries, one may assume that a very large proportion of the liver cancers are related to alcohol drinking. In countries where hepatitis B is still a common disease, it shares the responsibility of many primary liver cancers with alcohol. This was shown in Japan, (Oshima *et al.*, 1984) but was not found in Greece (Trichopoulos *et al.*, 1987). In a rather similar process, pancreatic cancer is possibly related to chronic pancreatitis, which is by itself a consequence of excessive drinking (Lowenfels, 1993). The matter is further discussed in the chapter on pancreas.

ALCOHOL AND BREAST CANCER

The relationship between breast cancer and alcohol consumption still remains a matter of controversy. There are, however, arguments in favour of the hypothesis. In three large cohort studies all published in the U.S.A. in 1987: Hiatt *et al.*, 1987; Schatzkin *et al.*, 1987; Willett *et al.*, 1987, an excess risk for breast cancer has been found, the relative risk being of the order of 2.5 for those drinking 15 g. of alcohol (one and a half drinks) a day (Willett *et al.*, 1987) or 3.3 for those indulging in six or more drinks a day (Hiatt *et al.*, 1988). This is indeed a rather moderate increase in comparison with the risks described above for cancer of the upper aerodigestive tract, but it refers to a cancer which is much more widespread and it would thus concern large numbers of patients.

Many more case-control studies have since produced controversial results and the problem must still be considered as unsolved. In 1988, the IARC concluded that more convincing evidence is still needed (IARC, 1988). More recently, an excellent review of the epidemiologic evidence (Rosenberg *et al.*, 1993) noted that the results of the studies have generally been null or positive.

BEER DRINKING AND CANCER OF THE RECTUM

An increased risk for rectal cancer has been described among Irish brewery workers known to receive a free ration of beer (Dean *et al.*, 1979). This provoked a certain emotion among the populations whose alcohol intake is mainly beer. A study of a similar design was also carried out among the Danish brewery workers (Jensen, 1979) and the danger of beer for rectal cancer could not be confirmed — while there was, as expected, an excess number of oesophageal, laryngeal and liver cancer deaths.

In the large cohort studies on alcoholics mentioned above (Schmidt and De Lint, 1972) no excess risk was observed for rectal cancer. Various case-control studies which investigated the possible risk factors for bowel cancer produced inconstant results (Tuyns, 1988); the relative risk of 1.3 or 1.5 described in the few that found an excess risk (Miller *et al.*, 1983) is not very convincing. More recently, however, several case-control studies in Australia (Kune *et al.*, 1987) and in the U.S. (Freudenheim *et al.*, 1990; Longnecker, 1990) all reported a weak association between beer drinking and rectal cancer.

ALCOHOL AND OTHER CANCERS

Other cancer sites have occasionally been suspected to be related to alcohol drinking: lung, urinary bladder, ovary and several others. These findings seem to be accidental and have not been confirmed by most well designed studies.

THE ALCOHOL CONSUMER AND THE RISK OF MULTIPLE CANCERS

The occurrence of simultaneous or successive cancers is sometimes encountered in clinical practice. In alcoholic patients, the risk of developing a cancer in any one of the target organs is so elevated, that such an event is rather frequent. This implies that the detection of a cancer at any level of the aerodigestive tract must immediately be followed by a complete and careful examination by the ENT surgeon of all the other relevant organs. There is no time limit to this surveillance. When a patient has been cured for one cancer, he is still likely to develop one at another site, even if he abstains from drinking — in which case, however, the risk is smaller than if he continues to abuse (Wynder *et al.*, 1969).

BIOLOGIC MECHANISMS

Is alcohol a "carcinogen"?

In the vocabulary of most cancer research workers, a carcinogen is a chemical substance (or a physical or biologic agent) which produces cancer in one or more animal species, when introduced parentally or per os or by injection. The existence of a dose-response effect is an argument in favour of carcinogenicity.

In laboratory animals, the experimentalist can freely play with mice, rats, guinea pigs or any other convenient animals. He may submit individuals of the selected species to increasing doses of the suspected chemical and try various routes of administration. If cancers appear more frequently among animals exposed to the product than in controls, the substance is said to be a carcinogen, whether or not the human observations are in line with these results. The absence of human data does not prevent many experimentalists calling a substance a carcinogen, when the evidence from experiments in animals is found to be sufficient.

In spite of repeated attempts to produce cancer in animals by ingestion of alcoholic beverages, experiments of this kind have always been unsuccessful. According to the strict criteria mentioned above, alcohol is thus not a carcinogen, but this is indeed a tricky way of altering the meaning of this word. If one sticks to the restrictive definition of the term, one should say that alcohol is not a carcinogen; it is a substance which, when ingested by humans, increases their risk of developing certain cancers. By putting things this way, one can avoid misunderstandings and unpleasant disputes with otherwise respectable purist colleagues!

ALCOHOL AS A POSSIBLE SOLVANT OF OTHER CARCINOGENS

Since ethanol does not produce cancer in animals, some investigators have worked on the hypothesis that substances accompanying ethanol in beverages might be the responsible agents. In addition to ethanol, hard liquors obtained by distillation usually contain alcohols of higher molecular weight, sometimes referred to as fusel oil. The administration of certain substances of the kind may produce cancer in rats (Gibel *et al.*, 1970). This, however could not explain why use of other alcoholic beverages obtained by fermentation, such as beer, wine or cider also increases the risk. At the early stage of the investigations in the West France provinces (Tuyns, 1970) it had been suspected that a local brandy derived from apple cider might contain specific carcinogenic substances. This, however, could not be confirmed and later studies showed that only the content in ethanol was of importance.

Since smoking is often associated with drinking, it has been hypothesized that alcohol would only enhance the role of carcinogens known to be present in tobacco smoke, such as nornicotine or other chemicals. In some studies on laryngeal cancer, the distribution of the observed cases provided some support to the theory (Wynder *et al.*, 1976). More recent observations on oesophageal cancer patients in Calvados (see Table 10.7) have shown, however, that even among non-smokers, the risk increases with increasing consumption of alcohol, thus demonstrating the independent role of alcohol. Passive smokers are likely to experience an increased risk similar to that of non-smokers.

Working on well identified and classical carcinogens, some Japanese research workers (Kuratsune *et al.*, 1971) noted that benzo[α]pyrene, a well known carcinogen, could accumulate in much greater amounts in the oesophageal cells when administered in diluted ethanol rather than in other solvents. They observed that by ingestion in an aqueous solution no cancer of the oesophagus would be produced, but when ingested in an alcoholic solution the same product could cause alterations of the oesophageal mucosa. They even succeeded in producing papillomas and carcinomas in mice with this approach (Horie *et al.*, 1965).

ALCOHOL AND NITROSAMINES

More recently, a new group of chemical substances producing cancer at various sites have been identified and extensively investigated: the nitrosamines. In contrast with most carcinogens described previously, some were found to be remarkably organotropic. Some turned out to increase the frequency of cancer in the progaster of experimental rodents (equivalent to oesophagus in man) even though the organ is rarely the seat of a spontaneous cancer in these animals. By administrating N Nitrosodiethylamine (NDEA) on two groups of mice respectively with and without alcohol, it was noted that an excess of squamous cell carcinomas of the forestomach appeared in animals that had received ethanol. (Griciute *et al.*, 1984). The same author found similar results by using N-nitrosodi-n-propylamine (NDPA), and with a cocktail NDMA + NDEA + NDPA (Griciute *et al.*, 1982). In several other experiments, other nitrosamines were tested but the addition of ethanol did not increase the number of tumours produced.

DISTURBED METABOLISM OF ALCOHOL

Acetaldehyde is the main metabolite of ethanol. It has been tested for carcinogenicity and found to produce cancer in the respiratory tract when inhaled (IARC, 1985). In alcoholics, the mechanism regulating the metabolism of ethanol are perturbed. In experimental animals, long-term exposure to ethanol enhances the clearance of the product (Lieber, 1970). It enhances its metabolism in microsomes (Lieber and Carli, 1968); this has been attributed to increased ethanol oxidation via cytochrome P450 system. (Lieber, 1970). Using baboons as experimental animals, it has been demonstrated that such changes result in liver damage: fatty liver, hepatitis (Lieber, 1975) fibrosis and cirrhosis (Lieber, 1985). Since in humans primary liver cancer is often associated with cirrhosis, it is not unrealistic to suggest that it is by these metabolic changes that ethanol would in the long term produce liver cancer. It would not explain, however, why most ethanol-related cancers occur in the upper aero-digestive tract; this suggests a more direct effect on the exposed mucosas.

CONCLUSIONS AND IMPLICATIONS

Regular consumption of alcoholic beverages increases the risk of developing cancer of the mouth, pharynx, larynx and oesophagus and the level of risk is proportional to average daily intake. This risk is combined with that related to smoking, another habit causing dependency. Among South-West European males, the contribution of these cancers to total cancer mortality and incidence is considerable. In countries with a fairly low consumption of alcohol, the patients who are true alcoholics usually die from alcoholism or from cirrhosis. Some of the very heavy consumers also die from one of the cancers discussed in this chapter, but such cases represent only a small fraction of the bulk of alcohol- related deaths.

In countries with a greater average consumption, this fraction is much greater, and the alcohol-related cancers often occur among individuals who are considered to be "reasonable" or "moderate" drinkers, with levels of consumption which are nevertheless large enough to increase sizeably their risk of developing such cancers. The concept of "moderate" drinking is obviously subjective and is subconsciously based on the belief in a threshold, a limit below which one can safely consume. Assuming that the existence of such a threshold could be scientifically demonstrated, then it is likely to be far below what many people would like to believe.

What is considered socially to be "reasonable" or "moderate" drinking thus varies enormously from one individual to another and also from one country to another within the EEC, for historical, cultural and economic reasons. In wine producing countries, the daily consumption of half a liter of wine (the equivalent of about 40g of ethanol) would generally be considered as "normal" and those who indulge in drinking even a little more would still be ranked as "moderate" drinkers. At such levels of consumption, people in the N-W countries of Europe would already be considered as "very heavy" consumers, if not as alcoholics.

In some countries, particularly in South-West Europe, the production of alcoholic beverages is an important economic and political issue. The size of the alcohol capital is enormous and its attitude governed by profits. The producers are all in favour of the efforts of anti-alcohol leagues to reduce "excessive" drinking. At the same time, however, they often encourage what they still consider to be "moderate" consumption, which indeed represents a large proportion of their sales and benefits. They even try to extend it to population strata so far protected by social and cultural barriers: women and youngsters have become their favourite targets. This kind of attitude is familiar to producers of other dangerous products; the tobacco companies are doing just the same.

In high risk countries, the problem is thus to protect people against the concept of "socially acceptable" and to replace it by that of "healthwise acceptable". The two concepts coincide more or less in N-W Europe, where people seem to be able to drink "sensibly" (Kendell, 1987) but they are largely divergent in the South. In South-West Europe, the "moderate" drinkers are far more numerous than the "excessive" drinkers but they contribute almost as many cancer cases as the latter group. The risks related to such "moderate" drinking are usually ignored and this is where health education could and should be developed.

Most efforts so far promoted by alcohologists are concerned with detection and treatment of alcoholics. This has also been the main objective of most national anti-alcoholic leagues. If we were able to decrease the number of excessive consumers, this would indeed result in an appreciable decrease of alcohol-related cancers. This may not be sufficient, however, to reduce the incidence of these cancers in South-West Europe, with their large number of "moderate" drinkers. More attention should be given to the ill effects of what people still consider to be a "moderate" and safe consumption.

Health education concepts on alcohol problems need to be revisited. The oversimplified scheme of "alcoholics" vs "non-alcoholics" may have to be modified. There is no sharp limit between the two: the risk curve is a continuous one. Apart from being scientifically justified, the concept that a greater consumption entails a greater risk of cancer (or of cirrhosis) is astonishingly well understood by lay people and it should be more largely utilized in anti-alcohol campaigns. The same holds true for the concept of multiplication of risks — particularly when it refers to the combination of alcohol and tobacco.

Within the countries of the EEC, considerable efforts have been made to fight smoking by various types of legislation on price policies and prohibiting smoking in public places

(Sasco, 1991). Some progress has been observed — more so in the UK, Denmark and Benelux countries than in SW Europe. Middle-aged males smoke less, but youngsters do not. Together with females, they are the present target of cigarette producers and consumption of tobacco in these groups increases in alarming proportions.

Alcohol consumption seems to follow the same evolution, at least in France, even though a substantial reduction of alcohol has been observed — the mechanisms of which are difficult to understand (Sulkunen, 1988). In Italy, Spain and Portugal, there is no sign of a similar decrease. More health education campaigns along the lines described above should be launched, and they should address several health risks together — mainly those related to tobacco and to alcohol.

A reduction of alcohol-related cancer morbidity is not merely wishful thinking. The Italian migrants to Canada, to Australia and to the US lowered their consumption and the incidence of these cancers has decreased (Geddes, 1993). In Brittany and Normandy, heavy drinking is a privilege of males but it is not socially acceptable for females. As a result, there are twenty times less cases among females tham among males, otherwise exposed to a similar environment (Tuyns, 1977). This shows what could be achieved in the prevention of alcohol-related cancers. It is not out of reach.

Bibliography

Addiction Research Foundation (1985). *Statistics On Alcohol and Drug Use in Canada and Other Countries*, Vol 1, Statistics on Alcohol use, Toronto, pp. 214–218.

Birch, J.D., Howe, G.R., Miller, A.E. and Semenciw, R. (1981). Tobacco, Alcohol, Asbestos and Nickel in the Etiology of Cancer of the Larynx: A Case-Control Study. *J.N.C.I.*, **67**:1219–1224.

Boffetta, P., Mashberg, A., Winkelmann, R. and Garfinkel, L. (1992). Carcinogenic effect of tobacco smoking and alcohol drinking on anatomic sites of the oral cavity and oropharynx. *Int. J. Cancer*, **52**:530–533.

Breslow, N.E. and Enstrom, J.E. (1974). Geographic correlations between mortality rates and alcohol-tobacco consumption in the United States. *J.N.C.I.*, **53**:631–639.

Dean, G., Mac Lennan, R., McLoughlin, H. and Shelley, E. (1979). Causes of death of blue-collar workers at a Dublin brewery, 1954–73. *Br. J. Cancer*, **40**:581–519.

Doll, R. and Peto, R. (1981). The cause of cancer: quantitative estimates of avoidable risks of cancer in the United States today. *J.N.C.I.*, **66**:1191–1308.

Doll, R., Forman, D., La Vecchia, C. and Woutersen, R. (1993). Alcoholic Beverages and Cancers of the Digestive tract and Larynx. In *Health Issues Related to Alcohol Consumption*, pp 125–166 (P. Verschueren, Ed.) ILSI Press, Washington.

Elwood, J.M., Pearson, J.C.G., Skippen, D.H. and Jackson, S.M. (1984). Alcohol, smoking and occupational factors in the aetiology of cancer of the oral cavity, pharynx and larynx. *Int. J. Cancer*, **34**:603–612.

Enstrom, J.E. (1975). Cancer mortality among Mormons. *Cancer*, **36**:825–841.

Enstrom, J.E. (1980). Cancer Mortality among Mormons in California during 1968–75. *J.N.C.I.*, **65**:1073–1082.

The Finnish Foundation for Alcohol Studies. (1977). International Statistics on Alcoholic Beverages. 1950–1972. The Finnish Foundation for Alcoholic Studies. **Vol. 27**, Helsinki.

Freudenheim, J.L., Graham, S., Marshall, J.R., Haughey, B.P. and Wilkinson, G. (1990). Lifetime Alcohol Intake and Risk of Rectal Cancer in Western New York. *Nutr. Cancer*, **13**:101–109.

Gibel, W. (1967). Experimentelle Untersuchungen zur Syncarzinogenese beim ösophaguskarzinom. *Arch. Geschwultsforsch.*, **30**:181–189.

Gibel, W., Lohs, Kh., Schremmer, K. and Wildner, G.P. (1970). Experimentelle Untersuchungen über toxische Wirkungen von Alkoholbeistoffen. *Dtsch. Gesundh. Wes.*, **25**:573–579.

Griciute, L., Castegnaro, M. and Bereziat, J.Cl. (1982). *Influence of aethyl alcohol on the carcinogenic activity of N-nitrosodi-n-propylamine*. In *N-nitroso Compounds: Occurrence and biologic effects*, pp. 643–648, [Bartsch, H., Castegnaro, M., O'Neill, I.E. and Okada, M. Eds] (IARC Scientific Publication No. 41). Lyon, IARC.

Griciute, L., Castegnaro, M. and Bereziat, J-C. (1984). *Influence of ethyl-alcohol on carcinogenesis induced with N-nitrosodiethylamine*. In Borsomyi, M., Day, N.E., Lapis, K. and Yamasaki, H. eds. *Models, Mechanisms and Etiology of Tumour Promotion* (IARC Scientific Publications No. 56). Lyon, International Agency for Research on Cancer, pp. 413–417.

Griciute, L., Castegnaro, M. and Bereziat, J-C. (1987). Influence of ethyl alcohol on carcinogenesis induced by volatile N-nitrosamines detected in alcoholic beverages. In *Relevance of N-Nitroso Compounds to Human Cancer: Exposures and Mechanisms.* pp. 264–265 [Bartsch, H., O'Neill, I.E. and Schulte-Hermann, R. Eds] (IARC Scientific Publications No. 84. IARC. Lyon.

Hakulinen, T., Lehtimäki, L., Lehtonen, M. and Teppo, L. (1974). Cancer morbidity among two male cohorts with increased alcohol consumption in Finland. *J.N.C.I.*, **52**:1711–1714.

Hiatt, R. Klatsky, A.L. and Armstrong, M.A. (1988). Alcohol consumption and the risk of breast cancer in a prepaid health plan. *Cancer Res.*, **48**:2284–2287.

Horie, A., Kohchi, S. and Kuratsune, M. (1965). Carcinogenesis in the oesophagus. II. Experimental production of oesophageal cancer by administration of ethanolic solutions of carcinogens. *Gann*, **56**:429–441.

International Agency for Research on Cancer (IARC) (1985). *IARC Monographs on the Evaluation of the Carcinogenic Risk to Humans.* Vol. 36. *Allyl Compounds, Acetaldehyde and others, Epoxides and Peroxides.*

International Agency for Research on Cancer (IARC) (1986). Tobacco Smoking. *IARC Monographs on the evaluation of the carcinogenic risk of chemicals to humans.* Vol. 38.

International Agency for Research on Cancer (IARC) (1988). Alcohol drinking. *IARC Monographs on the evaluation of the carcinogenic risks to humans.* Vol. 44.

International Agency for Research on Cancer (IARC) (1992). Cancer Incidence in Five Continents. Vol. VI. [D.M. Parkin, C.S. Muir, S.L. Whelan, Y.T. Gao, J. Ferlay and J. Powell Eds] *IARC Scient. Publ.* **120**.

International Agency for Research on Cancer (IARC) (1992). Atlas of Cancer Mortality in the European Economic Community. [M. Smans, C.S. Muir and P. Boyle, Eds]. *IARC Scient. Public.* No. 107.

Jensen, O.M. (1979). Cancer morbidity and causes of death among Danish brewery workers. *Int. J. Cancer*, **23**:454–463.

Kabat, G.C., Howson, C.P. and Wynder, E.L. (1986). Beer Consumption and Rectal Cancer. *Intern. J. Epid.*, **15**:494–501.

Kendell, R.E. (1987). Drinking sensibly. *Br. J. Addict.*, **82**:1279–1288.

King, M.E., Stavens, B.W. and Spector, A.A. (1977). Diet induced changes in plasma membranes; fatty acid composition affect the physical properties detected with spin-label probe. *Biochem.*, **16**:5280–5285.

Klatsky, A.L., Friedman,G.D. and Siegelaub, A.B. (1981). Alcohol and mortality: a ten-year Kaiser-Permanente experience. *Ann. Intern. Med.*, **95**:139–145.

Kune, S., Kune, G.A. and Watson, L.F. (1987). Case-Control Study of Alcoholic Beverages as Etiological Factors: The Melbourne Colorectal Cancer Study. *Nutr. Cancer,* **9**:43–56.

La Vecchia, C. and Negri, E. (1989). The role of alcohol in oesophageal cancer in non-smokers and of tobacco in non-drinkers. *Int. J. Cancer*, **43**:784–785.

La Vecchia, C., Negri, E., Carli, A., D'Avanzo, B. and Franceschi, S. (1987). A Case-control study of diet and gastric cancer in Northern Italy. *Int. J. Cancer*, **40**:484–489.

Lehmann, W., Raymond, L., Faggiano, F., Sancho-Garnier, H., Blanchet, Fr., Del Moral,A., Zubiri, L., Terracini, B., Berrino, F., Péquignot, G., Estève, J. and Tuyns, A. (1991). Cancer of the Endolarynx, Epilarynx and Hypopharynx in South-Western Europe. Assesment of Tumoral Origin and Risk Factors. In *Advances in Oto-Rhino-Laryngology* pp. 145–156 [Ed. C.R. Pfalz] Basel, Karger.

Lieber, C.S. (1984). Alcohol and the Liver. 1984 update. *Hepatology*, **4**:1243–1260.

Lieber, C.S. and DeCarli, L.M. (1968). Ethanol oxydation by hepatic microsomes: adaptive increase after ethanol feeding. *Science*, **162**:917–918

Lieber, C.S., DeCarli, L.M. and Rubin, E. (1975). Sequential production of fatty liver, hepatitis and cirrhosis in sub-human primates fed ethanol with adequate diet. *Proc. natl. Acad. Sci. USA*, **72**:437–441.

Longnecker, M.P. (1990). A case-control study of alcoholic beverage consumption in relation to risk of cancer of the right colon and rectum in men. *Cancer causes and control*, **1**:5–14.

Longnecker, M.P., Orza, M.J., Adams, M.E., Vioque, J. and Chalmers, T.C. (1990). A meta-analysis of alcoholic beverage consumption in relation to risk of colorectal cancer. *Cancer causes and control*, **1**:59–68

Lowenfels, A.B., Maisonneuve, P., Cavallini, G., Amman, R.W., Lankisch, P.G., Andersen, J.R., Dimagno, E.P., Andrén-Sandberg, Å., Domellöf, L. and the Intern. Pancreatic Study group. (1993). Pancreatitis and the risk of pancreatic cancer. *New Engl. J. Med.*, **328**:1433–1437.

Lyon, J.L., Klauber, M.R., Gardner, J.W. and Smart, C.R. (1976). Cancer Incidence in Mormons and non-Mormons in Utah, 1966–1970. *New Engl. J. of Med.*, **294**:129–133.

Miyaji, T. (1976). *Association of hepatocellular carcinoma with cirrhosis among autopsy cases in Japan during 14 years from 1958 to 1971.* In *Cancer in Asia* (T. Hirayama, ed.) *Gann Monograph on Cancer Research No. 18*, 129–149.

Miller, W.R., Howe, G.R., Jain, M., Craib, K.J.P. and Harrison, L. (1983). Food items and food groups as risk factors in a case-control study of diet and colo-rectal cancer. *Int. J. Cancer*, **32**:155–161.

Monson, R.R. and Lyon, J.L. (1975). Proportional mortality among alcoholics. *Cancer*, **36**:1077–1079.

Nicholls, P., Edwards, G. and Kyle, E. (1974). Alcoholics admitted to four hospitals in England. II. General and cause-specific mortality. *Quart. J. Stud. Alcohol.*, **35**:841–855.

Oshima, A., Tsukuma, H, Hiyama, T., Fujimoto, I.,Yamano, H. and Tanaka, M. (1984). Follow-up study of HBsAg-positive blood donors with special reference to the effect of drinking and smoking on development of liver cancer. *Int. J. Cancer*, **34**:775–779.

Péquignot, G., Tuyns, A.J. and Berta, J.L. (1978). Ascitic cirrhosis in relation to alcohol consumption. *Intern. J. Epidem.*, **7**:113–120.

Péquignot, G., Tuyns, A.J., Riboli, E. and Lowenfels, A. (1985). Résultats d'une enquête alimentaire dans le Calvados. Ration alimentaire, consommation de tabac et d'alcool. *Gastroenterol. Clin. Biol.*, **9**:422–433.

Péquignot, G. (1988). Some relevant research evidence from France. *Br. J. Addict.*, **83**:41–43.

Péquignot, G. Crosignani, P., Terracini, B., Ascunce, N., Zubiri, A., Raymond, L., Estève, J. and Tuyns, A. (1988). A comparative study of smoking, drinking and dietary habits in population samples in France, Italy, Spain and Switzerland. III. Consumption of Alcohol. *Rev, Epid. Santé Publ.*, **36**:177–185.

Phillips, R.L., Garfinkel, L., Kuzma, J.W., Beeson, W.L., Lotz, T. and Brin, B. (1980). Mortality among California Seventh-Day Adventists for selected cancer sites. *J.N.C.I.*, **65**:1097–1107.

Produktschap voor gedistilleerde dranken. (1986). How many alcoholic beverages are being consumed throughout the world? 25th ed. Produktschap voor gedistilleerde dranken. Schiedam.

Rezvani, A., Doyon, F. and Flamant, R. (1986). Atlas de la mortalité par cancer en France. Ed.de l'INSERM, Paris.

Riboli, E., Péquignot, G., Repetto, F., Axerio, M, Raymond, L., Boffetta, P. *et al.*, (1988). A comparative study of smoking, drinking and dietary habits in population samples in France, Italy, Spain and Switzerland. I. Study design and dietary habits. *Rev. Epid. Santé Publ.*, **36**:151–165.

Robinette, C.D., Hrubec, Z. and Fraumeni, J.F. Jr. (1979). Chronic alcoholism and subsequent mortality in World War 2 veterans. *Amer. J. Epidemiol.*, **109**:687–700.

Rothman, K.J. and Keller, A. (1972). The effect of joint exposure to alcohol and tobacco on risk of cancer of the mouth and pharynx. *J. Chron. Dis.*, **25**:711–716.

Rothman, K.J. (1978). The effect of alcohol consumption on risk of the head and neck cancers. *Laryngoscope*, **88** (suppl. 8):125–129.

Schatzkin, A., Jones, D.Y., Hoover, R.N., Taylor, P.R., Brinton, L.A., Ziegler, R.G., Harvey, E.B., Carter, C.L., Licitra, L.M., Dufour, M.C. and Larson, D.B. (1987). Alcohol consumption and breast cancer in the epidemiology follow-up study of the First National Health and Nutritional Examination Survey. *New Engl. J. Med.*, **316**:1169–1173.

Schmidt, W and De Lint, J. (1972). Causes of death of alcoholics. *Quart. J. Stud. Alcohol*, **33**:171–185.

Schmidt, W. and Popham, R.E. (1981). The role of drinking and smoking in mortality from cancer and other causes in male alcoholics. *Cancer*, **47**:1031–1041.

Schwartz, D., Lellouch, R., Flamant, R. and Denoix, P.F. (1962). Alcohol et cancer: Résultats d'une enquête rétrospective. *Rev. Fr. Etud. Clin Biol.*, **7**:590–604.

Sulkinen, P. (1988). A la recherche de la modernité. *Reports from the Social Research Institute on Alcohol Studies*. No. **178**.

Sundby, F. (1967). Alcoholism and Mortality. Nat. Inst. for Alcohol Research, Publ. no. 6. Universitetsforlaget. Oslo.

Systembolaget (Swedish Alcoholic Retailing Monopoly) (1986). Annual Report (Swed.), Stockholm.

Trichopoulos, D., Day, N.E., Kaklamani, E., Tzonou, A., Muñoz, N., Zavitsanos, X., Koumantaki, Y. and Trichopoulos, A. (1987). Hepatitis B virus, tobacco smoking and ethanol consumption in the etiology of hepatocellular carcinomas. *Intern. J. Cancer*, **39**:45–49.

Tuyns, A.J. (1970). Cancer of the oesophagus: Further evidence of the relationship to drinking habits in France. *Intern. J. Cancer*, **5**:152–156.

Tuyns, A.J. (1978). Alcohol et Cancer. Mon. hors série. Centre Int. de Rech. sur le Cancer.

Tuyns, A.J. (1982). Incidence trends of laryngeal cancer in relation to national alcohol and tobacco consumption. In: *Trends in Cancer Incidence. Causes and Practical Implications*, pp. 199–214. [K. Magnus, editor] Washington: Hemisphere.

Tuyns, A.J. (1982). Alcohol. In: *Cancer Epidemiology and Prevention*, pp. 293–303. [D. Schottenfeld and J.F. Fraumeni, editors] Philadelphia, Saunders.

Tuyns, A.J. (1983). Oesophageal cancer in non-smoking drinkers and in non-drinking smokers. *Int. J. Cancer*, **32**:443–444.

Tuyns, A.J. (1983). Protective effect of citrus fruit on esophageal cancer. *Nutrition and Cancer*, **5**:195–200.

Tuyns, A.J. (1988). The search for a "limit". *Br. J. Addict.*, **83**:35–36.

Tuyns, A.J. (1988). Beer consumption and rectal cancer. *Rev. Epidém. Santé. Publ.*, **36**:144–145.

Tuyns, A.J. (1989). Nutrition et cancer de l'oesophage. *Nutr. Clin. Métabol.*, **3**:119–121.

Tuyns, A.J. (1990). Alcohol related cancers in Mediterranean countries. *Tumori*, **76**:315–320.

Tuyns, A.J. (1990). Alcohol and cancer. *Proceedings of the Nutrition Society*, **48**:145–151.

Tuyns, A.J. (1991). Cancer et alcool: relations épidémiologiques. *Rev. Méd. Suisse Romande*, **111**:389–391.

Tuyns, A.J. (1991). Aetiology of head and neck cancer: tobacco, alcohol and diet. In *Advances in Oto-Rhino-Laryngology*. pp. 98–106 [C.P. Pfalz, Editor] Basel, Karger.

Tuyns, A.J. (1991). Alcohol and cancer. An instructive Association. *Br. J. Cancer*, **64**:415–416.

Tuyns, A.J. (1994). Laryngeal cancer. In *Trends in Cancer Incidence and Mortality*, pp. 159–173. (R. Doll, J.F. Fraumeni Jr. and C.S. Muir, Eds) Cold Spring Harbor Laboratory Press.

Tuyns, A.J. and Massé, L.M.F. (1973). Mortality from cancer of the oesophagus in brittany. *Int. J. Epidem.*, **2**:241–245.

Tuyns, A.J., Péquignot, G., Jensen, O.M. and Pomeau, Y. (1975). La consommation individuelle de boissons alcoolisées et de tabac dans un échantillon de la population en Ille et Vilaine. *Rev. Alcool*, **21**:105–150.

Tuyns, A.J., Péquignot, G. and Jensen, O.M. (1977). Le cancer de l'oesophage en Ille et Vilaine en fonction des niveaux de consommation d'alcool et de tabac. Des risques qui se multiplient. *Bull. Cancer*, **64**:45–60.

Tuyns, A.J., Péquignot, G. and Abbatucci, J.S. (1979). Oesophageal cancer and alcohol consumption: importance of type of beverage. *Int. J. Cancer*, **23**:443–447.

Tuyns, A.J. and Vernhes, J.C. (1981). La mortalité par cancer de l'oesophage dans les départements du Calvados et de l'Orne. *Gastr. Clin. Biol.*, **5**:257–265.

Tuyns, A.J., Péquignot, G., Gignoux, M. and Valla, A. (1982). Cancers of the digestive tract, alcohol and tobacco. *Int. J. Cancer*, **30**:9–11.

Tuyns, A.J., Hu, M.X. and Péquignot, G. (1983). Alcohol consumption patterns in the departement of Calvados (France) *Rev. Epidémiol. Santé Publ.*, **31**:179–197.

Tuyns, A.J. and Estève, J. (1983). Present and past alcohol consumption in Calvados (France). *Rev. Epid. Santé Publ.*, **31**:487–488.

Tuyns, A.J., Péquignot, G. and Estève, J. (1984). Greater risk of ascitic cirrhosis in females in relation to alcohol consumption. *Int. J. Cancer*, **13**:53–57.

Tuyns, A.J., Riboli, E., Doornbos, G. and Péquignot, G. (1987). Diet and oesophageal cancer in Calvados (France) *Nutrition and Cancer*, **9**:81–92.

Tuyns, A.J., Estève, J., Raymond, L., Berrino, F., Benhamou, E., Blanchet, F., Boffeta, P., Crosignani, P., Del Moral, A., Lehmann, W., Merletti, F., Péquignot, G., Riboli. E., Sancho-Garnier, H., Terracini, B. and Zubiri, L. (1988). Cancer of the larynx/hypopharynx, tobacco and alcohol. *Int. J. Cancer*, **41**:483–491.

Willett, W.C., Stampfer, M.J., Colditz, G.A., Rosner, B.A., Hennekens, C.H. and Speizer, F.E. (1987). Moderate alcohol consumption and the risk of breast cancer. *New Engl. J. Med.*, **316**:1174–1180.

Wynder, E.L. and Bross, I.J. (1961). A study of etiological factors in cancer of the esophagus. *Cancer*, **14**:389–414.

Wynder, E.L., Bross, I.J. and Feldman, R.L. (1957). A study of etiological factors in cancer of the mouth. *Cancer*, **10**:1300–1323.

Wynder, E.L., Lemon, F.R. and Bross, I.J. (1959). Cancer and coronary heart disease among the Seventh-day Adventists. *Cancer*, **12**:1016–1028.

Wynder, E.L., Dodo, H., Bloch, D.A., Gantt, R.C. and Moore, O.S. (1969). Epidemiologic investigation of multiple primary cancer of the upper alimentary and respiratory tract. I. A retrospective study. *Cancer*, **24**:730–739.

Wynder, E.L., Mabuchi, K., Maruchi, N. and Fortner, J.G. (1973). Epidemiology of the cancer of pancreas. *J.N.C.I.*, **50**:645–667.

Wynder, E.L., Covey, L.S., Mabouchi, K. and Mushinski, M. (1976). Environmental factors in cancer of the larynx. A second look. *Cancer*, **38**:1591–1601.

11 Alcohol-Related Adverse Social Consequences within the European Union

Esa Österberg

Social Research Institute of Alcohol Studies, Helsinki, Finland

This paper discusses alcohol-related adverse social consequences with a special reference to the EU countries. It first defines, and describes alcohol-related social problems. Next, it deals with the relationship between drinking and adverse social consequences. Data on the perception of alcohol problems and different social problems in the EU countries are presented. It then continues by discussing studies approaching the relationship between drinking and its numerous adverse consequences. Finally, some proposals for future action will be made.

Many studies show that the level of alcohol consumption is, in most cases, a highly accurate indicator of the problems related to prolonged heavy alcohol use. Changes in total alcohol consumption are also often related to the social consequences of drinking. Therefore, data on the annual per capita alcohol consumption should be reinforced by indicators of the style of drinking. One such measure might be the frequency of drunkenness. In this respect, general population surveys which ask questions about drinking patterns, drinking occasions, and the context in which drinking occurs, can be of great assistance.

INTRODUCTION

The discussion about the consumption of alcoholic beverages and its various consequences has mostly centred round the impact of continuous heavy drinking on health and round the relationship of the level of and changes in total alcohol consumption to public health (see eg. Bruun *et al.*, 1975; European Alcohol Action Plan, 1993; Verschuren, 1993; Edwards *et al.*, 1994). There is plenty of evidence that drinking alcohol causes many acute or chronic health problems to the drinkers themselves, and in some cases also to someone else. Therefore, there is no doubt that in the countries where alcohol is consumed in abundance, as EU countries (see e.g. Simpura, 1995), drinking endangers public health. But besides being a public health problem, drinking also causes many other problems which are not easily interpretable as related to health.

This paper discusses alcohol-related adverse social consequences with a special reference to the EU countries. The first task is to define, and to list and describe alcohol-related social problems. The next step is to deal in a more detailed way with the relationship between drinking and the adverse social consequences of drinking. After that some data of the perception of alcohol problems and different social problems in the EU countries are presented. The review then continues by discussing studies approaching the relationship between drinking and its numerous adverse consequences. Finally, some proposals for future action will be made.

ADVERSE SOCIAL CONSEQUENCES OF DRINKING

Problems experienced by the individual drinker can be divided into physical, psychological and social problems. Social consequences of drinking are composed of two elements: a particular drinking behaviour, and the reaction of someone else — a family member, a friend, a police officer, a work supervisor, and so on — to this drinking behaviour.

Alcohol-related social problems include, amongst others, decreased productivity or failure in work performance, absenteeism, dismissal and unemployment. Drinking can also result in many kinds of individual economic problems; for instance, spending too much money, debt, housing problems, or at the extreme, destitution. A spouse threatening to leave or breakdown of marriage are common outcomes of drinking in a family sphere, and there are many types of drinking-related impairment in other social relationships, too. The relationship between alcohol and crime is complex, but alcohol is directly or indirectly implicated in various types of belligerence and offences including crimes of violence and breaches of public order as well as drunken driving. Accidents, like motor vehicle crashes, falls, drownings, fire and burns as well as suicides are also commonly placed amongst alcohol-related social problems.

The problems which the drinker can inflict on other people commonly include a direct impact on the spouse and children and other acquaintances in terms of psychological or physical trauma, and educational, social and financial handicaps. There can also frequently be an element of inconvenience, damage or cost inflicted on members of the general public — the victims of drunken driving or violent crime, for instance, or the work mate who is involved in an alcohol-related industrial accident. Amongst these external effects of drinking one should also note the cost for society as a whole which accrues, for instance, as a result of the welfare and health services, insurance, and enforcement and penal costs associated with drinking and the cost resulting from loss of production or destroyed property. Finally, it is not improper to remind outselves that within the abstract listings lie degrees and varieties of unhappiness, loss, pain, deprivation and self-denial.

Above we have looked at different spheres of life and defined alcohol-related social consequences as problematic outcomes of drinking and the environment. We could also concentrate ourselves on the process of drinking and look at how different problems are related to drinking. For instance, in discussing consequences of drinking Klaus Mäkelä (1978) makes a distinction between drunken comportment or behavioural concomitants of drinking (belligerence, spending money, urinating in public, drunken driving), physiological consequences of drinking (passing out, hangover), events causally related to intoxication (accidents), behavioural after effects of drinking (staying away from work because of hangover, missing an appointment) and environmental reactions to any of these (police arrest, getting fired, wife leaving).

To be sure, many of the above mentioned alcohol-related social problems, including alcohol-related violence and accidents, also have a public health aspect. Furthermore, the scope of social consequences or problems is somewhat unclear; should all accidents, for instance, be viewed as social problems? It is true that there are some alcohol-related problems which do not require any direct social reactions to supervene, as for instance cirrhosis. Others, such as loss of job, imprisonment, the children being taken into care or the marriage breaking down are problems highly influenced in their causation by informal or formal social responses.

THE RELATIONSHIP BETWEEN DRINKING AND ITS SOCIAL CONSEQUENCES

The role of drinking can be assumed to be different with respect to various social complications. The prevalence of various alcohol-related social consequences is also apt to vary with regard to other factors, like gender, age, socio-demographic, cultural and historical factors. Moreover, social consequences of drinking are also often assumed to be more related to certain qualitative patterns of drinking than to the quantitative level of drinking.

In his review on social consequences of drinking Mäkelä (1978) brought together results from a number of studies pertaining to the relationship between the amount and patterns of alcohol intake and adverse social consequences of drinking. Mainly based on an analysis of survey data, he reported a generally positive association between alcohol consumption and the frequency of social problems (Mäkelä, 1978). For instance, a national Finnish survey of a representative sample of the population in 1968 found that 14% of the males aged 20–69 years with an annual alcohol consumption of less than one litre of pure alcohol had felt social drawbacks during their lifetime, whereas the corresponding proportion was 62% among those with an alcohol consumption of 20 litres or more per year. The most common problems in the latter category were arrests for drunkenness, staying away from work because of alcohol consumption and temporary economic problems. In a later analysis using interview data on drinking and its consequences, representative of the population between 15 and 69 years of age in Finland in 1984, Mäkelä and Mustonen (1988) were able to conclude that the majority of negative consequences of drinking showed a straight-line relationship to alcohol consumption and that a majority of social reactions to drinking increased as the square of the consumption level. Midanik (1995) has also reviewed the relationship between drinking and social consequences of drinking. The general finding is that the probability of social consequences rises with the level of drinking, however the latter is measured.

In a Canadian national survey of people aged 15 years and older, current drinkers were asked whether they have felt that their drinking had had a harmful effect on each of six areas on their life in the previous 12 months. For each life-area, the proportion reporting harm rises fairly steadily with increased volume of drinking, without a clear threshold of amount drunk below which drinkers are exempt from harm (Room *et al.*, 1994). In the sample as a whole, the proportion reporting their drinking had harmed two or more life-areas also rose fairly steadily with volume of drinking (Edwards *et al.*, 1994). A survey of New Zealand adults using the same questions as the Canadian survey likewise found roughly a straight-line relationship between volume drunk and the mean number of life-areas in which harm from drinking was reported. There were, however, some level-ling in the harm score at the highest category of drinking volume (Wyllie *et al.*, 1993).

In the US national survey in 1984 there was a statistically significant association between average daily alcohol consumption and intoxication, separately, and belligerence, social/family problems, work/financial problems, legal problems and physical problems. Gender, ethnicity, marital status and education were not confound variables for these asso-ciations. Belligerence, social/family problems and legal problems were more closely related to intoxication than to average alcohol consumption (Romelsjö, 1995). This indi-cates that many injurious social consequences of drinking are probably more closely related to a given pattern of drinking rather than to total alcohol consumption. Further-more, much of the variation in consequences remains unexplained even when there is detailed information about the frequency of drinking and the quantities consumed.

When they reach a given level of consumption, young people tend to run into severe trouble. This is presumably due to their drinking habits and the fact that inexperienced drinkers react more visibly than regular drinkers do to the same amount of alcohol. At the other end of the scale, the tolerance of chronically alcohol dependent individuals tends to decrease. The general impression obtained from literature is that the first signs of adverse social reactions appear at relatively low levels of drinking. At the other extreme, some individuals seem to be able to drink heavily for long periods without apparently encoun-tering social problems.

There are also gender differences in the social consequences of drinking. The bulk of this discrepancy is obviously explained by the fact that women tend to drink much less than men in most countries. It is, however, possible that, if the overall amount of intake and frequency of drunkenness were constant, the social consequences of drinking amongst men and women would still fluctuate because of gender-based differences in both behaviour and social control. Finally, social control influences the pattern of associ-ations between alcohol consumption levels, patterns of drinking and the social conse-quences of alcohol consumption.

Most societies have made drunken driving a crime as a result of an extensive body of research and other considerations. The proscribed blood alcohol level varies from country to country and does not necessarily coincide with the elevated risks of driving while intoxicated. The actual level-usually lying between 0.5 and 1.0 mg per mille litre — is, however, of great practical significance, since arrests and convictions for drunken driving are important amongst social consequences of drinking (Mäkelä *et al.,* 1981).

THE ROLE OF ALCOHOL IN DIFFERENT ADVERSE SOCIAL CONSEQUENCES

In their review Morawski, Moskalewicz and Wald (1991) show that alcohol consumption is associated with many problems in production. They discuss lowered productivity, absen-teeism, on-the-job accidents as well as personnel fluctuation and disturbances in interhu-man relations. An analysis of numerous research findings reveal that about 3 per cent of the working population have alcohol-related absences and alcohol abusers have two to five times more absences than their non-abusing colleagues (Morawski, Moskalewicz and Wald, 1991). Alcohol consumption may have a role in 3–4% of occupational related injuries, but higher figures have been reported. In West Germany, alcohol is estimated to be involved in 7–10% of all industrial accidents, while 32% of fatal industrial injury cases in Hamburg had a BAC of at least 0.5 mg per mille litre (Romelsjö, 1995).

The belief in a link between alcohol and crime has a long history. Laboratory research has produced evidence of links between pharmacologic effects of alcohol and aggressive behaviour. However, the fact that the relationship is complex is suggested by findings indicating that expectancies about the effects of alcohol may influence aggressive behaviour and that cultural, environmental and individual factors can influence the effects of drinking on aggression (Alcohol and Health, 1990). Therefore, the association between alcohol consumption and aggression is unclear. However, most scholars agree that a moderate alcohol intake, with a BAC of at least 0.5 mg per mille litre increases the tendency to aggressive behaviour, provided that the intoxicated person is provoked, e.g. by frustration. Most theorists would also agree with a simple model proposing that aggression is the result of an interaction between personal and situational factors, but would certainly disagree as to the relative importance of these factors.

Many studies have shown that alcohol misuse and alcoholism is associated with increased risk of suicide. Research indicates that 20 to 36 percent of suicide victims have a history of alcohol abuse or had been drinking shortly before their suicide (Alcohol and Health, 1990). Alcohol has been implicated as one important cause of unintentional injuries like motor vehicle injuries, falls, drowning, burns and fire. Drinking tends to increase the risk of accidents because it leads to reduced co-ordinations and balance, increased reaction time, impaired attention, perception and judgement. Partly because of drinking patterns, and partly because of lesser experience and tolerance, such casualties are especially common among younger adults in many societies and alcohol-related casualties are a substantial contributor to alcohol-related mortality, particularly when it is expressed in terms of years of life lost (Edwards *et al.*, 1994).

Motor vehicle crashes represent a leading cause of fatal accidents in many countries. Laboratory studies have shown that driving performance is reduced in a simulated driving test at a blood alcohol level of 0.2–0.3 mg per mille litre, and that there is a clear risk at over 0.5. The dose-response curve is exponential between blood alcohol concentration and risk of traffic accidents; the risk of crashing at 0.8 mg per mille litre is increased some 4 times, at 1.0 some 8 fold, and at 1.5 some 27 fold, compared to the risk with no alcohol in the blood (see e.g. Borkenstein *et al.*, 1964). Moreover, alcohol involvement is less common in nonfatal than in fatal traffic accidents.

Falls are also a prominent cause of non-fatal injuries in many countries, not least in the elderly. The proportion of fatal and non-fatal fall victims who had been drinking ranged from 21 to 77%, and from 18 to 53% respectively in a review of 21 studies on alcohol and unintentional injury published in 1947–1986 (Hingson and Howland, 1993). In three more recent studies 35–63% of persons fatally injured had been drinking. In five other studies 13–57% of persons injured in non-fatal falls had been drinking (Hingson and Howland, 1993). In a case-control study of 313 adult emergency-room patients who had suffered accidental falls, encompassing one summer week and one winter week in Helsinki, Finland, 60% had positive blood alcohol result and 53% had a BAC of over 2.0 mg per mille litre (Honkanen *et al.*, 1983).

The proportion of alcohol involvement in drowning has varied from 27 to 47% in 36 studies between 1950 and 1985 (Hingson and Howland, 1993). In eight subsequent studies, alcohol was identified in 21–47% of drowning deaths. Fire and burns constitute an important cause of injury and death. In an analysis of 32 studies published between 1947 and 1986, Hingson and Howland (1993) found that alcohol consumption was associated with an increased risk of fire and burns. In earlier review alcohol was involved in 9–86% of burn deaths. In five more recent US studies, alcohol was found in 12–61% of fatally injured burn victims (Hingson and Howland, 1993). The proportion of cases with alcohol involvement was higher among the fatal burns than in non-fatal ones.

Alcohol greatly increases the risk of exposure-related hypothermia and frostbite. Head injuries involve alcohol more often than other injuries. There is evidence that alcohol aggravates the prognosis of severe trauma. The impact of alcohol on the severity seems to vary with the cause of injury. Alcohol involvement in non-vehicular unintentional injuries is less well-documented for several reasons. There is a very diverse panorama of causes, these injuries are less dramatic and have less temporal variation than motor vehicle injuries, they are of less public interest, and legislative measures are less applicable in the control of these injuries.

Above we have covered a variety of adverse social consequences of alcohol consumption for the individual including unintentional accidents, all with different contributory causes and different mechanisms. There is profound empirical evidence that alcohol consumption is a contributory cause of most events in these fields. The cut-off point for increased risk is fairly well-known in some events, e.g. certain accidents, but less well-known for others, e.g. violence. A dose-response relationship is well established in most kinds of accidents and certain social complications, while the knowledge is scarce for violence and suicide. It is obvious that alcohol is but one of several contributory causes for the reviewed problems (Romelsjö, 1995).

PERCEPTION OF THE PROBLEM

Societies differ in what they regard as social problems and in the extent to which they attribute these problems to alcohol consumption. And societies change over time in terms of their readiness to attribute problems to drinking. Important national differences also exist in the division of labour among the authorities concerned with the management of alcohol problems; alcohol-related problems may be handled by the police, penal institutions, social authorities, or medical authorities. Moreover, besides their overall conceptualization of the adverse social consequences of drinking, countries also vary with regard to the details of their recording system.

Mäkelä and Viikari (1977) argue that, in modern societies, three principal ways of formulating "the social liquor question" can be distinguished. It can be formulated as a question of public order and security; as a problem of productivity; or as a question of public health. These cultural conceptualizations then have an influence both on the experiences of individual drinkers and on the official statistics on the consequences of drinking. If alcohol is treated as a problem of public order and security, the main responsibility for alcohol control falls upon the police and social authorities. If alcohol is treated as a problem of productivity, strict labour discipline is maintained, industrial alcohol programmes are launched, and the marginal alcoholic section of the population is relegated to skid row. A public health approach assigns the responsibility for the injurious effect of drink to public health authorities. Correspondingly, in the official statistics individual drinkers become registered as nuisances, for their poor performance at work, or as patients.

In the following we use the latest international survey conducted by the Brewers Association of Canada to get some idea of the perception of alcohol problems in different EU countries (Brazeau *et al.*, 1993). In some cases, we have supplemented this data with data from other sources, and in these cases we have indicated the source separately.

Austria.   In Austria the level of alcohol consumption is relatively high, and the country is not without its drinking problems. Variations in Austria's drinking patterns give rise to different alcohol-related problems in different parts of the country. The mortality rate from cirrhosis ranks among the highest in Europe. However, overall, it is believed that the problem has at least stabilized. Insofar as drinking and driving is concerned, 11.6 per cent of fatalities from traffic accidents were alcohol related in 1986.

Belgium.   The alcoholism rate in Belgium is generally considered to be relatively low. Sequential reports on cirrhosis death rates would seem to indicate that alcohol problems have been stable in Belgium since the mid-1970s. There is, however, a belief among health and government officials that alcohol problems remain very serious. Statistics indicate that alcohol is a factor in 30 per cent of traffic accidents, and in the case of fatal accidents, 40 per cent. It is estimated that 20 per cent of crimes are committed while under the influence of alcohol and it is believed that this increases to 40 per cent for violent crimes and vandalism. In addition, it is thought that six per cent of the Belgium work force have a drinking problem and alcohol is a factor in 30 per cent of the accidents in the work place. Concern has also been reflected in several studies on youth and alcohol consumption.

Denmark.   Data on cirrhosis deaths show an ongoing worsening alcohol problem. According to the International Survey of the Brewers Association of Canada, Danish statistics on the extent of alcoholic beverage misuse are inconsistent. The number of alcohol-related traffic accidents as a percentage of total traffic accidents increased from 12.3 in 1970 to 20.2 in 1987, and the number of alcohol-related traffic deaths as a percentage of total traffic deaths was 32% in 1987 (Moser, 1992).

Finland.   Finland has been one of the countries with the most controls on alcohol consumption during this century. Although the level of alcohol consumption has remained modest by international standards, alcohol-related problems have been quite severe. This is true especially with regard to the consequences of intoxication like arrests for drunkenness, violent crimes and alcohol poisonings. Some of the commonly used indicators on the extent of alcohol problems, such as alcohol-related traffic accidents and alcohol-related fatalities, amongst them alcohol poisonings and cirrhosis deaths, have increased in the late 1980s.

France.   A high incidence of alcoholic beverage misuse exists in France based on indices of alcoholism, cirrhosis rates, and alcohol-related traffic accidents and criminal offenses. However, some of these indicators e.g. cirrhosis death rates show that the situation is improving. Insofar as drunken driving is concerned, a study on accidents between

1977 and 1984 revealed that 38 per cent of those responsible for fatal road accidents were over legal blood alcohol limit. In other statistics 20 per cent of all serious crimes are attributed to excessive drinking.

Germany.   The death rate from cirrhosis has decreased in Germany in recent years. Despite this there seems to be a greater sensitivity to the problems of alcoholic beverage misuse. Awareness to the problems of alcohol have been heightened by churches and health organizations. In 1984, 21% of all traffic accident deaths were related to alcohol. In 1988, the corresponding figure was 18% (Moser, 1992).

Greece.   Greece is not included amongst the country reports in the international survey of the Brewers Association of Canada. As an answer to an inquiry in a study by Hermann Fahrenkrug (1991) the Greek Ministry sent five lines of regret that a public health policy on alcohol-related problems was not an issue in the country. It added as proof a statistic about the alcoholism mortality rate, which showed a total of only 24 victims of this disease in 1982!

Ireland.   The Irish have long been aware of the problems of alcohol misuse. There is a general belief that the Irish are heavy drinkers and that they have a high prevalence of alcoholism. It has been shown that up to 40% of deaths among drivers and 50% of those among pedestrians are related to blood alcohol levels above the legal limit (Moser, 1992). There is a general belief that alcohol-related problems have been on the increase in Ireland over the period coinciding with increases in consumption. This appears to be particularly the case for admissions to psychiatric hospital for alcoholism and alcoholic psychosis. At the same time, increases in public prosecutions for drunkenness, in alcohol-related crime and, particularly, in road accident fatalities, have been clearly evident (Davies and Walsh, 1983).

Italy.   The Ministry of Health has indicated that the extent of alcohol problems in Italy has only begun to be evaluated. Statistics on cirrhosis deaths per 100 000 population would indicate that while rates are high compared to many other countries, there appears to be a downward trend. Among the causes of death attributable to alcohol, the following are estimated: 80% of cirrhosis and of tumors of the mouth and oesophagus, 50% of homicides, 33% of tuberculosis of the respiratory system, 33% of traffic accidents and 25% of suicides (Moser, 1992).

Luxembourg.   Deaths from liver cirrhosis would seem to indicate that problems may be declining or at least have stabilized. It has been estimated that 50 per cent of homicides in Luxembourg are committed under the influence of alcohol and that 40 per cent of juvenile delinquency is alcohol related. Alcohol is held responsible for 25 per cent of divorces in Luxembourg and for 90 per cent of child abuse cases (Davies and Walsh, 1983).

Netherlands.   Alcohol misuse is thought to be relatively low in the Netherlands when compared to some other industrialized countries. Common indicators are, however, mixed as to whether problems are getting worse or stabilizing. The percentage of alcohol-related traffic fatalities has shown some improvement in recent years. The statistics on deaths from alcoholism and alcohol psychosis show a reverse trend. The most serious problem is a big increase in heavy drinking, with a concomitant increase in problems such as drunken driving, accidents in the workplace and at home, aggression and violence in bars during the weekends, admissions to general hospitals, psychiatric institutions and addiction clinics, violence in the family, costs of care and football hooliganism (Moser, 1992).

Portugal. Through application of the Jellinek and Ledermann formulas respectively, health officials in Portugal estimate that 4.2 per cent of the population are alcoholics and another eight per cent are excessive drinkers or consumers at risk. While cirrhosis mortality rates in Portugal have been among the highest in the world, the rate has shown some evidence of decline in recent years. It is generally recognized that the consumption of alcoholic beverages is the cause of serious problems: physical and mental disorders, family disturbances, accidents, violence and delinquency, loss of working capacity, premature death, suicide, and so on. About 50% of the deaths due to traffic accidents are estimated to be alcohol-related, as well as 25–30% of traffic accident injuries (Moser, 1992).

Spain. Although cirrhosis mortality is comparatively high in Spain, it has remained relatively stable from the late 1960s to the late 1980s. There is concern in Spain over the numbers and age of young people drinking alcoholic beverages. It is believed that a very substantial number of deaths in Spain can be attributed to alcohol. Indeed, it is projected that by the mid-1980s as many as one third of all Spanish deaths may be alcohol-related. One third of road accidents and 15 per cent of accidents at work are attributed to alcohol misuse (Davies and Walsh, 1983).

Sweden. Concern about alcoholic beverage misuse has existed in Sweden for many years and interest persists even though a number of indicators on the extent of misuse suggest that problems are trending downward from a peak reached in the late 1970s. Drunken driving is perceived to be one of the greatest problem areas connected with alcoholic beverage misuse. Drunkenness is another indicator in alcohol misuse. One problem that has been worsening is connected with crimes of violence. Drinking among young people has long been a concern in Sweden.

United Kingdom. On the basis of statistics on death from cirrhosis, alcohol-related deaths are considerably higher in Scotland than in England and Wales but appear to be increasing in both regions. Driving under the influence of alcohol and the consequent accidents and deaths are seen as highly disturbing problems in the United Kingdom. The impact of alcoholism on the family and home tends to be underestimated. Alcohol as a factor in family break-up, divorce and child abuse is receiving a considerable amount of attention in the United Kingdom at present (Moser, 1992).

It is easy to note that in the material referred to above health consequences have been dealt with more often and more thoughtfully than social consequences of drinking. Amongst social consequences of drinking, drunken driving is mentioned in nearly all country reports. Public drunkenness and problems of public order are also mentioned quite often as well as accidents and juvenile drinking. Family problems and problems with productivity are mentioned quite seldom.

APPROACHES TO THE RELATIONSHIP BETWEEN DRINKING AND ITS ADVERSE CONSEQUENCES

There are several approaches to the relationship between drinking and its numerous adverse social consequences. Firstly, there are studies in which the sample scrutinized is defined by some event or consequence related to alcohol. The drinking characteristics of the sample are then analyzed with the aim of determining the proportion of heavy drinkers, how many people meet a given clinical criterion of 'dependence', or simply how many people have an elevated blood alcohol level. Another type of study presents data on the incidence of different alcohol-related problems among known heavy drinkers or 'alcoholics'. Thirdly, there are investigations which present individual data on drinking and alcohol-related consequences among both clinical and general population samples. Fourthly, there are cross-regional and temporal studies of the relationship between drinking and its social consequences.

According to Mäkelä (1978) few consistent regional relationships between average level of alcohol consumption and social consequences of drinking are reported in the literature. The rate of road accidents might, however, correlate with the consumption level. The predominantly negative findings are probably partly due to the difficulty of getting comparable data for different jurisdictions. Regional comparisons are hampered by the fact that countries vary not only in the details of their control systems but also in their overall conceptualizations of the social consequences of drinking. Despite its technical and conceptual flaws, the available evidence indicates that there exist important cultural variations in the incidence of social consequences of drinking that are unrelated to the average level of consumption. The evidence available on instances of reduction in the consumption of alcohol, both temporary and permanent, and spontaneous as well as those caused by external circumstances, indicates that the decrease has been accompanied by a diminished intake among heavy drinkers and by a reduced frequency of obnoxious drinking occasions. On the other hand, according to the evidence available, at least a substantial part of the increase tends to be consumed in the same fashion as the earlier consumption. Therefore, potentially harmful drinking also tends to become more prevalent, whatever the characteristic consequences for each country and drinking culture might be (Mäkelä, 1978).

Until now, there have been few regional comparisons of the social consequences of drinking. What work has been done shows virtually no conclusive regional relationship between average consumption levels and the various social consequences of drinking. This finding is probably partly due to the difficulty in obtaining comparable data together with the problems encountered in planning research projects. Few temporal analyses of consumption levels, drinking patterns and consequences of drinking have been compiled (Giesbrecht *et al.*, 1983). The general conclusion to be drawn from such analyses is that changes in the total consumption of alcohol and drinking patterns are reflected in a range of harmful consequences of drinking. It should also be noted that cultural variations in drinking patterns are usually based on lasting historical traditions which are quite resistant to changes. The social consequences of drinking are therefore sometimes related to average consumption levels in temporal analyses and to drinking patterns in cross-sectional analyses.

Scandinavian Drinking Survey

The data for the Scandinavian Drinking Survey were collected in 1979 in Finland, Iceland, Norway and Sweden. These nations have relatively low levels of alcohol consumption compared to most other European countries. There are, however, clear differences between the four nations: in 1979 the consumption was highest in Finland (7.8 litres per adult), followed by Sweden (7.1), Norway (5.6) and Iceland (4.5).

The Scandinavian Drinking Survey questionnaire examined several types of adverse consequences of drinking (Mäkelä, 1981). There were no clear connections between the distributions of the answers related to negative consequences and those related to the total level of alcohol consumption. Iceland had the lowest per capita consumption but was the top country in reported consequences. It seems, therefore, that it is not possible to make reliable predictions of the extent of the negative consequences of drinking on the basis of a country's total alcohol consumption. On the other hand, it has been concluded that a higher level of annual consumption of respondents in each country was associated with a higher incidence of adverse consequences (Hauge and Irgens-Jensen, 1986). Consequently, at the same level of consumption, the average total of negative consequences was highest in Iceland, followed by Finland, Norway and Sweden in that order.

The Scandinavian Drinking Survey directed two sets of questions towards differences in drinking patterns (Simpura, 1981). First-hand experiences of intoxication and drinking occasions involving high consumption were more common in Iceland and Finland than in Norway and Sweden. In other words, the frequency of intoxication was very important in determining the frequency of adverse consequences of alcohol use. In each country there was a clear connection between annual alcohol consumption and the number of episodes of intoxication. When the frequency of intoxication remains constant there will be only minor differences in the incidence of injurious consequences in different countries. The information gathered in the Scandinavian Drinking Survey indicates that the drinking pattern itself, more precisely whether drinking alcohol leads to intoxication or not, is decisive for the social consequences of drinking. For most consequences, drinking patterns were more significant than total alcohol consumption. But the study also showed that other factors besides consumption play a role in relation to many of the adverse consequences of drinking (Hauge and Irgens-Jensen, 1986).

The International Study of Alcohol Control Experiences

The International Study of Alcohol Control Experiences (ISACE) presented an analysis of the social history of the post-war alcohol experiences of seven societies, namely California, Finland, Ireland, the Netherlands, Ontario, Poland and Switzerland (Mäkelä *et al.*, 1981; Single, Morgan and de Lint, 1981). ISACE was highly aware of the problems involved in comparing alcohol-related problems in several settings. Different societies, for instances, define social problems in different ways and also disagree about the extent to which these problems are related to alcohol (Mäkelä *et al.*, 1981).

ISACE's principal solution to the difficulty of comparing the nature and extent of alcohol-related problems in different societies was to seek measures on two dimensions: firstly, alcohol's role in problematic events or situations, and secondly, the cultural dimension in the definition of 'problems' and their attribution to alcohol. In practice, ISACE did not have access to anything near the optimum standard of data. The available time series came from four health and social statistical systems: mortality records, hospitalization records, statistics on arrests and convictions for public drunkenness, and road accident statistics. These data reflected differing mixtures of 'objective' reality and social definition and attribution. The available measures were thus severely limited as a means of describing and comparing alcohol problems in the seven societies studied.

Post-war alcohol consumption levels rose in every society studied by ISACE. Alcohol-related problems, on the other hand, showed a more complicated pattern. Increases in alcohol consumption were accompanied by increases in the incidence of many health ailments known to be causally related to prolonged drinking. Even so, the rate of increase varied from one disease and society to another. Evidence related to the consequences of single drinking occasions was less conclusive, but even in the societies in which conflicts related to drinking had increased in absolute terms, the rate of increase was lower than that in aggregate consumption. This can be seen as an indication of less conflict-prone patterns of drinking behaviour. Drunken driving is perhaps the only type of behaviour related to single drinking occasions which steadily gained in importance. The absolute number of alcohol-related road accidents increased in each of the societies studied, and when the overall accident rate fell, the proportion of all accidents in which alcohol played a part tended to rise.

The rate of increase of health ailments related to prolonged drinking tended to be higher than the rate of increase of conflicts related to single drinking occasions. Because of the different rate of growth in various types of drinking problems, variations between societies diminished. Nevertheless, persistent cultural differences exist. In Finland and Poland in particular, social conflicts related to drunken behaviour are still extremely important. The health consequences of single drinking occasions are similarly quite important in comparison to the health consequences of prolonged drinking (Österberg, 1990).

In broad terms, the findings of ISACE may be interpreted thus: Each society has certain specific cultural circumstances and drinking habits, and the range of alcohol-related problems varies accordingly. In cross-sectional comparisons, this — coupled with differences in the management of alcohol-related problems — leads to a situation in which there are few if any positive relationships between the consumption level and the incidence of specific alcohol-related problems at a particular time. Nevertheless, considering the historical experience of each cultural setting, problems are not unrelated to temporal variations in aggregate consumption. Even in a specific setting, the relationship between the consumption level and problems is by no means simple. First of all, patterns of drinking and drunken behaviour sometimes change. Secondly, many other factors besides drinking behaviour determine the rate and seriousness of alcohol problems. For instance, urban ecology influences the probability that public drunkenness will result in social conflicts, medical technology has an impact on the incidence of fatal delirium, and so on.

Discussion and conclusions

Per capita alcohol consumption is quite widely used as an indicator of the level of alcohol-related problems in different societies, and it is also employed as an indicator of changes in the level of the adverse consequences of drinking. Many studies show that the alcohol consumption level is, in most cases, a highly accurate indicator of the problems related to prolonged heavy alcohol use, such as cirrhosis mortality. Changes in total alcohol consumption are also often related to the social consequences of drinking.

Total alcohol consumption should, however, be augmented by other indicators. One promising way of increasing knowledge of the relationship between drinking and its injurious consequences is to collect general population data. Because of the many conceptual and technical difficulties connected with the composite indices commonly used in this kind of study, one should in future try to adopt less ambiguous measures. As the Scandinavian Drinking Survey shows, data on the annual per capita alcohol consumption should be reinforced by indicators of the style of drinking. One such measure might be the frequency of drunkenness. There are, however, technical difficulties in measuring the latter. Blood alcohol levels, for instance, vary with body weight and the speed of drinking; changes in behaviour depend on the blood alcohol concentration, the drinker's experience, tolerance and personality, and on the society in which he or she lives. Furthermore, many of the adverse consequences of drinking, such as alcohol poisoning, only occur at very high blood alcohol levels.

The measures used to describe the injurious consequences of alcohol use need to be more highly standardized. Most studies measure them on a lifetime basis because of the infrequency of serious social consequences. This does not take into account the fact that drinking and its consequences vary markedly over individuals' lifetimes. Even more difficult problems of interpretation arise from the use of rather heterogeneous composite measures which combine items from different spheres of life.

General population surveys are cumbersome and not very well suited to describing temporal changes in harmful consequences. The ISACE provides an example of another way to monitor and compare consequences in different societies and to study the relationship between drinking patterns and the consequences of drinking. It also shows that many problems connected with time series data gathered by different official authorities can be tackled in two ways. Firstly, it is always possible to study how such problems are defined, how the statistics are collected and how and why the activities of the authorities in question change over time. Secondly, such studies should not rely on too few indicators. On the contrary, interpretations should be based on all the available relevant indicators which give a coherent picture of the situation. It would also be important to collect data on the structure of consumption, because patterns of drinking and the dominant uses of alcohol tend to coincide with the favoured type of beverage. In wine producing countries, wine can be called a food; in the spirit producing countries alcohol is mainly used as an intoxicant; and beer drinking is traditionally connected with daily social contact. The connection between a specific type of beverage and drinking patterns, however, will not necessarily persist in a new cultural context, and changes in the structure of consumption do not form very good predictors of changes in drinking patterns. In this respect, general population surveys which ask questions about drinking occasions, and the context in which drinking occurs, can be of great assistance.

References

Alcohol and Health. From the secretary of health and human services. Seventh Special Report to the U.S. Congress. U.S. Department of Health and Human Services, January 1990.

Borkenstein, R.F., Crawther, R.F., Shumate, R.P., Ziel, W.B. and Zylman, R. (1964). The role of the drinking driver in traffic accidents. Bloomington, Indiana University Department of Police Administration.

Brazeau, R., Burr, N., Dewar, M. and Collins, H. (eds.) (1993). International Survey of Alcoholic Beverage Taxation and Control Policies. Eight Edition. Brewers Association of Canada, Ottawa.

Bruun, K., Edwards, G., Lumio, M., Mäkelä, K., Pan, L., Popham, R.E., Room, R., Schmidt, W., Skog, O.-J., Sulkunen, P. and Österberg, E. (1975). Alcohol Control Policies in Public Health Perspective. *The Finnish Foundation for Alcohol Studies, Vol 25*, Forssa.

Davies, P. and Dermot, W. (1983). Alcohol Problems and Alcohol Control in Europe, London: Croom Helm.

Edwards, G. Anderson, P. Babor, T.F. *et al.* (1994). Alcohol Policy and the Public Good. Oxford University Press, Oxford.

European Alcohol Action Plan. World Health Organization, Regional Committee for Europe, Copenhagen 1993.

Fahrenkrug, H. (1990). Alcohol control policy in the EC member states. *Contemporary Drug Problems,* **17,** 525–544.

Giesbrecht, N., Cahannes, M., Moskalewicz, J., Österberg, E. and Room, R. (eds.) (1983). Consequences of drinking. Trends in alcohol problem statistics in seven countries. *Addiction Research Foundation,* Toronto.

Hauge, R. and Irgens-Jensen, O. (1986). The relationship between alcohol consumption, alcohol intoxication and negative consequences of drinking in four Scandinavian countries. *British Journal of Addiction,* **81,** 513–524.

Hingson, R. and Howland, J. (1993). Alcohol and non-traffic unintended injuries. *British Journal of Addiction,* **88,** 877–883.

Honkanen, R., Ertama, L., Kuosmanen, P., Linnoila, M., Ahla, A. and Visuri, T. (1983). The role of alcohol in accidental falls. *Journal of Studies on Alcohol,* **44,** 231–245.

Mäkelä, K.: Level of consumption and social consequences of drinking. In: Israel, Y., Glaser, F.B. and Kalland, H., Popham, R., Smith, W. and Smart, R.G. (eds.) (1978). *Research Advances in Alcohol and Drug Problems, vol. 4. Plenum Press,* New York.

Mäkelä, K. and Mustonen, H. (1988). Positive and negative experiences related to drinking as a function of annual alcohol intake, *British Journal of Addiction,* **83,** 403–308.

Mäkelä, K. and Viikari, M. (1977). Notes on alcohol and the state. *Acta Sociologica,* **20,** 2, 155–179.

Mäkelä, K. Room, R. Single, E. *et al.* (1977). Alcohol, society, and the state. *Addiction Research Foundation,* Toronto.

Midanik, L.: Alcohol consumption and social consequences, dependence and positive benefits in general population surveys. In: Holder, H. and Edwards, G. eds. (1995). Alcohol and Public Policy: Evidence and Issues. Oxford University Press, Oxford.

Morawski, M., Moskalewicz, J. and Wald, I.: Economic costs of alcohol abuse, with special emphasis on productivity. In: Olaf Aasland (ed.): Expert meeting on the negative social consequences of alcohol use, Oslo, 27–31.8.1990, p. 266–299. Norwegian Ministry of Health and Social Affairs in collaboration with The United Nations Office at Vienna Centre for Social Development and Humanitarian Affairs, Oslo 1991.

Moser, J. (1992). Alcohol Problems, Policies and Programmes in Europe. *Eur/Hfa Target 17,* Copenhagen.

Österberg, E.: The relationship between alcohol consumption patterns and the harmful consequences of drinking. In: Plant, M. Goos, C. Keup, W. and Österberg, E. (eds.) Alcohol and drugs. Research and policy. Edinburgh University Press and World Health Organization, Regional Office for Europe, Edinburgh 1990.

Romelsjö, A.: The relationship between alcohol consumption and unintentional injury, violence, suicide and intergenerational effects. In: Holder, H. and Edwards, G. eds. (1995). Alcohol and Public Policy: Evidence and Issues. Oxford University Press, Oxford.

Simpura, J. (1981). Scandinavian Drinking Survey: Construction of alcohol intake. *National Institute for Alcohol Research,* Oslo.

Simpura, J. (1995). xxx (the chapter in this book).

Single, E., Morgan, P. and de Lint, J. (eds.) (1981). Alcohol, Society, and the State 2, The Social History of Control Policy in Seven Countries. *Addiction Research Foundation,* Toronto.

Verschuren, P.M. (executive ed.) (1981). Health Issues Related to Alcohol Consumption. *ILSI Press,* Washington.

Wyllie, A., Casswell, S. and Zhang, J.F. (June 1993). The Relationship between Alcohol Consumption and Alcohol-related Problems: New Zealand Survey Data. Paper presented at the 19th annual Alcohol Epidemiology Symposium, Kettil Bruun Society for Social and Epidemiological Research on Alcohol, Cracow, Poland, 7–11.

12 Conclusions

G. Edwards and T.J. Peters

1. Alcohol related harm is a major cause of morbidity and mortality and, with certain exceptions, looks set to increase: Consumption rates similarly are largely on the increase. The EC has a major responsibility to record accurately, reliably and consistently this data. In addition, co-ordination and support for health promotion and preventative measures is essential, particularly in view of the enormous resources available from the liquor trade aimed at promoting consumption. It is suggested that a fully resourced and mandated working party be assembled to address these issues with a remit to establish Institutes of Alcohol Misuse Prevention, Detection and Treatment.

2. Consumption, both qualitatively and quantitatively varies between countries and between various ethnic, socio-economic, and age groups within individual countries. These relate to genetic, cultural and environmental factors. These are areas receiving little attention in Europe, in contrast to the USA. A major inter-country collaborative research programme would clarify many of these issues providing invaluable information for health policy planners as indicated in paragraph one.

3. Although it is now clear that the widespread organ damage found in alcohol misusers is directly due to ethanol and/or its metabolites and not, as believed for several decades, due to a concomitant malnutrition, the importance of nutrition in the overall picture of alcohol abuse and, in particular, the therapeutic efficiency and outcome, have largely been neglected. It is also uncertain whether the usual nutritional indices, both biochemical and anthpomorphic, are applicable to chronic alcohol misusers. The latter is particularly relevant in view of the toxic effects of alcohol on the musculo-skeletal and dermatological systems. There is a clear need for the development of nutritional indices and a cross country standardisation of such measures.

4. Alcoholic liver disease is a major and increasing consequence of alcohol misuse. Treatment, particularly of cirrhosis and hepatitis, is currently unsatisfactory and a major research programme into the pathogenesis of alcoholic liver disease, including the basis for individual susceptibility, is urgently needed. There will be a major benefit in a collaborative EC programme in this and other genetic aspects of alcohol

195

misuse. Hepatic transplantation is increasingly being used in severe alcoholic liver disease and several ethical problems have emerged. These and other ethical issues concerning alcohol misuse should be debated in a European context and research in this area should be commissioned.

5. Alcoholic skin disease is a major hitherto neglected area of alcohol related harm, recently identified for the first time, as a major cause of morbidity in the UK. These studies should be confirmed and extended, on a collaborative international basis, particularly because the prevalence of various skin diseases themselves, varies across the EC. These studies would complement individual research programmes on pathogenic mechanisms.

6. HIV-related disease is an important group of syndromes with a high profile, both on research, detection and treatment agenda. The relation to alcohol misuse has been little studied apart from surveys of HIV in alcohol misusers. Of increasing importance is the prevalence of alcohol misuse in HIV positive subjects, especially gay men and those engaging in unsafe sex. Similarly, the importance of alcohol misuse on the prognosis of HIV-related syndromes is an important unanswered question. Although some work in the USA and in individual EC countries is being conducted in this area, collaborative multi-centre international studies would have added value. A related area of some importance is the biomedical importance of alcohol-mediated immune dysfunction.

7. Brain dysfunction, both acute and chronic, reversible and irreversible, are all hallmarks of alcohol misuse. Although the clinical syndromes are well described, pathogenesic mechanisms are poorly understood. Treatment strategy and, in particular, novel approaches are needed to overcome the increasing burden of neurological damage related to alcohol toxicity. Innovative approaches are needed and support in the Neuroscience Institutes investigating these problems should be enhanced.

8. Musculo-skeletal problems related to chronic alcohol misuse were first recognized as major complications a decade ago. In the intervening period the frequency of these complications and their potential reversibility with abstinence has been confirmed. Pathogenic mechanisms are at present under investigation in both man and the experimental animal. The importance of these complications as indicators of chronic ill health and, conversely, of undetected alcohol misuse remain to be identified as does the biological basis of individual susceptibility.

9. Pancreatic disease is an increasingly frequent complication of alcohol misusage, second only to liver damage but many questions such as the basis of individual susceptibility, pathogenesis of tissue damage and effective therapies remain unanswered.

10. Alcohol-related malignancy has been well described in clinical, epidemiological and experimented studies and, with tobacco usage, is a major cause of mortality. The importance of relatively moderate use of alcohol and tobacco to the overall incidence of malignancy has been little considered. These are major public health implications and the EC should take a vigorous role in limiting misuse.

11. Alcohol-related social consequences are the damaging effects most identified by the public and all, including representatives of the liquor trade, are concerned to reduce these adverse affects. As a consequence there are excellent opportunities for collaborative (and well funded) research in this area. Translation of the findings and implications in to public health measures are, however, patchy. There is an opportunity for the EC to co-ordinate and standardize such studies and to positively influence public opinion.

12. Over the past decade since the last EC supported Workshop was held in London, considerable progress has been made in individual laboratories, particularly in the USA, on the molecular genetics and biochemical basis of alcohol-related organ damage. There is, however, a need for concerted EC-supported programmes of research into these topics in Europe. The multiplicity of alcoholic beverages and their use, the ethnic variability and many dietary and environmental factors provide an ideal opportunity for making unique research contributions. Compared with the USA, the funding of alcohol-related research in Europe is limited. Similarly, funds for alcohol related problem research and treatment is much less than that for other diseases, e.g. drug abuse, HIV disease, although in quantitative terms, the social, medical and economic costs of alcohol related morbidity and mortality are orders of magnitude more important.

There is need for a NIAAA equivalent in Europe. Training in research methods, spanning the biomedical and psycho-social disciplines is an area that the EC could profitably target funds, accompanied by a parallel development of basic research programmes.

T.J. Peters